Care Ethics

The ethic of care has developed to become a body of theory that has expanded from its roots in social psychology to many other disciplines in the social sciences as well as the humanities. This work on care has informed both theory and practice by generating complex accounts of care ethics for multiple and intersecting kinds of relationships, and for a variety of domains and contexts. Its application now extends from the moral to the political realm, from personal to public relationships, from the local to the global, from feminine to feminist virtues and values, and from issues of gender to issues of power and oppression.

The developments in the theories and applications of care ethics over the past few decades make this book an appropriate and timely publication. It includes chapters by authors who are developing or expanding theories of care ethics and also by those who work on applying and extending insights from care ethics to practices and policies in personal and institutional settings. *Care Ethics* provides readers from different disciplines and professional groups with a substantial number of new theories and applications from both new and established authors.

This book was originally published as two special issues of *Ethics and Social Welfare*.

Christine M. Koggel is Harvey Wexler Chair in Philosophy, Departmental Chair and Majors Advisor, and Co-Director of the Center for International Studies at Bryn Mawr College, USA.

Joan Orme is Emeritus Professor of Social Work at the Glasgow School of Social Work, Scotland, UK.

Care Ethics
New Theories and Applications

Edited by
Christine M. Koggel and Joan Orme

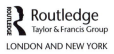

Routledge
Taylor & Francis Group

LONDON AND NEW YORK

First published 2013
by Routledge
2 Park Square, Milton Park, Abingdon, Oxon, OX14 4RN

Simultaneously published in the USA and Canada
by Routledge
711 Third Avenue, New York, NY 10017

Routledge is an imprint of the Taylor & Francis Group, an informa business

British Library Cataloguing in Publication Data
A catalogue record for this book is available from the British Library

ISBN13: 978-0-415-62330-8

Typeset in Helvetica
by Taylor & Francis Books

Publisher's Note
The publisher would like to make readers aware that the chapters in this book may be referred to as articles as they are identical to the articles published in the special issue. The publisher accepts responsibility for any inconsistencies that may have arisen in the course of preparing this volume for print.

Printed and bound in the United States of America by Publishers Graphics, LLC on sustainably sourced paper.

Table of Contents

CONTENTS

Citation Information

The following chapters were originally published in the journal *Ethics and Social Welfare*. When citing this material, please use the original issue information and page numbering for each article, as follows:

Chapter 2
Can the Ethics of Care Handle Violence?
Virginia Held
Ethics and Social Welfare, volume 4, number 2 (July 2010) pp. 115-129

Chapter 3
After Liberalism in World Politics? Towards an International Political Theory of Care
Fiona Robinson
Ethics and Social Welfare, volume 4, number 2 (July 2010) pp. 130-144

Chapter 4
Cosmopolitan Care
Sarah Clark Miller
Ethics and Social Welfare, volume 4, number 2 (July 2010) pp. 145-157

Chapter 5
Creating Caring Institutions: Politics, Plurality, and Purpose
Joan C. Tronto
Ethics and Social Welfare, volume 4, number 2 (July 2010) pp. 158-171

Chapter 6
Interweaving Caring and Economics in the Context of Place: Experiences of Northern and Rural Women Caregivers
Heather Peters, Jo-Anne Fiske, Dawn Hemingway, Anita Vaillancourt, Christina McLennan, Barb Keith and Anne Burrill
Ethics and Social Welfare, volume 4, number 2 (July 2010) pp. 172-187

Chapter 7
Gratitude and Caring Labor
Amy Mullin
Ethics and Social Welfare, volume 5, number 2 (June 2011) pp. 110-122

CITATION INFORMATION

Chapter 8

The Productivity of Care: Contextualizing Care in Situated Interaction and Shedding Light on its Latent Purposes
Alessandro Pratesi
Ethics and Social Welfare, volume 5, number 2 (June 2011) pp. 123-137

Chapter 9

The Individual in Social Care: The Ethics of Care and the 'Personalisation Agenda' in Services for Older People in England
Liz Lloyd
Ethics and Social Welfare, volume 4, number 2 (July 2010) pp. 188-200

Chapter 10

A Comparative Analysis of Personalisation: Balancing an Ethic of Care with User Empowerment
Kirstein Rummery
Ethics and Social Welfare, volume 5, number 2 (June 2011) pp. 138-152

Chapter 11

Abandoning Care? A Critical Perspective on Personalisation from an Ethic of Care
Marian Barnes
Ethics and Social Welfare, volume 5, number 2 (June 2011) pp. 153-167

Chapter 12

Care Ethics and Carers with Learning Disabilities: A Challenge to Dependence and Paternalism
Nicki Ward
Ethics and Social Welfare, volume 5, number 2 (June 2011) pp. 168-180

Chapter 13

Care Ethics in Residential Child Care: A Different Voice
Laura Steckley and Mark Smith
Ethics and Social Welfare, volume 5, number 2 (June 2011) pp. 181-195

Chapter 14

Care as Regulated and Care in the Obdurate World of Intimate Relations: Foster Care Divided?
Andrew Pithouse and Alyson Rees
Ethics and Social Welfare, volume 5, number 2 (June 2011) pp. 196-209

Chapter 15

An Ethic of Care in Nursing: Past, Present and Future Considerations
Martin Woods
Ethics and Social Welfare, volume 5, number 3 (September 2011) pp. 266-276

Chapter 16

Ethics and the Street-level Bureaucrat: Implementing Policy to Protect Elders from Abuse
Angie Ash
Ethics and Social Welfare, volume 4, number 2 (July 2010) pp. 201-209

CITATION INFORMATION

Chapter 17

Crossing the Divide between Theory and Practice: Research and an Ethic of Care
Lizzie Ward and Beatrice Gahagan
Ethics and Social Welfare, volume 4, number 2 (July 2010) pp. 210-216

Chapter 18

That Others Matter: The Moral Achievement - Care Ethics and Citizenship in Practice with People with Dementia
Tula Brannelly
Ethics and Social Welfare, volume 5, number 2 (June 2011) pp. 210-216

Chapter 19

The Daily Grind of the Forgotten Heroines: Experiences of HIV/AIDS Informal Caregivers in Botswana
Odireleng Jankey and Tirelo Modie-Moroka
Ethics and Social Welfare, volume 5, number 2 (June 2011) pp. 217-224

Introduction

Christine M. Koggel and Joan Orme

Introduction

When Carol Gilligan (1982) first introduced the ethic of care she did so from the discipline of psychology using empirical data that questioned Kohlberg's (1981) negative assumptions about the moral development of women. Gilligan argued that Kohlberg's research assumed a male model of moral reasoning and decision making, and that women were either left out of the studies all together or judged to have less ability to reason. Gilligan's uncovering of a 'different voice' has had broad implications in its challenge to mainstream moral theory in the liberal tradition. In contrast to accounts of universal principles and of the significance of impartiality, individual rights, consequences, and justice in consequentialist and deontological moral theories, the ethic of care emphasizes the importance of context, interdependence, relationships, and responsibilities to concrete others. In developments that followed, some debates centred on the extent to which care ethics are *feminist* ethics (Held 1995; Koehn 1998) relevant predominantly to interpersonal *caring* relationships (Noddings 1984) and the institutions based on these. Other theorists broadened the debate to the political realm (Tronto 1993; Sevenhuijsen 1998; Robinson 1999) or explored intersections between or the possible integration of care and justice in international relations and the global context (Held 2006).

The ethic of care has developed over the past few decades to become a body of theory that has expanded from its roots in social psychology to many other disciplines in the social sciences as well as the humanities. This work on care has informed both theory and practice by generating complex accounts of care ethics for multiple and intersecting kinds of relationships and for a variety of domains and contexts. Its application now extends from the moral to the political realm, from personal to public relationships, from the local to the global, from feminine to feminist virtues and values, and from issues of gender to issues of power and oppression more generally.

These theoretical developments have led to examinations of an ethic of care that challenge contemporary theories such as the capabilities approach, cosmopolitanism, global justice, international political theory, and virtue ethics (to name a few). Often these accounts begin with a feature of an ethic of care already present in Gilligan: the idea that individuals are not the isolated and abstract entities described in traditional liberal theory, but are fundamentally relational and interdependent. Care theorists who bring this feature to the forefront highlight our embeddedness in networks of relationships that intersect at various levels of the personal and political in ways that shape people's lives as well as the values, practices, policies, and institutions that affect them (Koggel, 1998). As it relates to political theory, this work on an ethic of care identifies the limitations of liberal accounts of the self, autonomy, justice, and equality and reconceives these concepts in relational terms (Downie and Llewellyn, 2012). The result is the envisioning of new theory, policies, and structures (Mahon and Robinson, 2011; Miller, 2011). All of these developments in theories and applications make care ethics an appropriate and timely topic for further exploration.

About this volume

The influence of care ethics is such that when the call went out for papers for a special issue of the journal *Ethics and Social Welfare* on *Care Ethics: New Theories and Applications*, the response was overwhelming. It was not just the volume of papers, but also the scope of the topics covered and the international spread. The areas covered went beyond what had been anticipated by highlighting the continuing applicability of care ethics to all aspects of human relations and organisation and involving responses both to theoretical challenges and to fast changing social circumstances. The richness of submissions led to the publication of two special issues on an ethic of care, and other papers appeared in other issues of the journal. The organising principle for the publication of the papers accepted was along the lines of those authors who worked on developing or expanding theories of care ethics and those who worked on applying and extending insights from care ethics to practices and policies in personal and institutional settings. This monograph combines the papers from the two special issues along with one other and maintains the distinction in its two parts: Part I, New Theories and Contemporary Issues and Part II, New Applications in Contemporary Contexts.

If we take a central feature of care ethics to be its attention to the specificity of contextual description and analysis, this division between theory and practice or policy may be somewhat artificial. While it is true that the papers in Part I, New Theories and Contemporary Issues, use issues and examples from real contexts and lives, they do so in order to illuminate the new theories that the individual authors attempt to articulate and develop. Some of these theorists returned to their early, substantive work that helped to develop the ethic of care in order to reflect on what was missing then, left unsaid, could be challenged, needed to be developed, given a new emphasis, or taken in new directions. An important point is that the authors' reflections, critiques, and broadening of their early work is now being done in the light of urgent and serious issues in a global context, ones that require paying attention to and addressing the needs of distant others in morally responsible ways. In other words, the global context highlights the very features of dependence and interdependence that were central from the very beginning, when Gilligan took relationships and responding to the needs of others as central to the moral reasoning underlying an ethic of care. In this collected volume, therefore, we not only have some of the most prominent care theorists reflecting on their own previous work on an ethic of care, we also have them in dialogue with other authors in the use that each makes of the work and insights of others to develop new theories and new applications for care ethics.

New Theories and Contemporary Issues

The papers in Part I investigate the broad implications for theoretical developments of care ethics for a variety of issues and contexts. Authors explore the relevance of care ethics to current issues such as war, terrorism, gender violence, and health care; to global concerns such as international law, economic globalization, poverty, and the global economic crisis; and to inequalities in a postcolonial context. In taking such a broad perspective we are widening the definitions of welfare to that of well fare. In other words, we are moving beyond an understanding of welfare that relates only to the services provided by the state, or by organisations on behalf of the state, to one which includes all relations and interventions that contribute to the well being, health, safety and security of individuals, communities and nations. It is testimony to the impact of care ethics over the decades that the focus of attention is so broad. The papers in Part I reflect these theoretical developments and applications, some of which broaden the discussion to the global context and issues in it, some of which focus on the effects of state and global economic policies on people in a specific context, and some of which illuminate how care ethics can avoid the pitfalls of current policy and envision new policies and structures.

Part I, therefore, includes authors that work with this broad understanding of welfare to delineate new theories and applications in the political realm. Virginia Held opens the volume by asking 'Can the Ethics of Care Handle Violence?'. She acknowledges that care ethics has been viewed as having little to offer in dealing with issues such as crime, war, terrorism, and violence against women. Held works with the two issues of violence against women and terrorism to develop an ethics of care that can acknowledge the need for law and its enforcements at the same time as it rejects law and enforcement as encompassing the whole of morality. The result is an account that can provide guidance in understanding and dealing with family violence and terrorism in ways that go beyond and may help supplant the need for justice. In the paper that follows, Fiona Robinson uses the current economic global crisis as an opportunity to challenge and rethink liberal and neo-liberal approaches that have dominated international political theory. By challenging the individualism of liberalism, Robinson uses insights of relationality, interdependence, and responsibilities to others to sketch an international political theory of care. The result is a political theory of care that is able to reveal the gendered and raced nature of caring and better address the real needs of others in a postcolonial context shaped by a global political economy. She discusses the earthquake in Haiti and its aftermath to illustrate features of an international political theory of care.

In 'Cosmopolitan Care', Sarah Clark Miller reflects on how care ethics can deal with another crisis that has demanded a global response: that of widespread violence in the Darfur region of Sudan and, specifically, of gender violence as a mechanism of war. She moves away from the usual focus on justifications for humanitarian intervention to sketch a cosmopolitan account of care that can do the crucial work of rebuilding the lives of women and communities affected by the devastation of gender violence by restoring and strengthening their ability to care for others. Unlike cosmopolitanism in the justice tradition, with its assumptions of individualism, universality and generality, cosmopolitan care emphasizes the importance of responding to others' needs in ways that are contextually sensitive and culturally attuned. Miller's call for strengthening institutions that reflect responsive and responsible care practices is given a theoretical framework in Joan Tronto's 'Creating Caring Institutions: Politics, Plurality, and Purpose'. Tronto extends her earlier work that brought care ethics into the realm of political theory and social policy by developing an account of what it would mean for institutions to provide good care. Accounts of institutions of care tend to model them on the family or the market, both of which are shown to fall short of providing good institutional care. Tronto uses key features of an ethic of care to delineate three elements of good care in an institutional context: the purpose of care, a recognition of power relations, and the need for pluralistic, particular tailoring of care to meet individuals' needs. In the paper that follows, Heather Peters et al. pick up on an aspect of Tronto's critique of a market model of care by examining how care in families and in caring institutions is affected by economic decline and the resulting government policies of cuts to these institutions and programs. They contextualize the effects of economic decline and these now popular cuts to federal and provincial funding by explaining what this means for people in northern, rural and remote communities in northern British Columbia, Canada.

The final two papers in Part I further expand the ethic of care in its academic and theoretical scope and also in its application to personal, public and political relationships. Focusing on gratitude, Amy Mullin identifies the particularities and vulnerabilities of caregivers and care-recipients and explores how these are shaped by social hierarchies and public institutions. She argues that a feminist ethics of care can usefully employ gratitude as a way to draw out morally significant aspects of care and highlight the importance not only of responding to specific needs but also of attending to the capacities of recipients of care. Alessandro Pratesi uses care ethics as a lens through which to examine the sociological aspects of care that can result in emotional and psychological exhaustion at the same time as it can be gratifying, rewarding and empowering. By situating an analysis in her study of the daily activities of caregivers, Pratesi uses care as a strategic site through which to understand the interactional mechanisms and explore the emotional dynamics of caregivers. These emotional and relational dynamics become a recurring theme in the papers that follow in Part II.

New Applications in Contemporary Contexts

While feminist accounts of theory and connections with care ethics in domains that were primarily and obviously relational continue, there is clear acknowledgement of the political impact and implications of the conditions in which care is provided (Williams, 2001) and of the relevance of care ethics to policy, analysis, and activism. Those conditions include contexts of paid and unpaid labour in caring domains. Yet in terms of the practice of care (in professions such as nursing and social work) there was initially surprisingly little attention to the implications of an ethic of care: practitioners who provided care assumed they understood care and deemed it an uncontested concept (Orme, 2002) and have only begun to explore the complexities in the last decade (Parton, 2003). In looking at new applications of an ethic of care, our particular interest in getting historical and contemporary examples or case studies of care ethics in social work, community work, and related social and health professions came to fruition. This was true as well in having authors explore the implications of both the ongoing need for a critical analysis of any policy initiative from the perspective of the ethic of care and the interconnections among relationships in more detail. Some of the work in this area of case studies and applications of care ethics to policy analysis and implementation is the focus of and reflected in the papers included in Part II of this volume, New Applications in Contemporary Contexts.

Part II, therefore, follows on Part I by building on the theoretical explorations of care ethics, but it does so in the context of examining their application in different areas of health and social care and in various domains and contexts. The first three papers provide a link between the political theory, agendas and policy, and the practice implications of caring. They also place a greater emphasis on the application of the ethic of care in domains that reflect the more traditional understanding of welfare. In the United Kingdom, the policy of personalisation has developed as a response to the activism of service user groups; that is to those who require the intervention of care services to facilitate daily living. This policy has been heralded as a means of granting more autonomy, but is highly contested. Critiques provided by Liz Lloyd argue that it has failed to incorporate the political and personal implications of care ethics. Lloyd focuses on how such policies construct individuals who are recipients of services. She uses the example of how the policy impacts on older people to argue that it fails to address interdependence, relationships, and responsibilities to concrete others, which are both fundamental to and a consequence of the application of the ethic of care.

The papers by Kirstein Rummery and Marian Barnes continue Lloyd's discussions of personalisation. Rummery recognises it as a global policy development and provides a comparative analysis of its introduction across Europe and the U.S. Her conclusions that personalisation is an 'under governed commodification of care' that leaves both carers and cared-for vulnerable, disempowered, and exploited are echoed by Barnes. Barnes explores the relationship between personalisation and care ethics by using analytic tools developed by care ethicists. Specifically, she uses Selma Sevenhuijsen's 'Trace' analysis to trace the normative frameworks in key policy documents and thereby unpack and challenge the assumptions underpinning the policy and practice formulations in England.

The four papers that follow move from theory through policy to practice by examining relations between caregivers and care-recipients and exploring answers to questions about what care demands in relationships of inequality and dependency as these are manifested in particular domains and contexts. Nicki Ward focuses on learning disabilities in the context of caring relations. In keeping with the relational approaches embedded in the ethic of care, she uses personal narrative to contextualise the experiences of people with learning disabilities. In exploring caring in unequal relations, she not only reprises many of the themes in the preceding papers, she also challenges binaries that make people dependent or independent. This leads her to argue for citizenship and social justice for people with learning disabilities. In the paper that follows, Laura Steckley and Mark Smith discuss unequal relationships in the context of child care practice in which caring is associated frequently with protection. They explore the implications of an ethic of care for residential child care, where care, protection and control are often interwoven – and confused. They argue that public care needs to move beyond its current instrumental focus to articulate a broader ontological purpose, informed by what is required to promote children's growth and flourishing. Staying in the area of child care but moving the focus from care in (and by) public institutions Andrew Pithouse and Alyson Rees look at relations of adults and children in foster care and the private setting of the home. They explore the tensions between foster care as an institution that has adopted a highly regulatory approach and foster care in the home that requires daily and ordinary practices that are relational, constitutive, and contextual. They argue that an analysis of the taken-for-granted and ordinary aspects of domestic life such as food, the body, and touch can help elucidate the care that is provided in and central to the 'nebulous mix of paid and unpaid fostering.' Explorations of the relevance of care ethics in welfare have been paralleled by a burgeoning interest in the nursing profession (see the special issue of *Nursing Ethics,* vol. 18 2011). However it is appropriate that Martin Woods' paper appears in this volume. It explores the application of care ethics to nursing and challenges assumptions that by virtue of providing practical care nurses demonstrate an ethic of care. He recognises the pressures from the changing organisational context of health provision and drawing on theories of care ethics he argues for the relational dimensions: care as a way of being and as a practice.

The final four papers in Part II are shorter pieces that examine ethical issues from the perspective of practitioners and those in receipt of welfare services, often drawing on participatory research The first is an essay by Angie Ash, which won first prize in the 2009 Jo Campling Memorial *Ethics and Social Welfare* Student Essay Competition. This essay, based on Ash's research, explores the gap between policy intention and implementation and practice in the area of elder abuse. She describes how she discovered 'the missing ethical voice' in her analysis, a voice subsequently provided by drawing on Tronto's work. Research practice with older people is the focus of the piece by Lizzie Ward and Beatrice Gahagan who use an ethic of care framework to respond to the ethical challenges of undertaking participatory research that attempts to involve and understand older people as genuine co-researchers.

The theme of voice and its importance in particular contexts of care is pursued in the shorter pieces by Tula Brannelly and by Odireleng Jankey and Tirelo Modie-Moroka. Brannelly reports on research that looks at the application of an ethic of care to situations where people cannot articulate their own care needs, older people with dementia. Her conclusions that an ethic of care strengthens the position for the negotiation of care between practitioners, service users and their families is vital if the voice of older people with mental health problems is to be heard. The Jankey and Modie-Moroka paper also reports on a piece of research that gives voice to those who are not heard or taken seriously, but in this case to those who provide caregiving to people diagnosed with HIV/AIDS in Botswana. It, therefore, reports on the direct experiences of caregiving, but importantly it also examines notions of care and an ethic of care in a cultural setting very different from the rest of the papers in this volume.

Conclusion

In sum we feel that the breadth of these papers devoted to exploring new theories and applications of care ethics is testimony to the work of the authors in this volume and to the continuing, and indeed growing relevance of the ethic of care. Collecting the work of the authors from the two special issues of *Ethics and Social Welfare* on *Care Ethics: New Theories and Applications* provides a rich source of scholarship and research on the ethics of care. This volume supports our assertion that care ethics has relevance to diverse academic disciplines and contemporary issues and to applications in many domains and contexts.

References

Gilligan, C. (1982) *In a Different Voice*, Harvard University Press, Cambridge Massachusetts & London.

Downie, J. and J. Llewellyn (eds.) (2012) *Being Relational: Reflections on Relational Theory and Health Law*, University of British Columbia Press, Vancouver.

Held, V. (ed) (1995) *Justice and Care: Essential Readings in Feminist Ethics*, Westview Press, Bolder CO and Oxford.

Held, V. (2006) *The Ethics of Care: Personal, Political, and Global*, Oxford University Press, Oxford.

Koehn, D. (1998) *Rethinking Feminist Ethics: Care, Trust and Empathy*, Routledge, London.

Koggel, C. (1998) *Perspectives on Equality: Constructing a Relational Theory*, Rowman & Littlefield. Lanham, MD.

Koggel, C. & J. Orme, (2010) 'Care Ethics: New Theories and Applications' *Ethics and Social Welfare* vol. 4 no. 2 pp. 188-200.

CARE ETHICS

Koggel, C. & J. Orme (2011) 'Care Ethics: New Theories and Applications: Part II' *Ethics and Social Welfare*, vol. 5 no. 2 pp. 107-09.

Kohlberg, L. (1981) *The Philosophy of Moral Development,* Harper Row, San Francisco.

Lloyd, L. (2010) 'The Individual in Social Care: The Ethics of Care and the 'Personalisation' Agenda in Services for Older People in England' *Ethics and Social Welfare* vol. 3 no. 2 pp. 188-200.

Mahone, R. and F. Robinson (eds.) (2011) *Feminist Ethics and Social Politics: Towards a New Global Political Economy of Care*, University of British Columbia Press, Vancouver.

Miller, S.C. (2011) *The Ethics of Need: Agency, Dignity, and Obligation*, Routledge, New York.

Noddings, N. (1984) *Caring: A Feminine Approach to Ethics* University of California Press, Berkeley.

Orme, J. (2002) 'Social Work: Gender, Care and Justice', *British Journal of Social Work*, Vol. 32, pp. 799-814.

Parton, N. (2003) 'Rethinking Professional Practice: the Contribution of Social Constructionism and the Feminist 'Ethic of Care'', *British Journal of Social Work*, Vol. 33, pp. 1-16.

Robinson, F. (1999) *Globalizing Care: Ethics, Feminist Theory and International Relations*, Westview Press, Boulder, CO.

Sevenhuijsen, S. (1998) *Citizenship and the Ethics of Care*, Routledge, London.

Sevenhuijsen, S. (2003) 'Trace: a method for normative policy analysis from an ethic of care', Paper prepared for the seminar Care and Public Policy, University of Bergen, 19-11 November.

Tronto, J. (1993) *Moral Boundaries. A Political Argument for an Ethic of Care*, Routledge, New York & London.

Williams, F. (2001) 'In and Beyond New Labour: Towards a New Political Ethic of Care', *Critical Social Policy*, Vol. 21, no. 4 pp. 467-493.

Can the Ethics of Care Handle Violence?

Virginia Held

It may be thought that the ethics of care has developed important insights into the moral values involved in the caring practices of family, friendship, and personal caregiving, but that the ethics of care has little to offer in dealing with violence. The violence of crime, terrorism, war, and violence against women in any context may seem beyond the ethics of care. Skepticism is certainly in order if it is suggested that we can deal with violence simply by caring. Violence seems to call for the harsh arm of law and enforcement, not the soft touch of care. Elsewhere I have discussed how the ethics of care would recommend respect for international law and how it would thus approach issues of military intervention. I will concentrate here on how the ethics of care can contribute guidance in dealing with family violence and in confronting terrorism.

It may be thought that the ethics of care has developed important insights into the moral values involved in the caring practices of family, friendship, and personal caregiving—both the values that can be found in existing practices, and guidance on how these practices should be improved—but that the ethics of care has little to offer in dealing with violence. The violence of crime, terrorism, war, and violence against women in any context may seem beyond the ethics of care.

Virginia Held is Distinguished Professor of Philosophy at the City University of New York, Graduate School, and Professor Emerita at Hunter College. Her book *The Ethics of Care: Personal, Political, and Global* was published by Oxford University Press in 2006. Among her other books are *The Public Interest and Individual Interests* (Basic Books, 1970); *Rights and Goods: Justifying Social Action* (Free Press, 1984, University of Chicago Press, 1989); *Feminist Morality: Transforming Culture, Society, and Politics* (University of Chicago Press, 1993); and *How Terrorism is Wrong: Morality and Political Violence* (Oxford University Press, 2008); as well as the edited collections *Property, Profits, and Economic Justice* (Wadsworth, 1980), and *Justice and Care: Essential Readings in Feminist Ethics* (Westview, 1995). She co-edited the collections *Philosophy and Political Action* with Kai Nielsen and Charles Parsons, (Oxford University Press, 1972) and *Philosophy, Morality, and International Affairs*, with Sidney Morgenbesser and Thomas Nagel (Oxford University Press, 1974). In 2001–2002 she was President of the Eastern Division of the American Philosophical Association. She has been a fellow at the Center for Advanced Study in the Behavioral Sciences, and has had Fulbright and Rockefeller fellowships. She has been on the editorial boards of many journals in the areas of philosophy and political theory, and has also taught at Yale, Dartmouth, UCLA, and Hamilton. She has two children and five grandchildren.

Skepticism is certainly in order if it is suggested that we can deal with violence simply by caring. Violence seems to call for the harsh arm of law and enforcement, not the soft touch of care. I will argue, nevertheless, that the ethics of care is a comprehensive morality that can offer guidance for problems of violence as it can for other problems.

In recent years I have worked on the ethics of care, on the one hand, and terrorism and political violence on the other. For some time I saw these two topics as poles apart, at something like the opposite ends of a continuum of human interaction. What could be less caring than terrorism, we might think, and what could require more avoidance of violence than caring for a helpless infant? Until recently I pursued these topics independently and did not even try to bring them together. Lately, however, I have been trying to see what the ethics of care can helpfully say about violence, especially political violence, and to see how even violence between groups and states can better be understood with the help of the ethics of care.

Elsewhere I have discussed how the ethics of care would recommend respect for international law and how it would thus approach issues of military intervention (Held 2008c). I will concentrate here on how the ethics of care can contribute guidance in dealing with family violence and in confronting terrorism.

In recent decades, the ethics of care has been developed into what is potentially a comprehensive moral outlook suitable for human relations generally. It can evaluate the relations that exist not only within families, between friends, and in small groups, but relations that are social and political on a large scale. It can provide guidance for how relations between human beings should develop even in the international arena and in the growing relations of global civil society. The ethics of care has developed in ways that show how it can address persons morally in their most distant as well as their closest relations.

For many issues in the domains of the legal or political, when these are seen as embedded within a wider network of relations between human beings, traditional and dominant moral theories may still be suitable. The deontological and consequentialist approaches of Kantian ethics and utilitarianism, for instance, may still be appropriate for many issues within the realm of the legal or political. From the perspective of the ethics of care, we can agree to treat certain issues in the ways they recommend. These theories, however, are less satisfactory than usually thought when expanded into comprehensive moral theories, as they have been. For violence arising within political conflict and being dealt with in political and legal ways, the more familiar approaches may often remain useful. For longer-term evaluations of political institutions and practices, however, the ethics of care may be more promising. It can offer guidance for dealing with states and non-state groups and the violence they often now employ, and for thinking about how the domains of the legal and political should be configured within wider societies such as a developing global one.

As it was originally developed, the approach of care was often seen as conflicting with the approach of justice, making them mutually exclusive. I have subsequently tried to show how they can be integrated if caring relations are seen as the wider and deeper network within which some relations can be dealt with in accordance with the principles of justice (Held 1995, 2006). To understand what this means I have suggested the analogy of friends engaged in a competitive game. When they play tennis, each tries above all to win, limited only by what the fair rules of the game require. If this approach were generalized to the whole of their relation, they would no longer be genuine friends, though it is suitable for limited interactions. Analogously, persons should be tied together as caring members of the same society, yet can agree to treat their limited legal interactions in ways that give priority to justice. When justice should then prevail in certain contexts, it need not oppose or cancel the care on which legal systems should be built.

To the ethics of care, the relations that are of special value are caring relations between persons. This is obvious to us at the personal level, where human life would not be able to continue without the care that has allowed each one of us to survive. But caring relations are not only valuable within families and among friends, they are important in a different way at the most general level of relations between all human beings. The ethics of care understands the value and necessity of caring labor and it emphasizes the values of empathy, sensitivity, trust, and responding to need. It cultivates practices such as the building of trust, and practices of responding to actual needs. At its most basic level it understands persons as interrelated, in contrast with the model of the independent, self-sufficient individual of liberal theory. The ethics of care as it has developed is increasingly appropriate for the wide but shallow human relations of global interactions as well as for the most personal and deepest human relations of care in families.

An appreciation of the value of care has grown out of feminist awareness of the enormous amount of overlooked but utterly necessary labor involved in bringing up children and caring for the ill. The ethics of care articulates especially the *values* involved in caring practices and it explores the guidance they provide. It also *evaluates* existing practices and understands that caring practices as they exist are usually in need of vast improvement. They usually take place in highly unsatisfactory social and political conditions that need fundamental restructuring to make them less unjust and inequitable.

The ethics of care has developed care as a value at least as important as justice, and it evaluates practices of care and of justice. It is based on experience that really is universal, the experience of having been cared for. No child can even survive without a lengthy period of care, and further care is needed for many years for adequate development. The ethics of care compares favorably with contractual views in regard to its potential appeal; contractual views of morality claim to be universal but are not thought to be so in many cultures. The ethics of care does not rest on religious views that are divisive, but on common experience. It promotes the values associated with care as fundamental, and offers strong grounds for countering violence. Whether it can adequately address the issues that arise in dealing with violence is often questioned.

I hope to indicate its promise for doing so in what follows.

Violence in the Family

Let's consider, first, violence in the family. How the ethics of care might not be satisfactory in dealing with domestic violence was raised as a problem by feminists in the early period of interest in the ethics of care. A battered woman who continues to care for and empathize with her batterer may increase the harms she and her children suffer and worsen the effects of his violent tendencies. What seems to be needed in the face of domestic violence is the superior force of law with its stern enforcement, not caring sympathy.

And yet, with a more developed view of care, the ethics of care can well handle such issues. If it is empirically evident, as it seems to be, that in situations of domestic violence prompt legal intervention to prevent further violence is more effective than postponing it and allowing the violence to escalate, the ethics of care would have no trouble recommending this.

Consider Marilyn Friedman's discussion of domestic violence and of how the law and professional caregivers should respond when women in abusive relationships refuse to press charges and are unwilling to leave the men who batter them. Evidence suggests, Friedman notes, that 'mandated legal procedures do tend to reduce the overall level of woman battering' (2003, p. 148; see also Hanna 1996). And yet, legal intervention against the wishes of the battered woman, who may not want her batterer to go to jail and leave her economically worse off or her and her children in even greater danger from his violent retaliation, can seem to 'revictimize' the woman, paternalistically reinforcing her lack of power.

Friedman argues on grounds of respect for the autonomy of abused women that the law should tend toward preventing domestic abuse through mandatory arrest and prosecution of batterers whether or not the victim cooperates, but that professional caregiving services should 'lean toward providing support for abused women', whether or not they stay in abusive relationships and hamper legal intervention (p. 141).

The same positions could as well be arrived at on the basis of the ethics of care. Friedman's argument shows, rightly, that the functions of the law and of professional support services are different, and that law is only one, and often not the most important, of the ways society can try to reduce the incidents and harms of violence. The ethics of care can recognize how mandatory legal proceedings may reduce future incidents of domestic violence and can support them. It can also recognize how shelters, counseling, and social support may be more effective in empowering women to leave or avoid abusive relationships and improve their lives. Care requires that women care for themselves as well as for others.

Recent studies show that arrest and prosecution may not be enough to deter batterers from returning to violence against their intimate partners (Sullivan 2006). If sentences are no more than probation, this may be inadequate. It has been found that when police action was not coordinated with other components of the social system, perpetrators actually increased their use of violence against women. To actually reduce recidivism, men need to be mandated into batterer intervention programs. In the words of Sullivan's discussion of what works and what does not, 'Findings strongly support the contention that men's use of violence against women ... is related to how the community responds to them. Lack of arrest, as well as arrests that lead to no sanctions, sends a clear signal to perpetrators that they can abuse their partners with impunity' (p. 203). Batterer intervention programs reeducate batterers through cognitive-behavioral efforts and coordinate with victim service programs to assure the safety of the women battered. Such findings are entirely consistent with the ethics of care, which would especially demand attention to how *best* to care for all involved in preventing family violence. Empirical evidence is crucial for determining this.

As services for battered women have become more professionalized, however, and such general policies as mandatory arrest instituted because they have been shown to be best for most cases, the voices of individual women have often been listened to less. Since every case is different, this can lead to responses that in some cases are less caring than they should be (Goodman & Epstein 2008). But then, once again, the ethics of care can provide the standards and values with which to criticize developed practices that need reform, in this area as in others.

Children who have been abused are at risk of becoming violent themselves, as partners and parents. A discussion by a number of experts explores ways of helping the victims of child maltreatment to develop satisfactorily (Fantuzzo *et al.* 2006). It has been shown that children making a successful transition from home to going to school for the first time strongly predicts satisfactory academic and social outcomes later. Children with various risk factors, such as having been maltreated, can be identified, and programs can intervene at this point. For instance, through special play sessions children who have difficulty engaging appropriately with others can be drawn into productive peer interactions and cooperative behavior can be reinforced. Such programs probably reduce the chances of children who have suffered from domestic violence becoming violent themselves. Clearly, values of care and responsiveness can guide such efforts.

Two authors discuss various evidence-based interventions to try to prevent the physical abuse of children. While admitting that there is not yet sufficient empirical evidence for any to be declared 'well-supported', the authors consider them promising. These treatments are: group parenting classes or parent support groups, anger management groups, family preservation and reunification programs, parent–child interaction therapy, and cognitive-behavioral therapy and family therapy. Parent–child interaction therapy can be shown to be 'highly effective in decreasing child behavior problems' (Chaffin & Schmidt 2006, p. 53) and is probably responsible for reduced physical abuse by parents. It trains parents using live coaching and teaches relationship-enhancing and discipline skills. We might see this as an example of how the ethics of care could be better than traditional moral theories at guiding how we ought to work to prevent family violence. Instead of emphasizing the punishment of violent parents, it would focus our attention on the relation between parent and child. It would understand child abuse as a failure of care, not just a harm to an individual.

In the caring upbringing of children, it can be understood that punishment may sometimes be needed. Comparable findings can be arrived at elsewhere. But the ethics of care would emphasize how seldom the punishments of the law should be needed if the work of care is adequately facilitated and provided for in all the earlier and other ways in which persons are shaped. For instance, in times and places of high unemployment and resulting high stress, the violence to which anger and frustration can lead increases. A caring society would take responsibility for reducing the stresses of workers abandoned to the uncertainties of unfettered markets. And it would provide adequately for all the other more caring ways in which those inclined toward violence can learn to live their lives nonviolently. A caring world would fundamentally transform the oppressive social structures that produce misery and increased violence for vast numbers of people throughout the world.

The ethics of care may be especially helpful in dealing with the backlash that acceptance of women's progress and of diverse gender identities seems to provoke. To counter the hostility, its sources need to be understood. Understanding the threatened sense of masculinity felt by young men with few social and economic prospects is important; care as well as firmness or punitive legal measures may be needed in efforts to deflect the resulting rage that can lead to violence (Held 2008a).

The ethics of care can acknowledge the need for law and its enforcements in their appropriate domain. Of course, rights need to be respected and violations of them dealt with. What the ethics of care rejects is the expansion of law and legalistic thinking to encompass the whole of morality, marginalizing care to private preference or nonmoral 'natural' inclination. To imagine justice and law as the basis for all of morality, as has been done with such dominant moral theories as Kantian ethics and utilitarianism, is mistaken from the point of view of the ethics of care. But this does not mean that the ethics of care would reject legal intervention in cases of domestic violence and other crime, or, as I argue, in preventing violence between groups and states. Care and concern for victims and potential victims will demand it.

Because of its feminist foundations, the ethics of care will assure that the enormous amount of violence against women that occurs—domestic violence, violence against women in wartime, in ethnic cleansing, and as a result of repression—will be attended to. Gail Mason examines the connections between violence and power, and the view that violence erupts especially when power is threatened or in danger of losing its hold. Violence is often an instrument of power, as when a government uses violence to suppress opposition. Mason's examples are especially of violence against lesbians and gay men, where violence makes 'a statement that to be homosexual is to be in danger of violence, or that to be a heterosexual male is to be a potential source of such danger'. Such statements and the knowledge they embody bolster 'existing systems of sexual order, and the power relations that infuse them' (2002, p. 133). Such systems, like political systems, need not use violence if they are not challenged. But their capacity to use violence can uphold their power.

If we consider the power of caregivers, however, we notice that situations of care are characteristically ones of asymmetric power: parents are far more powerful than children, nurses than patients. But this greater power has, or should have, little to do with the capacities of caregivers to use violence. It has to do with their abilities to respond to needs. Occasionally, or maybe not so infrequently, caregivers do become violent. But it is usually clear that when they do so they are violating the norms of caregiving and failing to act in accordance with the values of care (Ruddick 2002). The values of care demand that one achieve the upbringing of children and the treatment of patients with a variety of ways to influence those cared for without the violence that would harm them. Other areas of human activity could learn much from the way such practices of care exert influence nonviolently.

Liberal individualism sees a sharp break between the care that has a place in the household but not beyond it and the justice that should but often does not govern political and legal affairs. The ethics of care, in contrast, can see the strong relevance of the values involved in practices of care and those that ought to be influential in social and global realms beyond those of family and friendship (Engster 2007; Held 1993, 2006; Ruddick 2002; Tronto 1993, 2007).

Consider, however, how even in the context of care, violence may occasionally be called for. One may violently yank a child out of the path of an oncoming car even if it dislocates her shoulder. If a patient obtains a knife or gun and threatens to use it to kill someone, violent intervention may possibly be needed. The point of these uses of violence, however, will be to further the aims of care, not to destroy opponents.

In the international context, a 'humanitarian intervention' might comparably aim to advance the safety of a civilian population, not obliterate enemies. A military action might aim to restore the legal order of nonaggression between states, not destroy the evil.

A moral theory such as the ethics of care is needed to assure that we care enough about our fellow human beings to actually respect their rights and take appropriate account of their interests and especially that we refrain from aggressive violence. The ethics of care advises that we promote our policies and seek change and maintain order as nonviolently as possible.

Within both families and in a global context, to avoid paternalistic domination, care needs to be interpreted from the perspective of the recipient as well as of the provider. Care *can* be provided in ways that are domineering, oppressive, insensitive, and ineffective, but this is not *good* care. The ethics of care provides guidance for meeting the needs of persons, including needs for peace and security from violence, in ways that are liberating, effective, sensitive, and responsible.

Terrorism and Warfare

The relevance of the ethics of care to international relations has been recognized (Held 2006, chap. 10). An example is the work of Fiona Robinson, whose discussions of globalizing care examine how attention to care would further efforts to combat global poverty (1999, 2006). Mainstream international relations theory, and mainstream normative theory about international relations have resulted, she writes, 'in the creation of a global "culture of neglect" through a systematic devaluing of notions of interdependence, relatedness, and positive involvement in the lives of distant others' (1999, p. 165). With the ethics of care, overcoming poverty would be appropriately emphasized. But can the ethics of care deal with war, or terrorism? Surely here, the skeptic contends, the ethics of care is out of place. On the contrary, I think that the ethics of care is highly relevant in dealing even with violence between states and groups.

Let's consider terrorism specifically. What, if anything, can the ethics of care usefully say about the threat of terrorism? Carol Gould argues that terrorism exemplifies a failure to care. Of the 11 September 2001 attacks on the World Trade Center towers she says: 'there was not only the violation of rights but also what we might call a wholesale lack of human fellow-feeling, an absence of caring about or empathy with the potential victims on the part of the terrorists' (2004, p. 350).

Although we can agree, it needs also to be said that this is true of most violence, and especially of war. Yet many believe war can be just. It is inherent to violence that it disregards its victims. War, in the extent of its destruction and the numbers of its victims, is the ultimate example of the horrors of violence and disregard. Individual participants in terrorism as in war may mourn the victims they produce, but many will not. The failure of those involved in using terrorism to be guided by empathy may be no more pronounced than is that of those who advocate war to answer terrorism.

The ethics of care would guide us away from losing the capacity to empathize with the victims of violence, whatever the kind of violence. It would also ask us, with Gould, to better understand those who turn to violence. In learning how to reduce the appeal of violence, we need to be aware of the combination of humiliation and deprivation that motivates some to support and some to engage in acts of terrorism. We need to understand how governmental and economic policies damage and oppress persons and their cultures. Since terrorist groups cannot continue to exist without a continuing supply of recruits, understanding how to draw such recruits away from the path of violence is the most important factor in dealing with terrorism.

Answering terrorism with wider war is not only among the most uncaring of responses but is also among the least successful. It multiplies both new victims and new recruits. Louise Richardson's important book on terrorism reviews the history of fighting terrorism with military force and makes clear 'the lesson that has already been taught many times': states cannot translate overwhelming military force into victory over terrorists (2006, p. 180; see also Pape 2005).

In considering what US policy ought to be, we should begin by rejecting the blanket condemnations that demonize all terrorists as exceptionally irrational and exceptionally immoral. As political scientist Martha Crenshaw, who has studied terrorism for several decades, concludes: 'terrorism has been an important part of successful struggles for independence from foreign domination'. It is only rational that others learn from this experience. 'Terrorism', she continues, 'is a highly imitable innovation in violent tactics; it combines drama, symbolism, low cost, and ease of implementation ... Thus powerful models can stimulate the imitation of terrorists' (1983, p. 18).

Mia Bloom, another political scientist, reaches a comparable conclusion in her very useful study of suicide terrorism. She notes that

> although the individual bombers might be inspired by several—sometimes complementary—motives, the organizations that send the bombers do so because such attacks are an effective means to intimidate and demoralize the enemy ... [Such] organizations are rationally motivated and use violence to achieve their goals. The operations are carefully calculated and aimed at ending a foreign occupation, increasing the prestige of the organization that uses them, and leading to regional autonomy and/or independence. (2007, p. 3)

I have argued elsewhere that terrorism is not uniquely atrocious (Held 2008a). It is political violence that often, though not, I think, necessarily, targets civilians. It often aims to create sufficient fear to cause others than those attacked to change their policies. I have argued that it resembles guerrilla war or small war in the way it should be evaluated, but it is not the same as war. Terrorist groups use crime to achieve their political goals and can be responded to in the short term with the apprehension, trial, and punishment of those involved in ways that minimize the appeal of such violence. Responding with wider war magnifies not only the violence, with all its moral costs, but also the sympathy felt for the war's victims and the terrorist groups who claim to fight for them. In the longer term, responses need to involve diplomatic, political, social, and economic measures.

There have been claims that the United States is currently faced with a 'new kind of terrorism', such that no lessons of the past are relevant. Such views have served to support the misguided 'war on terrorism' of the administration of George W. Bush, but have been effectively refuted (Crenshaw 2008). To those familiar with the terrorism of the past, that of the present is largely a continuation.

Much is often made of the difference between intentionally targeting civilians, as terrorism often or on some definitions always does, and only killing civilians unintentionally, as does conventional warfare. In the view of those who think conventional warfare can be morally justified while terrorism never can, this distinction is crucial. Together with many others, I do not believe the distinction can bear the moral weight it has been assigned.

The distinction between targeting civilians intentionally and only killing them forseeably as collateral damage means little to those who identify with the dead. Even if terrorism does target civilians (in fact it often, as well, attacks military targets) it is usually far less deadly than conventional warfare. Conventional warfare may proclaim an intent to spare civilians, then yield to 'military necessity', bombing whole cities and all their inhabitants. Or, as weapons become more precise, states may target specific persons and only kill civilians inadvertently but in far greater numbers than those killed by terrorism. Over many years, the deaths of Palestinian children have been approximately eight times the deaths of Israeli children resulting from the conflict (Kristof 2008).

When the United States responded with military force in Iraq to what was claimed to be a terrorist threat posed by Saddam Hussein, it caused the deaths of some 10,000 civilians in just the initial invasion (Massing 2007, p. 87).[1] Since then, the war has led to the deaths of many tens of thousands and perhaps hundreds of thousands of civilians (Altman & Oppel 2008). Terrorism, in comparison, has killed relatively very small numbers. In conventional war, the killing of civilians often becomes routine and overlooked. Certainly, some terrorists commit atrocities that are absolutely horrendous. So do some armed forces members in the course of fighting wars. The goals of some terrorists are, without doubt, morally abhorrent. So are the goals of some who use ordinary military power. If, however, the objectives for which they are used are justifiable, the weapon of terrorism and how it is used are not necessarily more immoral than the weapon of conventional military force and how it is used.

Robin May Schott effectively argues against the just war tradition on which seeing a vast moral divide between terrorism and war usually rests. She finds that the just war tradition all too easily normalizes war, suggesting that provided certain limits are observed, war is morally acceptable (2008). She uses Kant to argue that war is never morally acceptable, but an ethics of care might even more reliably keep us from forgetting that war is always atrocious, even if sometimes better than its alternatives. Which terms one uses to make the distinction between war being sometimes necessary or better than its alternatives but never morally acceptable is somewhat arbitrary. The point to remember is that it should always be viewed as needing to be prevented, averted, avoided. If it has become better than capitulation against an aggressor or abdication of responsibility in the face of genocide, the situation already represents a massive moral failure.

One could argue that the problems of the just war tradition result more from the misuse of its norms, as by the administration of George W. Bush, rather than of the norms themselves which do require that war be a last resort. But the specific norms have been developed for conflicts between the armed forces of

---

1. Massing writes that "10,000 civilians at a minimum were killed during the invasion, the large majority victims of the coalition" (p. 87).

states. It is questionable whether they can be applied to the kinds of violence engaged in, for instance, by nonstate groups trying to achieve liberation from colonial oppression. The ethics of care can accept the underlying norms of the just war tradition such as the requirement that one's cause be just, and that the violence used must be proportional. It is better able to keep in mind the overriding context of caring relations between human beings that are so obviously shattered by war.

Those who use terrorism often believe they have no other way to resist unjust oppression, and sometimes this judgment may be correct. To the opponents of those with vastly superior power, terrorism is often seen as self-defense, or reprisal against attacks they have suffered, attacks by the strong on the weak.

It is not inherently better to use force or violence to maintain an existing political situation or territorial boundary than to use force or violence to change them. Stability has definite value, if it can be maintained without the undue use of force or violence. When it becomes sufficiently intolerable to enough people for it to be maintained only with severe repression, however, the use of force or violence to change the political situation or territorial boundary may be less unjustifiable than using them to maintain the intolerable situation. The better alternative in all such cases is to have guidelines to achieve such change through peaceful means, through negotiations, international judicial decisions, referenda and the like. But when the power resisting change refuses to employ such means, violence to change the situation may be better than violence to maintain it, if the new situation will be more just.

In the case of South Africa, apartheid was ended without civil war and with only a moderate use of violence by the opponents of apartheid. After decades of violent repression, the African National Congress and its leader Nelson Mandela were enabled by the white South African government to pursue their objectives politically. If, on the other hand, the repression had been further escalated and the ANC had resorted to further terrorism, we might judge that in view of the justifiability of ending apartheid, the violence used by the ANC was less unjustifiable than that used by the white South African government.

If it is sincerely believed that only force rather than argument will move an opponent, and that one's position and aim are clearly just, force applied through terrorism may be on a par with force applied through conventional arms in being resorted to in the first place. Sheikh Ahmad Yasin, founder of Hamas, who was assassinated by Israel in March 2004, said that 'Once we have warplanes and missiles, then we can think of changing our means of legitimate self-defense, but right now, we can only tackle the fire with our bare hands and sacrifice ourselves' (Bloom 2007, pp. 3–4). As expressed by the secretary-general of the Palestinian Islamic Jihad, summarized by Ehud Sprinzak, 'Our enemy possesses the most sophisticated weapons in the world and its army is trained to a very high standard ... We have nothing with which to repel killing and thuggery against us except the weapon of martyrdom ... [H]uman bombs cannot be defeated' (Bloom 2007, pp. 89–90).

In assessing the justifiability of the means used in violent conflict, the demand that opponents of states with armed forces and sophisticated weaponry fight the way such states do amounts to an argument that they should meet us on our own ground so that we can defeat them. From the point of view of a militarily weak opponent, it would be irrational as well as impossible to do this. As Lionel McPherson said of Michael Walzer's demand that native groups seeking liberation must 'earn' their freedom by confining their attacks to members of the armed forces and refraining from attacking anyone else: 'this reeks of ... condescension' (2008, p. 8). Terrorism is a weapon that helps to neutralize the enormous military power possessed by some states. Using this weapon can be the rational course of action for such states' opponents, and not clearly more immoral than war.

The ethics of care provides strong grounding for valuing nonviolence over violence in political conflict. Violence damages and destroys what care labors to create. Care instructs us to establish the means to curb, contain, prevent, and head off the violence that characteristically leads to more violent behavior. In bringing up children, this requires a long process of nurturing and education in order to cultivate nonviolent feelings, self-restraint, appropriate trust, and an understanding of the better alternatives to aggressive conflict. In interactions with others at some distance, the primary institutions with which to prevent and deal with violence are political and legal, and care can recommend acceptance of these institutions when appropriate even as it recognizes their limits. Moreover, it can suggest alternative ways of interacting that may prove more satisfactory, and these understandings can be matched at the international level. Sudden reactions that are themselves violent are much less effective at reducing violence than are patient, caring, long-term efforts.

With the guidance of the ethics of care, we would acknowledge that violence is an aspect of human reality that must be expected, but that we can successfully work to contain it. With care, we can decrease violence and the suffering and damage it brings about. Guided by the values of care, we would restrain rather than destroy those who become violent, we would inhibit violence as nonviolently as possible, and we would especially work to prevent violence rather than wipe out violent persons. As Sara Ruddick has recently written: 'Many mothers know what many military enthusiasts forget—the ability to destroy can shock and awe but compelling the will is subtle, ultimately cooperative work' (2009, p. 307).

The most important factor in dealing with terrorism is understanding how to draw potential recruits away from the path of violence. In Bloom's view, the key 'is to reduce [terrorists'] motivations for suicide bombings rather than their capabilities to carry them out ... There are no military solutions to terrorism' (2007, pp. 39–40). Vengeful retribution for insulted authority leads to reactions such as the 'war on terror'. The result of George W. Bush's such reaction has been a great increase of support for extremist groups, based on sympathy for the victims of US wars. The ethics of care's focus on how to reduce the appeal of terrorist groups to potential supporters would be more effective in reducing terrorism.

The ethics of care can help us to listen to the views of others and try to understand their points of view. Care inherently involves attentiveness to others and responding to needs, and its values prepare us to do what is needed to reduce and undermine trends toward violence. Those motivated by care will be open to the evidence that terrorism is not defeated by greater violence but by promoting other means through which those with political objectives can pursue their aims. When those aims are misguided, they can be defeated politically, and when they are legitimate they can be enabled (Barber 2004; Richardson 2006).

We should constantly and insistently remind ourselves and others that violence is often or usually counterproductive, and that there are nearly always better and more effective nonviolent ways of pursuing political objectives. Yet there are good reasons not to rule out as always unjustifiable all uses of violence (Hutchings 2007). The ethics of care, I believe, would agree. Some violence is usually thought defensible in the enforcement of justifiable law. Yet education, treatment, and negotiation can usually preclude much of the need for violent law enforcement. Protest that may become violent is often thought better than acquiescence in morally indefensible repression. Civil actions of various kinds, however, such as protests, demonstrations, and disobedience, together with clever and creative uses of the media, can often shame repressive opponents. Nonviolent opposition often has more chance of success than the violence that invites greater violence or repression that, though ineffective, can be politically popular.

The ethics of care would direct us to counter terrorism with policies that will not only be more caring in the ways that they themselves minimize violence but also more effective in undermining the violence of those opposing us, whoever we are.

Acknowledgements

An earlier version of this paper was presented at a conference on Philosophy and Everyday Life at the University of Oslo, Norway, 9–10 June 2008. I am grateful to Tove Pettersen and others for comments on that version, and to Christine Koggel and Joan Orme for subsequent comments. The paper is based in part on my books The Ethics of Care *and* How Terrorism is Wrong.

References

Altman, L. K. & Oppel, R. A. Jr (2008) 'W.H.O. Says Iraq Civilian Death Toll Higher than Cited', *New York Times*, 10 January, p. A14.
Barber, B. R. (2004) *Fear's Empire: War, Terrorism, and Democracy*, Norton, New York.
Bloom, M. (2007) *Dying to Kill: The Allure of Suicide Terror*, Columbia University Press, New York.
Chaffin, M. & Schmidt, S. (2006) 'An Evidence-based Perspective on Interventions to Stop or Prevent Child Abuse', in *Preventing Violence: Research and Evidence-based*

Intervention Strategies, ed. J. R. Lutzker, American Psychological Association, Washington, DC, 49–68.

Crenshaw, M. (ed.) (1983) *Terrorism, Legitimacy, and Power*, Wesleyan University Press, Middletown, CT, 117–136.

Crenshaw, M. (2008) 'The Debate over "New" vs. "Old" Terrorism', in *Values and Violence: Intangible Aspects of Terrorism*, eds I. A. Karawan, W. McCormack & S. E. Reynolds, Studies in Global Justice, Vol. 4, Springer, New York.

Engster, D. (2007) *The Heart of Justice: Care Ethics and Political Theory*, Oxford University Press, New York.

Fantuzzo, J. W., Bulotsky-Shearer, R. J. & McWayne, C. M. (2006) 'The Pursuit of Wellness for Victims of Child Maltreatment: A Model for Targeting Relevant Competencies, Contexts, and Contributors', in *Preventing Violence: Research and Evidence-based Intervention Strategies*, ed. J. R. Lutzker, American Psychological Association, Washington, DC, 69–91.

Friedman, M. (2003) *Autonomy, Gender, Politics*, Oxford University Press, New York.

Goodman, L. A. & Epstein, D. (2008) *Listening to Battered Woman: A Survivor-centered Approach to Advocacy, Mental Health, and Justice*, American Psychological Association, Washington, DC.

Gould, C. C. (2004) *Globalizing Democracy and Human Rights*, Cambridge University Press, New York.

Hanna, C. (1996) 'No Right to Choose: Mandated Victim Participation in Domestic Violence Prosecutions', *Harvard Law Review*, Vol. 109, no. 8, pp. 1849–910.

Held, V. (1989) *Rights and Goods: Justifying Social Action*, University of Chicago Press, Chicago.

Held, V. (1993) *Feminist Morality: Personal, Political, and Global*, University of Chicago Press, Chicago.

Held, V. (1995) 'The Meshing of Care and Justice', *Hypatia*, Vol. 10, no. 2, pp. 128–32.

Held, V. (2006) *The Ethics of Care: Personal, Political, and Global*, Oxford University Press, New York.

Held, V. (2008a) 'Gender Identity and the Ethics of Care in Globalized Society', in *Global Feminist Ethics: Feminist Ethics and Social Theory*, eds R. Whisnant & P. DesAutels, Rowman & Littlefield, Lanham, MD, 43–57.

Held, V. (2008b) *How Terrorism is Wrong: Morality and Political Violence*, Oxford University Press, New York.

Held, V. (2008c) 'Military Intervention and the Ethics of Care', *The Southern Journal of Philosophy*, Vol. XLVI, pp. 1–20.

Hutchings, K. (2007) 'Simone de Beauvoir and the Ambiguous Ethics of Political Violence', *Hypatia*, Vol. 22, pp. 111–32.

Kristof, N. D. (2008) 'Tough Love for Israel?', *New York Times*, 24 July, Op-ed page.

Mason, G. (2002) *The Spectacle of Violence: Homophobia, Gender and Knowledge*, Routledge, London.

Massing, M. (2007) 'Iraq: The Hidden Human Costs', *New York Review*, 20 December, pp. 82–87.

McPherson, L. (2008) Commentary for Central APA Symposium 'Is Terrorism Ever Justifiable?', Chicago, 17 April, unpublished typescript.

Pape, R. A. (2005) *Dying to Win: The Strategic Logic of Suicide Terrorism*, Random House, New York.

Richardson, L. (2006) *What Terrorists Want: Understanding the Enemy, Containing the Threat*, Random House, New York.

Robinson, F. (1999) *Globalizing Care: Ethics, Feminist Theory, and International Affairs*, Westview Press, Boulder.

Robinson, F. (2006) 'Care, Gender and Global Social Justice: Rethinking "Ethical Globalization"', *Journal of Global Ethics*, Vol. 2, pp. 5–25.

Ruddick, S. (2002) *Maternal Thinking: Toward a Politics of Peace*, Beacon Press, Boston.

Ruddick, S. (2009) 'On Maternal Thinking', *Women's Studies Quarterly*, Vol. 37, nos. 3–4, pp. 305–08.

Schott, R. M. (2008) 'Just War and the Problem of Evil', *Hypatia*, Vol. 23, pp. 122–40.

Sullivan, C. M. (2006) 'Intervention to Address Intimate Partner Violence: The Current State of the Field', in *Preventing Violence: Research and Evidence-based Intervention Strategies*, ed. J. R. Lutzker, American Psychological Association, Washington, DC, 195–212.

Tronto, J. C. (1993) *Moral Boundaries: A Political Argument for an Ethic of Care*, Routledge, New York.

Tronto, J. C. (2007) 'Is Peace Keeping Care Work?', in *Global Feminist Ethics: Feminist Ethics and Social Theory*, eds R. Whisnant & P. DesAutels, Rowman & Littlefield, Lanham, MD, 179–200.

After Liberalism in World Politics? Towards an International Political Theory of Care

Fiona Robinson

This paper explores the potential for an international political theory of care as an alternative to liberalism in the context of contemporary global politics. It argues that relationality and interdependence, and the responsibilities for and practices of care that arise therewith, are fundamental aspects of moral life and sites of political contestation that have been systematically denied and obfuscated under liberalism. A political theory of care brings into view the responsibilities and practices of care that sustain not just 'bare life' but all social life, from nuclear and extended families to local, national and transnational communities. It disrupts and challenges the individualism of liberalism, and the associated valorization of 'freedom', 'autonomy', and 'toleration'. Instead, it emphasizes an ontology of relationality and interdependence that accepts the existence of vulnerability without reifying particular individuals, groups or states as 'victims' or 'guardians'. Furthermore, by demonstrating the gendered and raced nature of caring in the contemporary world—from the household to the transnational level—an international political theory of care challenges our received assumptions about 'dependence' in world politics, and opens up space to interrogate politically not only gender but race and other aspects of inequality in the global political economy.

Political theories ... are intended to capture the conditions for justice. The relationships of dependency and care are viewed as standing outside these public domains. (Kittay 2001b, p. 47)

The principles of mutuality and interconnectedness provide a chance to rediscover politics as a practical interrogation of power. (Duffield 2007, p. 233)

Fiona Robinson is an associate professor and Director of Graduate Studies in the Department of Political Science, Carleton University, Canada.

Introduction

My book *Globalizing Care: Ethics, Feminist Theory and International Relations*, was published in 1999. My aim in that book was to offer a critique of dominant understandings of ethics in the discipline of international relations, and to consider the implications of a feminist ethics of care in the context of global politics (Robinson 1999a). At that time, the ethics of care went very much against the grain of contemporary international political theory. While critical approaches existed, the literature was dominated by what could be called the liberal 'global justice' industry. By that I am referring to the large body of work consisting mainly of deontological liberal and liberal contractualist accounts of justice. Most of this work took a universalist or 'cosmopolitan' position, but the liberal 'communitarian' critique of cosmopolitanism also played an important part in framing this literature. There were certainly some interventions from anti-foundationalist social theorists and some feminists at that time; by and large, however, normative theory in international relations in the 1990s was mapped along this axis, and almost completely dominated by liberal approaches.

These academic accounts were both reflected, and were mutually constitutive of, events in world politics. In a different 1999 publication—this time on liberalism in world politics—I argued that, despite the fact that liberalism had always played 'second fiddle' to realism in international relations, the recent end of the Cold War had brought with it an 'explicit and renewed commitment to liberalism on a global scale' (Robinson 1999b, p. 143). While it was accepted that liberal reform was ultimately limited by the presence of the states system, the importance of liberal values as a marker of legitimacy of state forms in that political climate could not be underestimated. Moreover, the global reach and power of the global capitalist economy was at its zenith at this time; liberalism had apparently won not just the day but the war itself. My purpose in writing this was not to applaud liberalism but to point out the astonishing lack of attention to what Wallerstein called the 'total self-contradiction' of liberal ideology (Wallerstein 1995, p. 161).

A decade later, the tide has turned somewhat. Perhaps not surprisingly, international relations theorists are turning their attention to the 'end of the liberal moment', citing key developments in the twenty-first century as evidence: the failure of liberal internationalism—most notably in the Darfur region of Sudan; the 'War on Terror' and its associated policies and practices with respect to 'security' and human rights; and, finally, the ongoing global financial and economic crisis, beginning in the autumn of 2008 and continuing today. In October 2009, the London School of Economics hosted the annual *Millennium* conference on international relations, this time titled 'After Liberalism'. This theme was emphasized in panel titles such as 'Liberalism and its Discontents'; 'The 'Post-liberal' World'; and 'RIP Neo-liberalism: 1979–2009'. Less evident from the panel or paper titles, however, was any clear indication of what would fill the gaping void left by the alleged demise of liberalism as a global ideology. If, indeed, the liberal moment is ending, what will, or should, take its place?

In this article I argue that we should be careful about heralding the demise of liberalism in world politics; indeed, liberal ontological categories and normative dispositions are remarkably persistent in contemporary international relations. Paradoxically, it is both the apparent crisis—especially of neo-liberalism—and the endurance of liberal values which point, at this time, to the need to articulate an international political theory of care as an alternative, critical political theory of global politics. To that end, I argue that relationality and interdependence, and the responsibilities for and practices of care that arise therewith, are fundamental aspects of moral life and sites of political contesta-tion that have been systematically denied and obfuscated under liberalism. An international political theory of care brings into view the responsibilities and practices of care that sustain not just 'bare life' but all social life, from nuclear and extended families to local, national and transnational communities. It disrupts and challenges the individualism of liberalism, and the associated valorization of 'freedom', 'autonomy', and 'toleration'. Instead, it emphasizes an ontology of relationality and interdependence that accepts the existence of vulnerability without reifying particular individuals, groups or states as 'victims' or 'guardians'. Through this lens, equality does not mean 'sameness' or 'equal opportunity'; rather, the focus is on ensuring that all people are able to give and receive care that is adequate to their needs as defined in the context of particular relationships and communities. Furthermore, by demonstrating the gendered and raced nature of caring in the contemporary world—from the household to the transnational level—an international political theory of care challenges our received assumptions about 'dependence' in world politics, and opens up space to interrogate politically not only gender but race and other aspects of inequality in the global political economy.[1]

Liberalism in International Political Theory

In *The Twenty-years Crisis*, E. H. Carr argues that the crisis of the late 1930s that led to the onset of the Second World War was brought about by a collapse of the edifice of 'liberal-idealist' thinking which had dominated international affairs in the inter-war period (Carr 1939, p. 62). The period from 1945 to 1989, by contrast, is generally regarded as being dominated by realism, which holds that states are the dominant actors in an anarchic system, and that power—in particular, the quest for security—is the central feature of interstate relation-ships. The period from 1989 to 2001, it could be argued, saw a shift back towards what came to be known not as 'idealism' (something clearly to be avoided in international politics) but 'liberal internationalism'.

---

1. The transnationalization of care refers to the flow of (mainly women) caregivers from low-income countries to wealthier countries. The concept of the 'global care chain' (Parrenas 2001) illustrates the effects of this migration, as women often leave their own children in the care of another female relative in their country of origin in order to seek opportunities abroad that will help them support those children.

There is no doubt that the end of the Cold War ushered in a period of rhetorical and policy commitment to the values of liberalism, including a strong belief in the possibility of achieving reform in the direction of something that might be called 'global liberalism'. Fukuyama's *The End of History* (1992) was a credo for the 1990s in the West, inspiring confidence in decisive interventions in the name of pursuing and achieving pro-liberalization policies around the world. From the Gulf War of 1990–91, to the even more decisive war of NATO with Yugoslavia over the fate of Kosovo, these events are held up as examples of 'liberal's wars': that is, wars fought 'predominantly in response to gross human rights violations and threats of genocide' (Brown 1999, p. 49). In the 1990s, these decisive victories were seen to reinforce the claim that, as Chris Brown puts it, '[t]here is no viable form of emancipatory politics except that which takes place within the basic liberal model' (Brown 1999, p. 51).

The post-Cold War linking of development and security, moreover, served to reinforce the moral rectitude of these interventions, and to entrench the alleged necessity of a liberal international politics that was universal in scope. While the events of September 2001 called other aspects of the liberal project into question, this linkage has been strengthened, rather than weakened, by the War on Terror. Development programs and initiatives are now routinely justified on the basis that they will help to mitigate exclusion and alienation, thereby delivering greater stability not only to the nation-state or region in question but also to the world as a whole (see Duffield 2007).

While these apparent sea changes from utopianism to realism to liberal internationalism do correspond at some level to the changing nature of international politics, they also serve to belie the continuity of the principles that have governed world politics since the beginning of the 'short' twentieth century. In other words, in emphasizing shifts from utopianism to realism back to liberalism (and, since 2001, back to realism) we obfuscate the extent to which liberal ideas of individual (state) autonomy, agency and contractarianism have always been at the heart of both the contemporary international system and the theories through which it is constituted. Thus, while some international relations theorists use 'liberalism' to refer simply to a belief in the ability of international institutions to promote cooperation and collectively manage conflict, a return to the foundational principles of liberalism allows us to see clearly how they underwrite not only the global political economy but also the legal and normative order upon which the international system rests.

The UN Charter rests on the idea of the sovereign equality of states based on the notions of territorial integrity and political autonomy. The Universal Declaration of Human Rights rests on the notion of the fundamental equality of all persons based on the idea of human dignity which, in turn, rests on the idea of individual autonomy. While it is indeed the case that these two documents display the tensions surrounding the doctrines of state sovereignty and individual rights, it could similarly be argued that these two ideas are mutually constitutive and reinforcing, especially in the so-called 'human rights era' since 1945 (see Reus-Smit 2001). Seen in this way, it would seem that despite the apparent end of the liberal moment as displayed in events and trends internationally since 2001, the ontological and normative categories of liberalism are remarkably persistent. Challenging the dominance of liberalism will require that we reflect critically on our most basic ideas about subjectivity, personhood and equality that form the basis of the dominant understandings of the nature of politics, and what counts as politics, both within and beyond states.

Liberalism has successfully constructed a series of dichotomies at both the domestic and the international levels that shape these definitions. While the most enduring and prevalent of these is the 'public/private' dichotomy, other, related dichotomies include 'autonomy and dependence', 'sovereignty and intervention', 'self-determination and imperialism'. These dichotomies both shape the direction of world politics and limit our vision in the search for solutions to endemic suffering and violence around the globe.

The End of the Liberal Moment?

In spite of my argument above that liberalism is built into the most basic political theoretical ideas which inform our views of how the international system works, it may indeed be the case that, for strategic reasons, the contemporary political landscape is ripe for the articulation of alternatives to liberalism. While the end of the Cold War brought inquiries into what justice would look like in a 'post-socialist' world, most of those speculations were drowned out by the resounding triumphal cries of liberals everywhere. Moreover, while the period immediately following September 2001 challenged the West's apparent invincibility, any suggestion that part of the problem might stem from 'our' way of doing things, and the manner in which we have sought to export this way around the world, was prohibited. But while decades of continued underdevelopment in the poorest regions of the world may not be enough to cause world leaders and international financial institutions to question the governance of the global economy, it may be that the global economic crisis of the last part of this decade will finally achieve that.

The current global economic crisis has not only affirmed the view of critics but has also shaken the resolve of many of those who continued to believe in the long-term rectitude of neo-liberalism. But while there is a growing consensus that unadulterated neo-liberalism may ultimately be in *no one's* interests, even the roughest outline of a solution to the perils of a neo-liberal, deregulated global economy is far from evident today. Traditional ideological categories seem neither to resonate nor apply in the contemporary context. Consider the infamous bailouts of 2009—from Wall Street to General Motors, the US and other governments around the world poured money into failing banks, corporations and entire industries that are currently regarded as the lifeblood of the global economy. Almost equal amounts of derision was heaped on these bailouts from both the right and the left; while the former saw them as representing a move towards 'socialism' in the form of a state-run economy, the latter pronounced the bailouts to be a clear example of the state acting in support of capital, and the interests of the wealthy.

Of course, critics have been decrying the effects of neo-liberalism on huge swathes of the world's population for decades. Throughout the 1990s, it became increasingly clear that structural adjustment and stabilization policies (SAPs) undertaken by international financial institutions including the IMF and, to a lesser extent, the World Bank, had the effect of exacerbating the conditions of poverty and suffering for large numbers of the populations of many developing countries. While the scaling back of social provision for health and education is often recognized as a 'gender issue', this has, by and large, served to keep it at the margins of the debate. Embedded in the ontological categories and normative discourse of liberalism, care is consigned to the 'private sphere' occupied by women, rather than occupying a central place in the search for solutions.

Thus, while some may portray the end of the liberal moment as happening suddenly and without warning, perhaps in the events of 11 September 2001, and solidified by the global financial crisis beginning in September 2008, many others would argue that the contradictions in post-Cold War liberalism existed for some time, even during the apparent 'heyday' of liberalism. Given the lack of credibility attached to most versions of 'socialism' since 1989, some of the strongest and most promising voices speaking out against liberalism—and neo-liberal economics in particular—have been those of feminists. In 1997, Nancy Fraser's study of justice and the 'post-socialist' condition addressed 'the crumbling of the old gender order', focusing on the increase in women's paid employment outside the home in most countries, changing family structures and new household arrangements (Fraser 1997, p. 41).

In a radical yet under-recognized argument, Fraser puts forward a model of the citizen as Universal Caregiver. Rather than aiming to make women more like men—in other words, to make everyone Universal Breadwinners—the aim is to re-vision the ideal-typical citizen as a Universal Caregiver. This, she admits, would require the wholesale redesign of all social institutions—including changes to the nature and structure of paid labour to make space for caregiving activities. Building on this argument, Alison Weir proposes an enlargement of this model to encompass a 'larger feminist imagination'; rather than focusing specifically on the achievement of gender equity in the nation-state, Weir argues for a shift in focus which directly addresses the global inequities of the global care chains (Weir 2005, p. 312).

While the emphasis in the work of Fraser and Weir described above is, quite rightly, gender equity, it is worth noting that the failure of states and other institutions to address these changes is a problem not only for women and their equity with men, but for families, communities, and sometimes even entire nation-states. Certainly, it is women, especially poor women and women of colour, who shoulder the burden of care for their own families or for families in income-rich countries overseas. Care workers of all kinds are underpaid and 'burnt out', leading to a decline in the quality of care. Those who migrate for care work often become 'second-class citizens' in the countries where they reside, while contributing to the care deficit in their own—often income-poor—countries.

In the context of neo-liberal restructuring and the scaling back of social spending, it is also the case that many men suffer the psychological and material burden of knowing that their 'male wage' is often insufficient for family survival. Many of these men, moreover, remain precluded from taking on caring roles due to dominant cultural norms of gender and constructions of masculinity. This exclusion from both traditional and non-traditional roles may be responsible for a rising incidence of masculinized violence—on a continuum from 'intimate' violence to forms of warfare within and among states. At the global level, both neo-liberalism and militarism are characterized by a refusal to acknowledge interdependence, vulnerability and the public role for caring practices in creating societies that are less prone to conflict and less reliant on violence as a solution to social problems. As Colleen O'Manique argues, feminists must move beyond a focus on 'male domination' towards an examination of a system of extreme masculine characteristics, which are reflected in the valorization and celebration of war and violent masculinity, and the devalorization of the labour of social reproduction more typically performed by women (O'Manique 2006, p. 174).

While theorizing about the relationship between care, masculinity and violence is important, there are also dangers of which to be aware in making such associations. Blaming individual, poor men for the widespread crisis of social reproduction obfuscates the way in which both women's *and* men's roles in care are governed by liberal and masculinist assumptions regarding the nature of care and caregiving. Indeed, these strategies may be seen as neo-liberal governance practices, whereby the 'responsibilizing' of men serves to further entrench the privatization of caring, while ensuring that, as Bedford puts it, a 'whole range of possibilities less focused on privatized loving' are left aside (Bedford 2008, pp. 100, 103). Rather than allowing our analyses of hegemonic masculinities to target specific groups of men in ways that are overtly raced and classed, we should consider the effects of norms of masculinity at the level of structures, norms and institutions: in national budgeting; the making and implementing of legislation governing intimate violence and 'intimate labour', and the relationship between the two; and in the still-powerful influence of national and global cultures of militarism. Perhaps most importantly, we should consider the powerful effects of not only the substance but also the form of masculinist logic on our thinking and theorizing about world politics; as Kimberly Hutchings has argued, if what masculinity *is* is rooted in what it *does*, then it is not any particular instantiation of masculinity which feminist scholarship needs to challenge but the work of evaluation and exclusion that it accomplishes in our frameworks for understanding the world (Hutchings 2008, pp. 28–29; emphasis in original).

I would argue that a critical, feminist ethics of care can help us navigate the contemporary landscape of international politics by disrupting a series of familiar oppositions, including those of individual and society, right and left. In her critique of Third Way discourse in Britain, Selma Sevenhuijsen argues that the discourse, in spite of its claims, remained marked by oppositions between the individual and society. By contrast, a feminist ethic of care denies the ontological distinction between individuals and society. Instead, it provides an 'alternative view on the creation of social ties compared to that of the building of bridges between individuals and society' (Sevenhuijsen 2000, p. 9).

A critical care ethics emphasizes the universality of the need to give and receive care, and critiques the near-universal undervaluing of the practices and labour of care and those who perform them. However, unlike most 'universalist' international political theories, this theory rejects epistemological foundation-alism, denies the existence of 'universal' principles of politics or justice, and eschews abstract appeals to 'human nature' as a foundation for theoretical or normative commitments. Instead, care should be seen as a critical theory of world politics that challenges traditional understandings of 'private', 'public' and 'international' by revealing how hidden dependencies support political economies, as well as how the social constructions of gender and race are constitutive of the value we place on caring practices, and how these assessments affect dominant understandings of 'autonomy', 'equality', 'labour' and 'citizenship'.

An international political theory of care has enormous potential to transcend the dichotomous ideologies and politics that have consistently dogged radical critiques of liberalism—including feminist critiques—for decades. But in order for this potential to be realized, care theorists must highlight the gendered and raced nature of the discourses and practices of care; at the same time, however, they must continue to emphasize the wide relevance of care ethics for families, communities and states. Despite the arguments of Fraser and countless others regarding the centrality of care work in the daily lives and identity of all peoples, the idea of 'care' remains marginal in political theory (and even more marginal in *international* political theory). I would suggest that this is due to the way in which ideas related to care are consistently framed by the politics of gender equality and women's emancipation. Tied to this, analyses of the (international) politics of care are usually regarded as addressing a peripheral issue area, rather than the central core of politics.

A fully developed international political theory of care rests not on a normative injunction to care; indeed, this moral position is already covered by liberal discourses of humanitarianism, which call upon the benevolent, auton-omous global North to keep peace, build security and 'develop' the dependent, impoverished global South. A critical feminist ethics of care grows out of a recognition of the role of power in constructing relations of dependence, upholding the myths of autonomy and concealing the needs and responsibilities of care. Thus, it recognizes the complex interdependence and relationality that characterize relations among states, institutions and individuals even in distant geopolitical regions.

Autonomy, Dependence and Power

In their revealing and insightful genealogy of 'dependency' in the US welfare state, Nancy Fraser and Linda Gordon show that the discourse of dependency affects not only the social politics of 'welfare' in that country but also how it maps onto a 'whole series of hierarchical oppositions' that define contemporary culture:

> Fear of dependency ... posits an ideal, independent personality in contrast to which those considered dependent are deviant. This contrast bears traces of a sexual division of labor that assigns men primary responsibility as providers or breadwinners and women primary responsibility as caretakers and nurturers and then treats the derivative personality patterns as fundamental ... In this way, the opposition between the independent personality and the dependent personality maps onto a whole series of hierarchical oppositions and dichotomies that are central in modern culture: masculine/feminine, public/private; work/care; success/love; individual/community; economy/family and competitive/self-sacrificing. (Fraser & Gordon 1994, p. 332)

They argue convincingly for the need to question our received valuations and definitions of dependence and independence in order to allow new, emancipatory social visions to emerge (Fraser & Gordon 1994, p. 332).

Despite its central place in the construction and constitution of world politics, the notion of 'dependence' has not received much attention in international political theory. Juridically speaking, dependence is regarded as a relic of the past—something that ceased to exist with the demise of colonialism following the Second World War. 'Dependency' theory—that version of neo-Marxism which regards 'underdevelopment' in the periphery as the inevitable and ongoing result of 'development' in the core—is regarded in international relations as a theory of 'development', and thus as not only outdated but largely outside of its disciplinary boundaries. Of course, postcolonial and decolonial theorists have argued convincingly that forms of economic and cultural neo-colonialism govern the relations between the global North and the global South in spite of the end of formal systems of imperialism. Despite their potentially enormous contribution to our understanding of contemporary world politics, these approaches have yet to permeate the mainstream of both international relations theory and international political theory.

The task of redefining the nature of, and relationship between, autonomy and dependence has been a central theoretical task of most feminist care ethicists. As Eva Kittay has argued, 'as long as we continue to occlude the existence of dependency, our political theory excludes ... those who are temporarily or permanently dependent and are so inevitably ... those whose labour is devoted to the care of dependents ... and the moral social and political importance of relationships of dependency rooted in the facts of human vulnerability and frailty' (Kittay 2001a, p. 529). While refocusing our attention in these directions is an important antidote to liberal theory, it is also crucial that we keep in view the agency of those who are dependent, and the ways in which various forms of dependency are socially constructed by existing norms, institutions and structures. Indeed, it may be that the lenses of postcolonial theory have important contributions to make to an international political theory of care. For example, while the government and people of Haiti may be temporarily and inevitably dependent on donor countries, especially after the recent earthquake, this fact should not blind us to the agency of Haitians in responding not only to the 'crisis' but also in their everyday struggles with poverty. Moreover, the ongoing engagement of the international community with Haiti should reflect not just benevolence but also a recognition of the common history of colonialism, slavery, occupation and 'development'—a history that is shared by most states. Placing existing relationships in a wider and longer historical perspective also reminds us that relations of dependence are subject to constant change. Seen in this way, our responsibilities to help alleviate poverty and deprivation arise not out of charity or even contemporary obligations of 'development' or 'cosmopolitan justice' but out of a common history and an interdependent future.

This perspective is crucial if care is to avoid slipping into what Uma Narayan has called 'paternalistic care' (Narayan 1995, p. 135). Narayan draws our attention to the existence of a colonialist care discourse whose terms have some resonance with those of some contemporary strands of the ethic of care (Narayan 1995, pp. 133–34). As she explains:

> This suggests that strands in contemporary care discourse that stress that we are all essentially interdependent and in relationship, while important, do not go far enough if they fail to worry about the accounts that are given of these interdependencies and relationships ... While aspects of care discourse have the potential virtue of calling attention to vulnerabilities that mark relationships between differently situated persons, care discourse also run the risk of being used to ideological ends where these 'differences' are defined in self-serving ways by the dominant and powerful. (Narayan 1995, p. 136)

At the international level, an ethics of care must not be seen to translate simply into benevolent and humanitarian practices through which the strong states and organizations that make up the international community 'care for' weaker, vulnerable populations. Rather, it means that the focus of attention is on attending to the needs, rights and interest of people as both givers *and* receivers of care. While I would eschew a strongly normative care ethics, the critical potential of the ethics of care goes beyond the ontological arguments about relationality. Also crucial to care ethics is the argument that practices of care are the basic substance of morality. Thus, recognition of responsibilities to particular others, and an understanding of the nature of those responsibilities are just the first steps. The next steps involve sustained attention to people not as autonomous rights-bearers but as relational subjects who are both givers and receivers of care.

These ideas may be applied to our moral understandings of contemporary humanitarian situations. In the light of the recent earthquake, 'Haiti' is constructed as a vulnerable population in need of benevolence and care. But a critical ethics of care reveals the moral and practical complexity of care in this context. A critical ethics of care asks 'what are the care needs in this context?' and 'how are these needs being met?' Answering these questions requires attention not just to the most basic, immediate care needs of those in grave physical condition—the needs of 'bare life'—but also to the wider landscape of care in this context. It asks how relationships and communities that previously attended to care have been dismantled by events, and what can be done to repair or rebuild those relations, or to find alternative means of providing care. It considers the distribution of the material, physical and emotional burdens of care, and how these are affected by constructions of gender and race. While recognizing that the negotiation of care provision is fundamentally political, it does not shrink from an explicit consideration of power relations in this context. Contrary to widespread perceptions, rights and interests are important aspects of a critical ethics of care. Rights are crucial in the context of both giving and receiving of care; however, they must always be understood relationally and always as embedded in and realized through existing social and political arrangements. Considering the complex landscape of relations and responsibilities of care in this way is not a short-term process; rather, it is an ongoing task of practical ethics which must always be cognizant of the past, the present and the short- and long-term future. This is in contrast to the way in which 'moral issues' are usually considered in international relations, where there is an emphasis on moments of crisis—as in the statist, militarized, gendered discourses of humanitarian intervention (see Robinson 2009), and in many accounts of the ethics of globalization, which focus on the accelerating speed of interactions in the contemporary world.

A critical feminist ethics of care can form the basis for a new international political theory which disrupts the dichotomy between autonomy and dependence, as well as challenging our conventional views of which individuals, groups or states are 'dependent' on which others, and how. Recognition of the increasing dependence of the North on the South for the provision of care work challenges conventional understandings of the South as 'dependent' on the North. When viewed through a critical care lens, what Saskia Sassen calls 'counter-geographies' of globalization are revealed. Sassen's analysis uncovers the systemic connections between poor migrant women (often represented as a burden rather than a resource) and significant sources for profit and government revenue enhancement. The lines of dependency, from this perspective, are striking:

> ... I use the notion of feminization of survival to refer to the fact that households and whole communities are increasingly *dependent* on women for their survival. It is important to emphasize that governments too are *dependent* on their earnings as well as enterprises where profit making exists at the margins of the 'licit' economy. (Sassen 2002, p. 258; emphasis added)

The aim of this line of argumentation is not simply to turn the autonomy–dependency dichotomy on its head; on the contrary, it is to demonstrate that the nature and extent of dependence and interdependence in social, political and economic life is constantly shifting and evolving, with different kinds of costs and benefits for different actors. As the example above illustrates, moreover, the relationships between dependence and power are not always clear. While income-rich states and individual families within those states may be dependent upon migrant women to fill the gaps in care provision in their countries, the migrant women themselves are rarely empowered by this relationship. To say this is not to underestimate the agency of these women, or the sacrifices they make in order to provide for their children. But in spite of this they remain embedded in a wider, structural inequality in which gendered, racialized care work is globally undervalued.

Shades of dependence and interdependence, moreover, are never simple or limited to a single sphere or scale. The critical lens of care allows us to see how apparently simple dependence is in fact constituted by and mediated through a range of structural and normative conditions—in the context of households, communities and the global political economy. An ethics of care that is not attuned to power relations—to the ways in which power operates through discourses and practices of care—runs the risk of reproducing these dichotomies. A critical ethics of care, however, destabilizes the dichotomy between a benevolent, autonomous global North and a dependent global South. As Mark Duffield has argued in his analysis of development and security, there is an urgent need to move away from the view of development as a 'one-way process between the provider and beneficiary'. This, he argues, is a process that emphasizes differences in power and distance, with providers in places of safety, and beneficiaries in zones of crisis (Duffield 2007, p. 233). A critical ethics of care 'focuses on interdependence and coexistence and the limits to these and makes apparent the potential connections and disconnections between respon-sibility, care and power, at a variety of scales' (Raghuram et al. 2009, p. 10).

As I have sought to emphasize, concentrating on ways in which to facilitate care among a variety of actors within and across borders is not the same thing as valorizing a caring morality or arguing for its superiority relative to the morality of rights or justice. Rather, it is about using the alternative ontological lenses of interdependence and relationality to reveal the extent to which the practices of care and responsibility, and the moral negotiation and deliberation which surround them, play an important role not only in the day-to-day lives of families and communities but also in the workings of collective actors, including states in the international system. This exercise also reveals the material and discursive bases upon which decisions about responsibilities for care are reached, and invites a critical inquiry into the ideational norms and political economy of gender and race that govern care.

Conclusion: Towards an International Political Theory of Care

In this article I have argued that contemporary conditions in world politics and the global economy have opened up discursive space to articulate a new international political theory that challenges the hegemony of liberalism. In particular, a critical theory of care disrupts the dichotomies—public/private; national/international; autonomy/dependence—that constitute and govern political life. On this view, interdependence is a defining feature of social life; it shapes and defines identity and influences well-being. Interdependence is not 'natural' nor is it simply a 'private' condition; rather, it is created by and mediated through social and political institutions. Vulnerability and dependence, moreover, are features of all human subjects as well as many social groupings at some point; levels of vulnerability, and the implication of vulnerability are, in part, a reflection of existing power relations in the context of relationships. Thus, if women, and especially women of colour, appear to be less autonomous than men, it is because of the ways in which their dependence has been constructed through norms of race and gender and their relationship to caring labour.

Autonomy, self-determination and individual rights and freedoms are neither 'natural' nor sustainable in the long term. While rights to secure independence and a meaningful voice in politics are strategically and discursively important for individuals and groups, true autonomy for *all* can only be achieved and sustained in and through fostering societies which value interdependence and acknowledge the vulnerability of all (Williams 2000, p. 481). An international political theory of care does not prescribe a duty among states to care for one another; nor does it proclaim a universal 'right' to care. It is not a normative theory in the sense that it prescribes how actors ought to act. Nor is it a conventional theory of global justice which focuses on the procedures for the fair distribution of goods (Tronto 2010). As Joan Tronto puts it, we need to remember that politics is about power not only in the distributive sense, but also in the sense of the creation or assumption of a capacity to act (Tronto 2010). Thus, there is a need to question the necessity behind certain practices, and consider what kinds of material and discursive structures serve to keep these practices in place.

An international political theory of care focuses on the permanent background of giving and receiving care that is central to preventing crises, and responding to crises when they do occur. As Virginia Held has suggested, in societies increasingly influenced by the values of care, the need for law and coercion would not disappear, but their use might become progressively more limited if our focus is shifted to the adequacy of relations of care on a *day-to-day basis* (Held 2006, p. 153). While care ethics is not an ethics of pacifism, it takes seriously the effects of the feminization of caring practices and the valorization of hegemonic forms of masculinity. Challenging the discursive and material arrangements that feminize care and legitimize masculine violence is a crucial critical resource of an international political theory of care.

A political theory of care argues that a focus on the nature, allocation and fulfillment of care policies should be the substantive focus of political deliberations (Tronto 2010). From this perspective, it becomes possible to draw lines of connection among apparently diverse international issues: global health crises and pandemics; 'refugee crises'; humanitarian emergencies;

'failed' states; peacebuilding; environmental security. In all these cases, these 'crises' and their effects on the security of real people can be temporally and spatially expanded in order to place them within a wider context of the protracted and multi-dimensional disintegration of networks of care.

References

Bedford, K. (2008) 'Governing Intimacy at the World Bank', in *Global Governance: Feminist Perspectives*, eds S. Rai & G. Waylen, Palgrave, London, pp. 84–106.

Brown, C. (1999) 'History Ends, Worlds Collide', *Review of International Studies* (special issue), Vol. 25, no. 5, pp. 41–58.

Carr, E. H. (1939) *The Twenty-years Crisis: An Introduction to the Study of International Relations*, Macmillan, London.

Duffield, M. (2007) *Development, Security and Unending War: Governing the World of Peoples*, Polity Press, Cambridge.

Fraser, N. (1997) *Justice Interruptus: Critical Reflections on the "Postsocialist" Condition*, Routledge, New York.

Fraser, N. & Gordon, L. (1994) 'A Genealogy of Dependency: Tracing a Keyword of the U.S. Welfare State', *Signs*, Vol. 19, no. 2, pp. 309–36.

Fukuyama, F. (1992) *The End of History and the Last Man*, Free Press, New York.

Held, V. (2006) *The Ethics of Care: Personal, Political, and Global*, Oxford University Press, Oxford.

Hutchings, K. (2008) 'Cognitive Short Cuts', in *Rethinking the Man Question: Sex, Gender and Violence in International Relations*, eds J. Parpart & M. Zalewski, Zed Books, London, pp. 23–46.

Kittay, E. F. (2001a) 'A Feminist Public Ethic of Care Meets the New Communitarian Family Policy', *Ethics*, Vol. 111, no. 3, pp. 523–47.

Kittay, E. F. (2001b) 'From Welfare to a Public Ethic of Care', in *Women and Welfare: Theory and Practice in the United States and Europe*, eds N. J. Hirschmann & U. Liebert, Rutgers University Press, New Brunswick, NJ, pp. 38–64.

Narayan, U. (1995) 'Colonialism and its Others: Consideration on Rights and Care Discourses', *Hypatia*, Vol. 10, no. 2, pp. 133–40.

O'Manique, C. (2006) 'The "Securitization" of HIV/AIDS in Sub-Saharan Africa: A Critical Feminist Lens', in *A Decade of Human Security: Global Governance and the New Multilateralisms*, eds S. Maclean, D. Black & T. Shaw, Ashgate, Aldershot, pp. 161–78.

Parrenas, R. S. (2001) *Servants of Globalization: Women, Migration and Domestic Work*, Stanford University Press, Stanford.

Raghuram, P., Madge, C. & Noxolo, P. (2009) 'Rethinking Responsibility and Care for a Postcolonial World', *Geoforum*, Vol. 40, no. 1, pp. 5–13.

Reus-Smit, C. (2001) 'Human Rights and the Social Construction of Sovereignty', *Review of International Studies*, Vol. 27, no. 4, pp. 519–38.

Robinson, F. (1999a) *'Globalizing Care: Ethics, Feminist Theory and International Relations'*, Westview Press, Boulder.

Robinson, F. (1999b) 'Globalizing Liberalism? Morality and Legitimacy in a Liberal Global Order', in *Politics and Globalization: Knowledge, Ethics, Agency*, ed. M. Shaw, Routledge, London, pp. 143–56.

Robinson, F. (2009) 'Feminist Ethics and Global Security Governance', in *The Ethics of Global Governance*, ed. A. Franceschet, Lynne Rienner, Boulder, pp. 103–118.

Sassen, S. (2002) '"Women's Burden": Counter-geographies of Globalization and the Feminization of Survival', *Nordic Journal of International Law*, Vol. 71, no. 2, pp. 255–73.

Sevenhuijsen, S. (2000) 'Caring in the Third Way: The Relation between Obligation, Responsibility and Care in Third Way Discourse', *Critical Social Policy*, Vol. 20, no. 1, pp. 5–37.

Tronto, J. (forthcoming 2010) 'A Democratic Feminist Ethics of Care and Global Care Workers: Citizenship and Responsibility', in *The Ethics and Social Politics of Care: Transnational Perspectives*, eds R. Mahon & F. Robinson, University of British Columbia Press, Vancouver.

Wallerstein, I. (1995) *After Liberalism*, The New Press, New York.

Weir, A. (2005) 'The Global Universal Caregiver: Imagining Women's Liberation in the New Millennium', *Constellations*, Vol. 12, no. 3, pp. 308–30.

Williams, F. (2000) 'In and beyond New Labour: Towards a New Political Ethics of Care', *Critical Social Policy*, Vol. 21, no. 4, pp. 467–93.

Cosmopolitan Care

Sarah Clark Miller

I develop the foundation for cosmopolitan care, an underexplored variety of moral cosmopolitanism. I begin by offering a characterization of contemporary cosmopolitanism from the justice tradition. Rather than discussing the political, economic or cultural aspects of cosmopolitanism, I instead address its moral dimensions. I then employ a feminist philosophical perspective to provide a critical evaluation of the moral foundations of cosmopolitan justice, with an eye toward demonstrating the need for an alternative account of moral cosmopolitanism as cosmopolitan care. After providing an explanation of how care ethics in connection with Kantian ethics generates a duty to care, I consider one main feature of cosmopolitan care, namely the theory of obligation it endorses. In developing this account, I place special emphasis on the practical ramifications of the theory by using it to analyze gender violence in conflict zones.

During the past two decades, care ethics has advanced beyond critique to become an established moral theory in its own right. It has done this through the refiguring of existing mainstream moral theories, as well as through more original and inventive efforts. Where does care ethics find itself today? What major contributions to philosophy is it poised to make? Which new directions are open to care ethicists both as theoreticians and as practitioners? The focus of this paper—contemporary philosophical discussions of cosmopolitanism—constitutes one main area ripe for care ethics' distinctive blend of critical and constructive engagement. In current discussions of cosmopolitan ethics, justice-based theories dominate the philosophical landscape (Appiah 2005; Beitz 1999; Caney 2005; Moellendorf 2002; Nussbaum 2006; Pogge 1989, 2002; Tan 2004). To date, only a few theorists have made advances in the direction of developing a sustained theory of cosmopolitan care (Engster 2007; Robinson 1999; Slote 2007a, b; Held 2005, 2008). Taking a critical approach to cosmopolitanism is certainly not a new move. Scholars from various perspectives have offered multiple critiques.[1] Care ethics, however, offers a somewhat distinctive angle of criticism that deserves further exploration. After determining the limitations of cosmopolitan justice from a care ethics perspective, I will counter with an alternative cosmopolitan moral formulation that care ethics generates. In brief, the shortcomings of predominant theories of moral cosmopolitanism as cosmopolitan justice currently on offer open a space for moral cosmopolitanism as cosmopolitan care.

My account of the important contributions that care ethics can make to cosmopolitan conversations advances in four main movements. I begin by offering a characterization of contemporary cosmopolitanism. Rather than discussing the political, economic, or cultural aspects of cosmopolitanism, I instead address its moral dimensions. I then employ a feminist philosophical perspective to provide a critical evaluation of the moral foundations of cosmopolitanism as understood from the justice perspective, with an eye toward demonstrating the need for an alternative account of moral cosmopolitanism as cosmopolitan care. After providing an explanation of how care ethics in connection with Kantian ethics generates a duty to care, I consider one main feature of cosmopolitan care, namely the theory of obligation it endorses. In developing this account, I place special emphasis on the practical ramifications of the theory by using it to analyze gender violence in conflict zones.

The Limitations of Moral Cosmopolitanism as Cosmopolitan Justice

The need for a care-based theory of cosmopolitanism emerges clearly against the backdrop of cosmopolitan theories of justice. Contemporary scholarly discussions of cosmopolitanism offer up multiple main approaches, many of which, though important, are not my current focus, which is instead the moral dimension of cosmopolitanism. Several main commitments are emblematic of moral cosmopolitanism in the justice tradition. Most notably, moral cosmopolitanism evidences a fundamental commitment to the equal moral worth of all human beings and to the use of impartiality in the process of moral judgment. Exactly how those commitments are enacted depends on the particular variety of moral cosmopolitanism under consideration. Such varieties are identifiable through their underlying philosophical commitments as Utilitarian, Kantian, Rawlsian, or Aristotelian, for example. A critical assessment of each of these subfields is not within the aims of the present effort. Identification and critical evaluation of the features held in common among them, however, will prove vital to the task of establishing cosmopolitan care as a viable alternative theory. By employing feminist philosophy as a critical lens through which to evaluate cosmopolitan justice, the need for a feminist account of moral cosmopolitanism based in cosmopolitan care clearly emerges.

---

1. Some important examples of such critical work include Lu (2000) and Scarry (2002).

Perhaps most obviously, any account of the moral foundations of cosmopolitanism must incorporate a form of moral regard for all of humanity. Beneath this allegiance to humanity, however, rests a prior allegiance 'to what is morally good—and that which, being good, I can commend as such to all human beings', as Martha Nussbaum has underscored (Nussbaum 2002, p. 5). Here the cosmopolitan's moral universalism shines through. The primary allegiance that the moral cosmopolitan holds is to principles or values, and more specifically, to the good and the right. It is worth noting that Nussbaum articulates this as an allegiance to 'justice and right' (Nussbaum 2002, p. 5), which evidences the justice-based nature of her approach. This strong identification with justice as a fundamental, guiding value epitomizes many contemporary approaches to moral cosmopolitanism as cosmopolitan justice. In addition to a primary allegiance to the moral principles of justice and right, moral cosmopolitans in the justice tradition adhere to three related principles, namely individualism, universality, and generality, as Thomas Pogge sets forth in a well-known essay entitled 'Cosmopolitanism and Sovereignty' (Pogge 1992). Individuality for Pogge means that individuals are the most significant units of moral concern. Collectivities, such as familial, national, or cultural groups, qualify only as indirect units of moral concern. The idea behind Pogge's conception of universality echoes a sentiment expressed by Nussbaum above: the equal moral standing of all persons. The third notion, generality, dictates that the equal moral standing of persons is a concern for all moral agents.

When reflecting on Nussbaum's and Pogge's contributions collectively, another important way of articulating a main conceptual thread of moral cosmopolitanism emerges. Moral cosmopolitanism involves a requirement of impartiality in moral judgment and structures of obligation. Cosmopolitan justice is deeply rooted in impartiality, which renders the ties of partiality questionable. Affective ties of family, friendship and fellowship, as well as geographical ties of nation and culture, find limited legitimate moral expression in a cosmopolitan justice framework. Under justice, moral cosmopolitans are to render moral judgments apart from the connections of partiality. Various modes of relatedness that give rise to special obligations, be they a matter of proximity, emotion or identity, are, to some degree, morally questionable. Special obligations gain little traction within this approach. At best, they are obligations of secondary importance. At worst, they are matters of suspicion.

With this general picture of moral cosmopolitanism in the justice tradition in mind, I now take a critical turn to evaluate moral cosmopolitanism through the lens of feminist critique. More specifically, my aim is to bring insights from care ethics to bear on the model of cosmopolitan justice. Four main criticisms occupy my attention. Care ethicists find fault with predominant versions of moral cosmopolitanism for their hyper-individualism, idealization, abstraction, and acontextuality. While I will treat each of these criticisms in turn, the conceptual overlap between some of them will be apparent at points. Aspects of this discussion will at moments have a familiar ring for those knowledgeable about the earlier justice–care debates, as some tensions that are present in the general normative discord between these perspectives plays out in a similar fashion at the cosmopolitan level.

One of the most distinctive contributions of care ethics has been its emphasis on relationships, both in terms of the relational nurturing and generating of moral agents and the intrinsic moral worth of relationships. Care ethicists would charge that the individualism at the heart of current accounts of moral cosmopolitanism amounts to a hyper-individualism. In the context of cosmopo-litan justice, the individual is the ultimate unit of moral concern, a view challenged by the foundational moral importance that care ethicists ascribe to human relationships. The atomistic, disconnected social ontology characteristic of the modern philosophical period, of which feminist theorists have been highly critical, reemerges, or perhaps carries over to contemporary theories of cosmopolitan justice, where individuals somehow separated from the relation-ships in which they are intertwined function as primary normative units. Care ethicists counter the hyper-individualism of cosmopolitan justice with their view of the primary moral importance of human interdependence and of the moral self-in-connection. From this vantage point, it is not possible to understand the moral self apart from the relationships in which it is embedded. From the cosmopolitan care perspective, a theory that fails to appreciate the primary normative significance of human interdependence—as cosmopolitan justice appears to do—is not a viable normative approach. Proponents of cosmopolitan care render interdependence the most morally salient feature of humanity. In this regard, cosmopolitan care and cosmopolitan justice are interestingly both varieties of moral universalism in form, though obviously the content of that universalism differs dramatically.

In addition to the hyper-individualism of cosmopolitan justice, care ethicists reveal that the typical moral agent of this normative stance is an idealized version of humanity, one that denies our shared vulnerability and finitude. The rational abilities featured in both Kantian and Rawlsian versions of cosmopoli-tanism demonstrate this trend rather clearly, with their emphasis on human reason and autonomy (O'Neill 1986, 2000; Rawls 1999). Cosmopolitan care ethicists approach matters of global responsibility with full awareness of the limitations that human beings face as always finite and often dependent creatures. In the cosmopolitan care framework, dependency relations are deserving of special moral attention, given the pivotal role that relations of dependency play in cultivating both moral reason and autonomy. Foremost in formulations of global responsibility from this perspective will be the needs and suffering of moral agents. Moreover, beyond guaranteeing that others' needs are met, cosmopolitan care makes the importance of care primary in the sense of ensuring the ability of moral agents to care, that is, to ensure that caring relations can happen in practice on the ground. This is a slightly different structure of obligation than the obligation to meet another's needs. It amounts to an obligation to support persons' abilities to meet others' needs, that is, to ensure that they can care.

The intertwined nature of the two final criticisms of cosmopolitan justice, targeting its abstraction and acontextuality, generally recommends treating these two complaints together. For the purposes of clarity, however, an initial attempt to disentangle the two concepts may be useful. The trouble with the abstraction at the core of moral cosmopolitanism is a problem primarily regarding the characterization of the persons on the receiving end of cosmopolitan obligations of justice. The problem of acontextuality, by contrast, is a problem with the nature of moral agents' deliberation that cosmopolitan justice recommends.

As already established, the moral cosmopolitan holds a primary commitment to the principles of justice and right, which many varieties of cosmopolitanism often express as an honoring of obligations to other humans because of the abstract humanity shared between them, that is, apart from the features that distinguish them one from another. Such a degree of abstraction willfully ignores the embeddedness of moral agents in at least two significant respects: first, as persons situated in a nexus of human relationships and second as persons with specific identities. Absent these features, care ethicists would argue, the moral self becomes an unrecognizable wisp of moral abstraction. In addition to the damage that such abstraction does to the moral self, the abstraction inherent in impartiality—the basis for moral judgment in cosmopolitan justice—skews the nature of moral responsibility by undervaluing contextual features. In contrast, care ethicists argue that moral reasoning functions best when it incorporates the rich details of persons' lives. How better to respond to another's needs and suffering than with a robust sense of the circumstances of their lives, that is, of their situatedness? Thus, cosmopolitan care advocates a widening of the requirements of moral epistemology such that moral agents might engage in a contextually sensitive version of moral judgment. It connects moral agents with the details of the lives of needy individuals. In short, at the heart of cosmopolitan care theory, one finds strong skills of moral perception that improve on the process of moral deliberation that accompanies cosmopolitan justice.

Caring through Duty

Gaining an overview of cosmopolitan justice and advancing a critique of its main tenets from a care perspective are worthwhile tasks. What such an approach does not do, however, is demonstrate the distinctive, positive contribution that care ethics can make on the cosmopolitan level. In the context of the critical engagement with cosmopolitan justice above, I was able to gesture toward some of the main aspects of a cosmopolitan care theory. Providing a complete theory of cosmopolitan care, though a worthy enterprise, is beyond the scope of this paper. Developing one main feature of such a theory, however, is possible and can provide a clear sense of what constitutes cosmopolitan care. To this end, I will focus on a discussion of the obligations that a cosmopolitan care theory entails.

The notion that care ethics could generate cosmopolitan *obligations* might at first seem strange. Care ethics has not often been known as a champion of moral duties. Common conceptions of this moral theory often render it indebted to sentimentalist or virtue-based theories, rather than the deontological tradition. I have argued elsewhere (Miller 2005, 2006, forthcoming, April 2011) that placing Kantian and care ethics in a symbiotic relationship with one another can generate a duty to care.[2] One of care ethics' great contributions to the field of ethical theory is the drawing of attention to the moral significance of human vulnerability, dependence and need. Humans are vulnerable in ways that we cannot predict or prevent. We begin our lives in a tremendous state of dependency and may return to this state throughout the course of our lives. We experience needs consistently, even when living in contexts of relative plenitude. These three features point to the necessity of receiving others' care to survive as human beings. Beyond survival concerns, care is a necessity for flourishing and for living the good life. The universal nature of this claim underscores our interdependence as a feature of fundamental moral importance. A normative analysis of the significance of our interdependent state results in a required moral response to human vulnerability, need and dependence.

This moral response is the duty to care, a sketch of which I will provide here. As finite and interdependent moral agents, we are required to respond to others' fundamental needs. Representative fundamental needs include obvious ones such as the need for food, clean water, and shelter, as well as what are perhaps less obvious needs, such as the need for social recognition.[3] Fundamental needs occur when a person's agency, or potential agency, is under significant threat. When people fail to have their fundamental needs met, the result can be significant harm and a curtailment of their powers of self-determination. The duty to care, therefore, is a duty intertwined not only with human need but also human agency, which I understand to be the ability to act freely so as to achieve self-determined ends of personal significance through rational, emotional and relational means. The scope of the duty to care is universal, meaning that all people are required to care, not simply those who are inclined to do so, either 'naturally' or through social conditioning. This duty is not overly onerous, however, in the sense of requiring moral agents to respond to every single need of which they have knowledge, as such a requirement would limit the well-being of

---

2. Cf. Engster (2005, 2007) and Manning (2002).
3. The related literature offers multiple lists of needs (e.g. lists by Terleckyj, Drewnowski, and Offe), which are nicely captured in Braybrooke's helpful list compilation (1987, pp. 35–38). Not all such lists, however, have agency as their focus, as mine does. While conducting a comparative analysis of lists of human needs is not a primary task of this article, consideration of the distinction between my approach and one other well-known one does merit comment. Martha Nussbaum famously offers a list of 'Central Human Functional Capabilities' (2000, pp. 78–80). Although some overlap does exist between our lists, I believe that our approaches differ in terms of their main focus and aim. That which I identify as fundamental needs are necessary for agency. They are what people need in order to function as self-determining agents in their lives. In contrast, what Nussbaum develops is a list of human capabilities, with a main focus on the capabilities that are necessary for achieving flourishing or to live a truly human life.

moral agents by causing them to experience needs themselves. Thus, a large degree of self-sacrifice is not required. The burden of response is thus limited by attention to the needs of the one who cares. The duty does not require and in fact prohibits moral agents from responding to others in a way that creates fundamental needs in them. Exactly when and how moral agents respond under the duty to care is a matter of flexibility. In this formulation, moral judgment, in connection with context, necessarily plays a large role in determining exactly when and how moral agents must meet others' needs.

The duty to care is a moral requirement designed not to foster dependence but rather self-determination. By addressing persons' experiences of needs that compromise their agency, the aim of caregivers enacting the duty to care is to help cultivate, maintain or restore agency and self-determination.[4] This means that the form of care giving that the duty to care requires will be care that respectfully acknowledges the abilities of those in need to set and realize their self-determined ends and life goals. Often, though admittedly not always, those in need will be best positioned to understand and articulate what they need. Respect for moral agents' powers of self-determination, as well as their sense of what leads to their happiness, is a vital component of the duty to care.

A point of apparent tension between care ethics and the duty to care concerns the role of emotion in the context of duty. The moral relevance of emotion has often been seen as a central component of care ethics and is one key element of what sets this ethic apart from other normative theories. In contrast, the duty to care does not require moral agents who perform the duty to experience any particular feeling for those whose needs they meet. This is because emotion cannot be a matter of obligation. Moral agents can be obligated to act in certain ways toward others, but they cannot be obligated to experience certain emotions toward those for whom they care. While acknowledging the importance of care ethicists' assertion that good care of intimates often involves significant emotional attachments between care giver and care receiver, the duty to care opens up the possibility of a different model of care between distant strangers, a model particularly relevant to reformulating moral cosmopolitanism from the perspective of care ethics.

The Obligations of Cosmopolitan Care

Structures of obligation are a cornerstone of many theories of moral cosmopolitanism. One useful step toward developing cosmopolitan care is, therefore, to

---

4. Of course, there will be limitations on the extent to which fostering agency and self-determination is possible in certain cases. The degree of human abilities spans a wide spectrum. Some individuals are not able to exhibit full agency and may not be self-determining. The duty to care is not designed to respond to such examples. My intent in developing the duty to care is not to exclude such individuals and their needs from the realm of moral consideration. A different avenue of argumentation, however, may be more productive for establishing a structure of obligation designed to meet their needs. One possible route would be an argument from human dignity.

envisage what account of global obligation this theory might recommend. What obligations does the cosmopolitan care theory entail? A guiding background interest that informs this question is the desire to determine the significance of feminist philosophy for discussions of global responsibility. The feminist emphasis on concepts such as need, vulnerability, interdependence and care transforms the justice-centered cosmopolitan discourse.

From the start, I want to acknowledge the importance of ensuring that the cosmopolitan care account of obligation does not remain solely in a theoretical register. Were that to be the case, critics could rightfully wonder to what extent this theory is practically applicable. They might query what exactly the global duty to care requires of real people in terms of the difficult details of practical response. Thus, clearly demonstrating the practical ramifications of the theory for current, real-world situations of need is a priority. Moreover, this emphasis seems particularly fitting, given the importance of concrete contexts to care ethics. To this end, I interweave an examination of an issue of great importance to the global community—violence against women and girls in conflict situations—with the development of the theoretical account of cosmopolitan care obligations. The specific instance of gender violence in conflict zones that I will address will be the ongoing sexual violence perpetrated against women and girls in the Darfur region of Sudan. What obligations of response do distant strangers have in light of this unfolding crisis? The global duty to care serves as one illuminating approach to this matter. In taking the different path of examining global responsibility in the context of situations of conflict and gender violence, instead of the more traditional issues of global hunger and poverty, for example, my aim is threefold: first, to employ cosmopolitan care to address an issue of specifically feminist interest; second, to advance a productive engagement with an area of international crisis that has thus far received inadequate attention; and third, to demonstrate the distinctive contribution that cosmopolitan care can make to the moral cosmopolitan scholarship.

An account of the recent events in Darfur makes clear why this particular case requires further attention and analysis. Although media reports of violence in the Darfur region of Sudan recently died down as attention turned to Southern Sudan and the regional and national elections in April 2010, civilian populations are still immensely vulnerable. Six years of conflict have left an estimated 300,000 people dead and 2.7 million internally displaced persons (IDPs).[5] Summarizing the complicated history of the war is a daunting task. An overview shows conflict that began in 2003 between government and militia groups, on the one hand, and rebels representing black African ethnic groups—the Fur, Masalit, and Zaghawa—on the other. The rebels charge that the Sudanese Arab government in Khartoum has repeatedly neglected the needs and interests of its people in an

---

5. Exact numbers of the dead and displaced are not available. One reputable source, John Holmes, United Nations Under-Secretary-General for Humanitarian Affairs, provided the estimate of 300,000 deaths as a result of the Darfur conflict to a meeting of the United Nations Security Council in New York in April 2008 (*BBC News* 2008). It is likely that the numbers have climbed since then.

active campaign to weaken those groups.[6] At the time of writing this article, widespread, coordinated violence against civilian populations appears to be lessening. It is necessary to note that there have been past periods of decreased violence, such as in 2007, that then were followed by increased escalation, as in 2008 (Polgreen 2008). Scholar Eric Reeves (2010) remarked in January 2010 that

> [a]midst the various comments and commentary arguing that war is over in Darfur, that there are only remnants of previous violence … several recent reports suggest that human security and humanitarian assistance are deeply imperiled. The gradual shift in international attention to the crises in Southern Sudan and Sudan's national elections … [has obscured] the immense dangers that continue to confront civilians throughout Darfur.

Setting divergent views of the current situation to one side, the picture that emerges from the recent history in Darfur is a clearer matter. Since 2003, the Khartoum government and Janjaweed militiamen have systematically brutalized civilian populations bearing the same ethnic identity as the rebels through both aerial and ground assaults. These assaults have led most to flee to IDP camps, where the cycle of violence, brutalization and deprivation continues. Many in the camps lack access to basic necessities, such as clean water, food, medical supplies and adequate shelter (Civet 2005; Sanders 2009).

Against this backdrop of brutalization, a specific picture of extensive violence against women and girls emerges. It will be impossible to gain an accurate count of the women and girls who have been violated in Darfur until further security is brought to the region. Current estimates place the number at roughly 10,000 women and girls raped since 2003.[7] Reports indicate that both Janjaweed militiamen and Sudanese government actors (e.g., members of the military) have perpetrated these crimes, which many claim have been encouraged or even directly organized by the Khartoum government (Robertson 2009). The age span of victims is broad—young girls and old women alike have reported assaults. Common methods of attack include beating victims with whips, sticks and axes, branding them, and penetrating them with penises, as well as with objects such as bottles and sticks. Raping family members in front of one another is a common practice, as are gang rape and sexual slavery. Reports of ethnically and racially fuelled assaults abound from survivors, who claim that assailants have referred to them as 'slave'

---

6. As is true with many national populations, the inner workings of the ethnic and racial differences are somewhat complicated. This is particularly so in Darfur, a region in which the assignment of ethnicity has been fluid, a situation resulting from substantial patterns of intermarriage between Arab herding communities and non-Arab farming communities. Beyond issues of ethnicity, the role of race in the conflict is deeply complex and contested. One way to characterize this complexity is to examine the tension between two competing sets of claims: (1) reports from many Darfuri women and girls that their attackers spoke of wanting to infiltrate the bloodline of their group by impregnating them so they would give birth to light-skinned babies and (2) critical claims that the Western media have oversimplified the conflict as one between races or between lighter- and darker-skinned peoples (Coates 2004).

7. For a recent and excellent study of sexual violence in Darfur, please see Physicians for Human Rights (2009).

and 'black dog', for example, and have expressed wanting to exterminate the groups from which they come (Gingerich & Leaning 2004; Amnesty International 2004). A 2009 report by Physicians for Human Rights offers further proof of such claims:

> Some women reported that the Janjaweed yelled racial slurs, announcing their intention to exterminate the non-Arabs of Darfur as well as their intent to take their land and their intent to make the women give birth to Arab children. Women from different ethnic groups and different parts of Darfur note that the Janjaweed taunted them calling them '*Slaves*' or '*Nuba*', '*We will kill all of the slaves!*' '*This is not your land—it is ours!*' and '*We will make you have Arab children!*' (p. 52)

Reports such as these support the notion that beyond being a weapon of war, rape in Darfur may in fact be a tool of genocide.[8]

With this disturbing picture of gender violence in Darfur in place, I turn now to an analysis of Darfur through obligations of cosmopolitan care, here rendered as a global duty to care. Clearly displaying its intellectual heritage, a first aspect of the global duty to care to note is how it requires moral agents to focus not only on meeting others' needs but also on restoring or bolstering the agency of those in need. The significance of agency to self-determination is one facet of why this move is important. An equally prominent angle, however, has to do with empowering individuals and communities to be able to engage in caring practices themselves, that is, to maintain, restore or strengthen their ability to care for others.[9] That the act of rape creates great suffering and need is abundantly apparent. The focus on how it disrupts the ability to care is an underexplored yet very significant aspect of the harm of rape. Rape in Darfur destroys caretaking abilities in several respects. The stigma rape victims suffer severs familial ties. Rape survivors in IDP camps struggle daily to provide basic necessities for their children, a situation demonstrated through the risk of further sexual assault they hazard when traveling outside the camps to collect firewood for cooking. Most notably, rape used in the service of genocide obliterates larger patterns of care within entire communities. Framing obligations to aid others through the issue of their ability to care provides a much-needed shift in focus concerning what moral agents enacting the global duty to care must do to respond adequately to crises of gender violence in conflict zones.

The global duty to care also emphasizes the importance of respecting both local caretaking practices and understandings of need. This requires moral agents to respond in ways that are contextually sensitive and culturally attuned. The practice of care is always necessarily located in a complex social-political context. Responding to distant others through the duty to care may often involve not meeting their needs directly but rather supporting the specific caring

---

8. An arrest warrant has already been issued for the president of Sudan, Omar al-Bashir, on seven charges of crimes against humanity and war crimes. International Criminal Court judges named rape as an aspect of those charges in the indictment. Whether he will face charges of genocide remains unclear. On 3 February 2010 the ICC's appeal chamber overturned a ruling that maintained that there was insufficient proof to bring charges of genocide (Black 2010).
9. Cf. West (2003, 2004).

practices they themselves endorse so as to improve their ability to care for one another. The strong emphasis on context sensitivity in the global duty to care is apparent here. Cross-cultural caretaking must prioritize respecting others' cultural particularity. Regarding needs specifically, while certain needs are universal, the way people experience them on the ground may differ. This draws attention to the striking interaction of the concept of empowerment and the global duty to care. Regarding rape survivors in Darfur, approaching the crisis with a mind to empowering communities to care for rape survivors, as well as empowering the survivors themselves by paying heed to the needs they understand themselves to experience, is crucial. Caring in such a fashion also evidences respect for those who are suffering and in need. While there may be different modes of assistance and intervention, the expressive function of such forms of care is meant to affirm the dignity of persons.

Care as an obligation pertaining to global situations readily moves beyond requirements of meeting needs by sending material aid. This is true in a couple of respects. Empowerment of others' caretaking abilities in a situation like Darfur may involve a solidarity component, in accordance with which fulfilling the global duty to care necessitates the involvement of people situated outside of the crisis in efforts to raise awareness in their home communities about the violence in Darfur. Such efforts can build networks of solidarity and create openings for supportive political action, such as advocating for various forms of intervention in the Darfur situation at present or for women to play a strong role in future justice and reparation activities. This is a moment that demonstrates ways in which cosmopolitan care can involve the blending of the ethical and the political, or perhaps the evolution of the ethical into the political. The moral cosmopolitanism of cosmopolitan care may, in fact, require a response that is political, rather than moral, in nature.

A second main way in which the global duty to care expands beyond more traditional duties of aid is in the requirement that moral agents develop a critical awareness of where they are situated in terms of global power structures, as well as how they might inadvertently contribute to the creation of distant need, suffering and oppression. Mounting a case for this more extended form of global responsibility is perhaps easier when considering global poverty. In some corners it is no longer at all a controversial claim that the wealth of the global North is built on the poverty and suffering of the global South. Establishing something like a causal relationship in cases of gender violence in conflict situations happening elsewhere, however, requires a more subtle approach. Clearly, certain specific assailants are directly responsible for the acts of rape they commit. We may also readily grant that government officials who either order mass raping of civilians (as may be the case in Darfur) or who turn a blind eye to it, bear a significant degree of responsibility, too. But how could a distant stranger who has never set foot in Sudan be implicated in a structure of responsibility? In requiring moral agents to analyze the role they play in global oppression, the global duty to care pushes moral agents to determine their role in the oppression of women globally, linking local situations of oppression in which they may be complicit to larger patterns of gender oppression. They must critically evaluate and then seek to change their role in patterns of gender domination both locally and globally.

The ground I have covered here in examining gender violence in Darfur illustrates only one possible application of cosmopolitan care to contemporary global issues. Further work must be done not only to explore additional applications of cosmopolitan care to real-world situations but also to advance the important task of establishing an overarching theory of cosmopolitan care, as well as its exact relationship to cosmopolitan justice. Hopefully, this discussion of the global duty to care has gone some length in showing the promise of this approach, in both theory and practice. Twenty years into the collective care ethics project, cosmopolitan care demonstrates the ongoing critical and constructive possibilities within this area of normative philosophy.

Acknowledgements

I would like to express my gratitude to Christine Koggel for her helpful philosophical and editorial guidance.

References

Amnesty International (2004) *Sudan, Darfur: Rape as a Weapon of War: Sexual Violence and its Consequences*, 19 July, AI Index: AFR 54/076/2004, available at: <http://www.amnesty.org/en/library/info/AFR54/076/2004> (accessed 10 February 2010).

Appiah, K. A. (2005) *The Ethics of Identity*, Princeton University Press, Princeton.

BBC News (2008) 'Darfur Deaths "Could be 300,000"', 23 April, available at: <http://news.bbc.co.uk> (accessed 9 February 2010).

Beitz, C. (1999) *Political Theory and International Relations*, 2nd edn, Princeton University Press, Princeton.

Black, I. (2010) 'Genocide Charge Put Back on Arrest Warrant against Sudan President', 3 February, available at: <http://guardian.co.uk> (accessed 10 February 2010).

Braybrooke, D. (1987) *Meeting Needs*, Princeton University Press, Princeton.

Caney, S. (2005) *Justice beyond Borders: A Global Political Theory*, Oxford University Press, New York.

Civet, N. (2005) 'The Humanitarian Situation in Darfur, Sudan', statement made to the United Nations Security Council 'Arria Formula' Meeting, 27 July.

Coates, T. (2004) 'Black, White, Read', *Village Voice*, 21 September, available at: <http://www.villagevoice.com/2004-09-21/news/black-white-read/1> (accessed 16 January 2010).

Engster, D. (2005) 'Rethinking Care Theory: The Practice of Caring and the Obligation to Care', *Hypatia*, Vol. 20, no. 3, pp. 50–74.

Engster, D. (2007) *The Heart of Justice: Care Ethics and Political Theory*, Oxford University Press, New York.

Gingerich, T. & Leaning, J. (2004) 'The Use of Rape as a Weapon of War in the Conflict in Darfur, Sudan', Program on Humanitarian Crises and Human Rights, François-Xavier Bagnoud Center for Health and Human Rights, Harvard School of Public Health.

Held, V. (2005) *The Ethics of Care: Personal, Political, and Global*, Oxford University Press, Oxford.

CARE ETHICS

Held, V. (2008) 'Gender Identity and the Ethics of Care in Globalized Society', in *Global Feminist Ethics*, eds R. Whisnant & P. DesAutels, Rowman & Littlefield, Lanham, MD, pp. 43–58.

Lu, C. (2000) 'The One and Many Faces of Cosmopolitanism', *Journal of Political Philosophy*, Vol. 8, no. 2, pp. 244–67.

Manning, R. C. (2002) *Speaking from the Heart: A Feminist Perspective on Ethics*, Rowman & Littlefield, Lanham, MD.

Miller, S. C. (2005) 'A Kantian Ethic of Care?', in *Feminist Interventions in Ethics and Politics: Feminist Ethics and Social Theory*, eds B. Andrew, J. Keller & L. Schwartzman, Rowman & Littlefield, Lanham, MD, pp. 111–27.

Miller, S. C. (2006) 'Need, Care and Obligation', in *The Philosophy of Need*, ed. S. Reader, Cambridge University Press, Cambridge, pp. 163–85.

Miller, S. C. (forthcoming, April 2011) *The Ethics of Need: Agency, Dignity, Obligation*, Routledge.

Moellendorf, D. (2002) *Cosmopolitan Justice*, Westview Press, New York.

Nussbaum, M. (2000) *Women and Human Development*, Cambridge University Press, Cambridge.

Nussbaum, M. (2002) 'Patriotism and Cosmopolitanism', in *For Love of Country*, ed. J. Cohen, Beacon Press, Boston, pp. 3–17.

Nussbaum, M. (2006) *Frontiers of Justice: Disability, Nationality, Species Membership*, Harvard University Press, Cambridge, MA.

O'Neill, O. (1986) *Faces of Hunger: An Essay on Poverty, Justice and Development*, Allen & Unwin, Boston.

O'Neill, O. (2000) *Bounds of Justice*, Cambridge University Press, New York.

Physicians for Human Rights, in partnership with the Harvard Health Initiative (2009) 'Nowhere to Turn: Failure to Protect, Support and Assure Justice for Darfuri Women and Children', May.

Pogge, T. (1989) *Realizing Rawls*, Cornell University Press, Ithaca, NY.

Pogge, T. (1992) 'Cosmopolitanism and Sovereignty', *Ethics*, Vol. 103, no. 1, pp. 48–75.

Pogge, T. (2002) *World Poverty and Human Rights: Cosmopolitan Responsibilities and Reforms*, Polity Press, Cambridge.

Polgreen, L. (2008) 'Scorched-Earth Strategy Returns to Darfur', *New York Times*, 2 March, available at: <http://www.nytimes.com> (accessed 25 January 2010).

Rawls, J. (1999) *The Law of Peoples*, Harvard University Press, Cambridge, MA.

Reeves, E. (2010) 'Civilians at Risk: Human Security and Humanitarian Aid in Darfur', available at: <sudanreeves.org> (accessed 10 February 2010).

Robertson, N. (2009) 'Sudan Soldier: "They Told me to Kill, to Rape Children"', *CNN*, 5 March, available at: <http://www.cnn.com> (accessed 8 February 2010).

Robinson, F. (1999) *Globalizing Care: Ethics, Feminist Theory, and International Relations*, Westview Press, Boulder.

Sanders, E. (2009) 'Camps in Darfur Struggle with Aid Groups' Exit', *Los Angeles Times*, 17 March, available at: <http://www.latimes.com> (accessed 29 January 2010).

Scarry, E. (2002) 'The Difficulty of Imagining Other People', in *For Love of Country*, ed. J. Cohen, Beacon Press, Boston, pp. 98–110.

Slote, M. (2007a) *The Ethics of Care and Empathy*, Routledge, New York.

Slote, M. (2007b) 'Global Caring, Global Justice', paper presented at the Eastern Division Meeting of the American Philosophical Association, 30 December.

Tan, K. (2004) *Justice without Borders*, Cambridge University Press, Cambridge.

West, R. L. (2003) 'Do We Have a Right to Care?', in *The Subject of Care: Feminist Perspectives on Dependency*, eds E. K. Feder & E. F. Kittay, Rowman & Littlefield, Lanham, MD, pp. 88–114.

West, R. L. (2004) 'A Right to Care', *Boston Review*, Vol. 29, no. 2, available at: <http://www.bostonreview.net> (accessed 10 February 2010).

Creating Caring Institutions: Politics, Plurality, and Purpose

Joan C. Tronto

How do we know which institutions provide good care? Some scholars argue that the best way to think about care institutions is to model them upon the family or the market. This paper argues, on the contrary, that when we make explicit some background conditions of good family care, we can apply what we know to better institutionalized caring. After considering elements of bad and good care, from an institutional perspective, the paper argues that good care in an institutional context has three central foci: the purpose of care, a recognition of power relations, and the need for pluralistic, particular tailoring of care to meet individuals' needs. These elements further require political space within institutions to address such concerns.

In the actions of all men, and especially of princes who are not subject to a court of appeal, we must always look to the end [*se guarda al fine*]. (*The Prince*, Book XVIII, Machiavelli 1979, p. 51)

Framing the Question

In recent years, scholars have made convincing arguments about the need for robust care policies (Engster 2007; Folbre 2001; Hankivsky 2004; Held 2006; Heymann 2000; Williams 1999, 2001) and have provided evaluations of the effectiveness of various policies (Gornick *et al.* 2005). But public policies, as well as less formal care practices, all work through institutions. If we are committed to policies to improve care we need also to be able to answer the question: how can we tell which institutions provide good care? A high school teacher told me

Joan C. Tronto is Professor of Political Science at the University of Minnesota, USA.

that she can tell the quality of a school she has entered within 10 minutes of being in the building. 'How?' I asked. 'Oh', she replied, 'you can just tell which buildings have caring principals and teachers.' While I am sure that this teacher is correct, those of us without such tacit knowledge, and, more generally, citizens in a democratic society, also want to be able to judge whether institutions provide good care. Is there a way to articulate the basis for such judgments more systematically? To provide some guidelines is the goal of this essay.

Scholars such as Nel Noddings (2002) argue that the best way to think about care institutions is to model them upon the family. Noddings quotes Lisbeth Schorr to support her point. Schorr concluded, in reviewing social welfare programs that benefit children, 'In their responsiveness and willingness to hang in there, effective programs are more like families than bureaucracies' (Schorr 1997, p. 231). On the contrary, I shall argue that while we can turn to family life to intuit some key elements of good care, to provide good care in an institutional context requires that we make explicit certain elements of care that go unspoken and that we take for granted in the family setting.

In recent years, one response to 'defamilization' of care (Lewis 1997) has been to turn increasingly to the market. As consumers, patients, parents, casual observers, we often can and do pass judgments about the quality of care in various institutional settings. In adopting many of the patterns of market life in 'the New Public Management' (Page 2005), managers in care institutions also have been trying to parse out the effectiveness of institutionalized care. They use such tools as measurements of 'customer satisfaction' and the introduction of competition as ways to assure that public services are being well provided. Cottage industries provide evaluations of 'patient satisfaction', or 'customer satisfaction', and these evaluations are justified, especially by their effect on the bottom line. A recent survey of patient satisfaction with nursing, for example, began by noting that as patients become more like consumers, profits are affected by the quality of the 'patient satisfaction' (Wagner & Bear 2009). Universities struggle to measure teaching effectiveness as well (Preskill & Russ-Eft 2005). But satisfying consumers may not be the same thing as providing care adequately. Market assumptions about the consumer—that she is rational, autonomous, capable of making a choice, and possessed of adequate information to do so—may not characterize the situation of people in care settings. In measuring patient satisfaction with nursing, for example, the questionnaires are only to be filled out by the patient, not by a family member. Surely, though, family members can provide insight into the quality of nursing care that might be more or equally useful to the evaluation by the patient. Such assumptions necessarily undermine the prospects for observing and improving care. Similarly, competition may be useful in goading public service providers to compete against one another, but it does not establish standards for care, only that one provider is better than another. If all are undesirable, a market mechanism cannot provide an alternative unless someone else decides to enter the market. Given its complexity, low rate of return, and labor-intensive nature of care provision, market solutions are unlikely to emerge from such competition. Perhaps, then, the market is not the starting place for analyzing the adequacy of care.

Instead of using consumer-like measures of good care, then, I shall start from the assumptions of those who are skeptical about institutional care as an alternative to family care. To do so, I shall make explicit some dimensions of family care that are usually left in the background. Families, I shall argue, already make certain assumptions about the purposes of care, about meeting the particular needs of individuals, and about the internal allocation of power. In formal care institutions, however, there may well be conflicting approaches to purpose, particularity, and power arrangements. As a result, care institutions need to have formal practices in place that will create the space for evaluating and reviewing how well the institution meets its caring obligations by being highly explicit about its pursuit of purposes, how it copes with particularity, and how power is used within the organization. From this set of initial concerns, we will be in a better position to evaluate whether care institutions are caring well.

Changing Institutionalized Contexts for Care

Berenice Fisher and I have described care in general in these terms:

> On the most general level, we suggest that caring be viewed as a species activity that includes everything that we do to maintain, continue, and repair our 'world' so that we can live in it as well as possible. That world includes our bodies, our selves, and our environment, all of which we seek to interweave in a complex, life-sustaining web. (Fisher & Tronto 1990, p. 40; Tronto 1993, p. 103)

In the context of institutional care, obviously some care issues are more relevant than others; self-care, for example, does not usually happen in institutional contexts. Nevertheless, while institutional caring is generally provided for the people who Robert Goodin has described as 'the vulnerable' (Goodin 1985), it is still useful to recall the complex and multi-dimensional nature of care proposed by Fisher and Tronto. By describing four phases of care—*caring about*, i.e. recognizing a need for care; *caring for*, i.e. taking responsibility to meet that need; *care giving*, i.e. the actual physical work of providing care; and, finally, *care receiving*, i.e. the evaluation of how well the care provided had met the caring need—we have highlighted many points where conflict, power relations, inconsistencies, and competing purposes and divergent ideas about good care could affect care processes. We have further argued that a care process that was integral and holistic, in which these phases somehow fit together, approached more closely ideal or good care. In her research, Fisher discovered that caring often seems to consist of something 'extra' (Fisher 1990). If caring is the 'extra', then how can we ever discuss it in institutional terms? It would seem that for institutions to provide 'extra' is already to move it from the status of 'extra' to 'routine'.

In foregrounding care as a kind of human activity, we followed many early feminist scholars of care such as Noddings (1984) and Ruddick (1989) in emphasizing care as a purposive practice. But as I have also noted, care is likely to face two dangers, namely those of paternalism, in which care givers assume that they know better than care receivers what those care receivers need, and parochialism, in which care givers develop preferences for care receivers who are closer to them (Tronto 1993). If we bring these two global, political concerns about caring down to the level of more concrete caring relationships, then the problems addressed by caring are the problems of power and particularity. Thus, all forms of caring, institutional as well as personal, require that attention be paid to purpose, power, and particularity. Identifying these three as the critical elements for assessing practices of care grows out of any understanding that takes care as a *relational practice*. Among others, Christine Koggel (1998) and Jennifer Nedelsky (2008) have insisted that we recognize caring as *relational*.

In part because most people's explicit experiences of being in care relationships are rooted in the family, we often take family care as paradigmatic of all care relations. The current phenomenon of shifting care from household to market, state, or non-profit organization is a shift in the *kind* of institutionalized care, because the family, though it often appears 'natural', is also a social institution with a particular history and structure. In recent years, feminist explorations of the nature of the family and care within it have made clear that all such arrangements are deeply embedded in their own times and places (Hays 1996; Ruddick 1995).

But is it still useful to think about this mythic family? What is it that makes family care so desirable? In the first instance, family care seems somewhat automatic. No one questions seriously the *purpose* of family care: helping the members of the family to flourish together and, often in our culture, as individuals. In the second instance, while this care appears to be automatic, in fact, family care rests upon clearly understood lines of *power* and obligation: children and parents, spouses, aunts and uncles, servants, know what they owe to one another. In the third instance, family care is highly *particularistic*: each family evolves its own ways of doing certain things, and part of the pleasure in being cared for by someone in one's own family is that the family member is likely to understand and act to accommodate those peculiarities.

The family was not always such a paradise, but it was the realm where most caring work was done. We should not be too nostalgic for the family, however. While changes in care through the growth of public institutions correspond to the diminishment of the family as the primary institution of care, these changes are also tied to many other changes in the nature of modern life. Until professional health structures grew, for example, people expected to live and die in their homes. Until antibiotics, death was often caused by fast-moving infections as well as by long-term chronic illness. Until recently, children of all but the most privileged classes were expected not to be educated but to become workers and often at a very early age. The field, mine, or work-house served as day care and schools. Whether these earlier modes are more desirable is not such an easy question.

Leaving aside our sentimental views of the family, though, the challenge is whether more public social institutions can be similarly arranged so that they provide the same elements of care that the family ideally provided. I will suggest that the same three elements can be present, but not in the same way. While the beauty of relationships in the mythic, glorified family was that they did not need discussion, they evolved out of the ongoing interactions among the personalities in the household. Thus, they could be taken for granted. In any other institution these aspects of care within the institution need to be worked out consciously. This does not make these elements less achievable, but it does mean that they become more visible and require a deliberate, political process to enact them. These three elements, then, are: first, a clear account of power in the care relationship and thus a recognition of the need for a *politics* of care at every level; second, a way for care to remain *particularistic and pluralistic*; and third, that care should have clear, defined, acceptable *purposes*.

As we think about institutional settings for care, we rarely invoke similar language about purposefulness or about power and particularity. As managerial experts have often advised, organizations that focus on the outcome of their work, rather than their profits, often work better. As Richard Ellsworth puts the point: 'A clearly articulated and properly formulated purpose—one that members of the organization understand and value—provides continuity and constancy while placing the need to adapt to changing customer needs at the heart of the company's shared values' (Ellsworth 2002, p. 5). At a second level, if we think about this idea in terms of care, we might reformulate it: care institutions have to think about the nature of the caring process as a whole in order to guide their actions. This requirement does not only demand that the 'needs' of the 'customers' come first but also that the needs of care workers, the allocation of responsibility and proper assessment also happen within the organization.

Indeed, thinking about the organization's purpose quickly requires us to notice the complexity of care, and that of all those people involved in the organization of care. Even Ellsworth's facile formulation of the requisites for 'leading with purpose' disclose that there has to have been a lengthy process by which the members of the organization have come to understand their common purpose and how best to act upon it. Thus, to imagine a world organized to care well requires that we focus on three things: *politics*: recognition and debate/dialogue of relations of power within and outside the organization of competitive and dominative power and agreement of common purpose; *particularity and plurality*: attention to human activities as particular and admitting of other possible ways of doing them and to diverse humans having diverse preferences about how needs might be met; and *purposiveness*: awareness and discussion of the ends and purposes of care. If we keep these aspects of care in mind then we will be able to determine how to think through institutions using the 'logics of care' (Waerness 1984a, b, 1990) that they require.

Seven Warning Signs that Institutions Are Not Caring Well

Nevertheless, it is also fairly easy to see when institutions are not caring well. At the present moment, when the costliness of labor-intensive care is foremost in the minds of citizens (Razavi 2007), we frequently hear about abusive or inadequate forms of care. We can even recognize more system-atically what such forms of bad care look like: they are callous, inadequate, rigid. Perhaps it would be useful to list seven warning signs of bad institutional care. When care is situated according to any of these seven assumptions, it is likely to be bad care because it lacks in adequate accounts of power, purpose, and plurality.

(1) Misfortune causes the need for care.

In the minds of most people, care is a concern for those who are vulnerable (Goodin 1985) or dependent. In truth, all human beings require care, all the time. Some are able to care better for themselves. Others are able to command the caring labor of others as 'personal service', so while they could clean up after themselves, for example, they hire others to do that work for them so that they can do something less tedious (cf. Waerness 1990). As long as the image of the 'autonomous career man' (Walker 1999) continues to exist, then those who are perceived as needing care are marginalized. It is, as many have observed, most recently Knijn and Kremer (1997), quite remarkable that this image of the breadwinning, autonomous adult male so dominates the way that we conceive of citizens because it so obviously does not describe how any humans are for all of their lives. A perspective that recognizes humans throughout the life cycle and with many different capacities and needs better describes people in society and better shapes the needs for institutional care.

(2) Needs are taken as given within the organization.

The process of determining *needs* is one of the foremost political struggles of any account of care (cf. Fraser 1989). Until recently, needs-talk was rarely taken as seriously as rights-talk. Michael Ignatieff, for example, has argued against replacing rights with needs (Ignatieff 1984), though his argument presumes that it is easy to discern the meaning of rights in specific situations. Needs, which are much more contested and unclear conceptually, raise many questions. Who should determine the needs of those who 'need' care? On one level, we expect people to be able to determine their own needs. On a second level, though, professional expertise may be necessary to make certain determinations of needs. There is a problem if the professional expert differs from the care receiver in what is needed. Further, professionals might have their own agendas in determining others' needs. Who then should be entrusted with such determinations? 'Impartial' observers? Philosophers, such as Martha Nussbaum

(Nussbaum & World Institute for Development Economics Research 1987), who believe they have a better account of basic human needs?

Recognizing this complexity, then, allows us to draw this conclusion: any agency or institution that presumes that needs are fixed is likely to be mistaken and to inflict harm in trying to meet such needs. A number of feminist authors have supported some version of a 'communicative ethics' to guarantee that such needs interpretations will go on well (Sevenhuijsen 1998). Nevertheless, even such a commitment is no guarantee that the process will be workable (Bickford 1996). Further, the 'needs' expressed by less advantaged people may be manipulated or distorted (Cruikshank 1994).

(3)   Care is considered a commodity, not a process.

Clare Ungerson (1997) has written extensively about the problem of the commodification of care. Usually, the problem of commodification is associated with a certain degree of dissatisfaction with the way that care is provided: here, as in the classic Marxist framework, the problem with commodification is that it is alienating. There is an analytical difference between providing cash within care relationships and the problem of alienation, though Ungerson is probably correct that in the framework of a capitalist society the danger of alienation is great when money is introduced. Nevertheless, it is possible to imagine a system in which alienation does not occur even though money has entered the equation. Diemut Bubeck's work to try to describe care in terms of exploitation points to some of the ways in which care is different from providing other commodities (Bubeck 1995).

There is a great danger in thinking of care as a commodity, as purchased services, rather than as a process. It seems to me that when we begin to talk in terms of commodification we too quickly begin to slip into thinking of the concomitant notion of *scarcity*. Now, I would not deny for a second the idea that there are more needs for care than can ever be met. But that is not the same thing as thinking of care as a scarce thing. If we think of care as a scarce thing then we are likely to imagine that care is *best* distributed by the market mechanism. If we think of care as scarce, then we are likely to think of care as a zero-sum provision. While it is true that care requires copious amounts of time, it is not the case that to increase care necessarily means that one decreases something else. The usual view that arises from thinking of care as commodity is to see any increase in caring time as a cut in time for another activity. If activities such as paid work can be arranged flexibly, then it may be possible to increase both care and other activities. But to do so requires flexibility, creative thinking, and going beyond the zero-sum model. This, it seems to me, is the greatest danger of the model of care as commodity (Xenos 1989).

This model, thinking of ourselves first as consumers (perhaps more insidiously as 'informed' consumers), is most objectionable to me because it seems to deny people the right to make judgments about their needs. But the only way to counter such forces is to provide alternative judgments, sources of legitimacy, information. These seem to me to be the essential activities of rhetorical, moral, or political, or still better, *public* space.

(4) Care receivers are excluded from making judgments because they lack expertise.

Often, recipients are looked upon as incompetent because they are dependent. Many thinkers have written about the problems of this understanding of dependency and independence (Kittay 1999; Scully 2008; Silvers 1995). Yet the problem remains a real one. People in wheelchairs are addressed as children, there is virtually no discussion of the need to exclude the mentally incapaci-tated, and so forth. Given the direction of power in institutionalized settings, where experts arrange processes of care for less-skilled care workers to carry out, there is virtually no role for the voice of the cared-for individuals in providing for their own care. Indeed, any suggestions that they might make to thinking about care are likely to be taken to be resistance or obstruction.

(5) Care is narrowed to care giving, rather than understanding the full process of care, which includes attentiveness to needs and the allocation of responsibility.

Although the language of care giver and care receiver is now widely used, these general terms have only come into existence relatively recently with the theoretical writings by feminist scholars on care. Note, though, that in our willingness to accept these labels, we have in part replicated the public/private split by *not* naming explicitly those who are involved in the care process through the two broader phases of care: paying attention and therefore being care attentive in the first place, and assuming responsibility. I propose that any account of institutional care that fails to name explicitly the 'care-attentives' and the 'care-responsibles' allows those people, and their roles in caring, to pass unnoticed. Such not-naming contributes to the process of 'naturalizing' care relations, and to blaming the care givers who may have inadequate resources etc.

(6) Care givers see organizational requirements as hindrances to, rather than support for, care.

Many care-giving institutions split hands-on care giving from higher 'manage-ment' functions. Managers are generally better compensated than direct care workers, and their work is less subject to control. Frequently, institutions cut budgets by cutting direct care workers, not managers. Care givers frequently complain that they have inadequate resources for their tasks at hand. When care givers find themselves saying that they care despite the pressures and requirements of the organization, the institution has a diminished capacity to provide good care. Many managerial rules may be necessary for the smooth functioning of organizations, but when they come into conflict with the provision of care, it is time to rethink them.

(7)   Care work is distributed along lines of class, caste, gender, race.

One of the main ways in which societies are able to distinguish among castes is by the kind of caring work that people do. The devalued work of dealing with pollution is in most cultures reserved for the least socially appreciated. It is difficult to determine whether care work is poorly compensated because its denizens tend to be the less privileged in society, or whether, given the relative unattractive nature of care positions, people who face discrimination else-where in the workforce become care workers. In either case, regardless of cause, the fact that care is still disproportionately the work of the less well-off and more marginal groups in society reflects care's secondary status in society.

Another dimension of this problem is that care is often a result of the irresponsibility and the non-responsiveness of the privileged. Bubeck (1995) has argued, for example, that not only is care gendered but it is also gendered in part because the kinds of practices that care entails, such as paying attention to the needs of others, are viewed as impediments to the project of masculinity in our culture.

What all of these seven warning signs point to, though, is one common conclusion: the intersection of purpose, power, and plurality make it very likely that one unintended consequence of institutional care will be that one or more of these dimensions of what constitutes 'good' care will drop out of the care that institutions provide. Is there a way to bring such purpose, properly balanced power, and attention to particularity back into caring practices if they are organized institutionally? It is possible to do so, but only if we conscientiously create ways for such conflicts to be recognized and resolved in their institutional settings.

Creating Space for Resolving Conflict: What Would We Wish For?

From such harmful possibilities and realities in existing caring institutions it is easy to see what we would wish for within caring institutions. Or is it? At first thought, we might expect caring to be seamless in an institutional setting and to provide integrated, holistic care. We might wish, for example, that caring have some of these characteristics:

- No one's social opportunities or 'life chances' would be constrained by gender, by sexual orientation, by race, by imposed creed. Such a view incorporates the wishes of the goals of inclusive citizenship and social cohesion.
- People would be free to live with and to affiliate with others in intimate arrangements of their own choosing (beyond a minimal age: Marge Piercy suggests in her utopian *Woman on the Edge of Time* that children at 13 be

permitted to choose their own names and mothers (Piercy 1976)). Some of the caring work in society would be organized so that intimates could share such arrangements, but other possible arrangements would also exist.

- All personal service work would be well paid, so that no class distinctions marked the necessity to do caring work or the privilege of receiving it (cf. Waerness 1990).

- Social institutions and practices would be organized so that vulnerable people as well as able-bodied strong, healthy, normative adults can be accommodated. People think about the needs of others, but everyone also has the capacity to state what their own needs are (cf. Fraser on the 'politics of needs interpretation (Fraser 1989)). There are multiple systems for meeting needs, and individual inclination allows people to choose which way they will meet their needs.

- We would want those who were caring for us to be happy about the fact that they were giving us care. They would find care rewarding, on both personal and, if necessary, economic grounds (either by the amount they were paid, or by some alternative means of economic provision so that they were not concerned about the 'opportunity cost' of caring.)

- We would not want to be cared for according to some set model of standardization. That is, we would want care to rest upon a thick model of our own sensibilities (e.g. respectful of our senses of physical modesty, propriety, spiritual life, etc.) and our real needs.

- We would want some way to acknowledge both the pleasures and frustrations of receiving both good and bad care and we would want to share our judgments with people who would understand them.

- We would want the caring work that we do to have these same qualities of being rewarding, fulfilling, well received, and we would want the chance to share our judgments and experiences about people who knew enough about caring work to make such sharing worthwhile.

- We would not want to be asked to do so much caring work ourselves that there was no space in our lives outside of the circles of care.

But the reality is that care is rarely without serious problems and conflicts. Consider some examples:

A daughter whose aged mother has become very frail with osteoporosis, but who refuses to be institutionalized, because where she is the institutions that offer assisted living refuse to allow pets and this mother's life would be greatly diminished by being cut off from her dog. Here, the problem is that institutions treat people in standard ways and have their own expediencies.

The manager of a firm that provides home help aides hears complaints that the home health aide whom she has sent to take care of a frail and elderly woman may have taken a small amount of money from the dresser-top. There is a shortage of aides: should she be fired? At first, we might want to excuse such bad behavior if it occurs; caring work is so poorly paid that the workers are in short supply and almost as vulnerable as the people they are assisting. But: was the money taken or mislaid? Did the aide take it? Or is the elderly client forgetful, anxious about money and therefore accusative, and if we cannot get to the 'truth' of the matter, how shall we resolve this situation?

As these examples make clear, even with the best of intentions and purposes, even with institutions that strive to be adaptable, problems in providing care continue to arise. This leads me to the final point of this paper.

While it may seem desirable to try to resolve care problems by an a priori reference to organizational purpose, to a desire for holism in the care process, and for making the situation more family-like, in fact institutional care is better understood in the context of conflict. As such, care institutions need explicit institutional arrangements to help to resolve conflict as it arises.

The complication is that in institutions of care there are many sets and levels of needs. This possibility of conflicting ends within institutions is a long-established problem with viewing institutions as single-purposed and single-minded. Just as all individuals have many ends, so too individuals within organizations have different ends and organizations have many ends.

Furthermore, what we think of as 'needs' changes. They change over time for particular individuals, they change as techniques of medical intervention change, they change as societies expand their sense of what should be cared for, and they change as groups make new, expanded or diminished demands on the political order. The demands placed upon institutions change. Within institutions, as the particular individuals within the institution change, they have different needs. Workers within institutions have their own needs. There is a large discussion of how professionals create and assess needs (Culpitt 1992). Determining needs is complicated.

Where all of this change leads, I think, is to a simple premise: no caring institution in a democratic society (I include the family) can function well without an explicit locus for the needs-interpretation struggle, that is, without a 'rhetorical space' (Code 1995) or a 'moral space' (Walker 1998) or a *political space* within which this essential part of caring can occur. Thus, one important criterion for investigating institutions includes: how does the institution come to understand its needs? How does it negotiate needs within itself? Which needs are taken as legitimate? How are responsibilities within the organization allocated? Who actually gives the care? How are the reception and effectiveness of care work evaluated?

In a democratic society, furthermore, we would expect these institutions to function democratically, that is, to take into consideration the needs and perspectives of all within the institution. In practical terms, this requirement dictates that hierarchies become flattened in caring institutions. This is more easily said than done, but the end result is that the contradictory needs of institutions can be more easily organized.

For example, home-health care workers, whose work is dispersed within the separate households of the many clients that they see, need to be brought together, as part of their official and paid duties, to compare notes, raise questions about the kinds of problems we mentioned above, and provided with an opportunity to resolve them. They need, furthermore, to be able to have some input in the ways that institutional controls above them are implemented.

Conclusion

If I am right about the complex intersections of purpose, power, and plurality, then rather than expecting other social institutions to be more family-like in providing automatic ways to meet needs, the chances are good that the best forms of institutional care will be those which are highly deliberate and explicit about how to best meet the needs of the people who they serve. This requirement in turn requires that such institutions must build in adequate and well conceived space within which to resolve such conflict, within the organization, among the institutional workers and their clients, and more broadly as the institution interacts in a complex world in order to resolve such conflicts. Non-family care can be outstanding in its quality, but only if organizations that provide care also care about their own ways of working.

To put this final point more forcefully, let us return to Machiavelli's point that we must 'look to the end'. For in the last analysis, what institutional care makes clear is that the determination of the end of institutional care must itself be resolved through a political process that considers the needs, contributions, and prospects of many different actors. Under these conditions, care becomes contested in many ways, but social provision for care is likely to be better.

References

Bickford, S. (1996) *The Dissonance of Democracy: Listening, Conflict, and Citizenship*, Cornell University Press, Ithaca, NY.

Bubeck, D. (1995) *Care, Justice and Gender*, Oxford University Press, Oxford.

Code, L. (1995) *Rhetorical Spaces: Essays on Gendered Locations*, Routledge, New York.

Cruikshank, B. (1994) 'The Will to Power: Technologies of Citizenship and the War on Poverty', *Socialist Review*, Vol. 23, no. 4, pp. 29–35.

Culpitt, I. (1992) 'Citizenship and "Moral Generosity": Social Needs, Privatization and Social Service Contracting', in *Welfare and Citizenship: Beyond the Crisis of the Welfare State?*, ed. I. Culpitt, Sage, London, pp. 48–95.

Ellsworth, R. R. (2002) *Leading with Purpose: The New Corporate Realities*, Stanford University Press, Stanford.

Engster, D. (2007) *The Heart of Justice: Care Ethics and Political Theory*, Oxford University Press, New York.

Fisher, B. (1990) 'Alice in the Human Services: A Feminist Analysis of Women in the Caring Professions', in *Circles of Care: Work and Identity in Women's Lives*, ed. B. Fisher, SUNY Press, Albany, pp. 108–31.

Fisher, B. & Tronto, J. (1990) 'Toward a Feminist Theory of Caring', in *Circles of Care*, eds E. Abel & M. Nelson, SUNY Press, Albany, NY, pp. 36–54.

Folbre, N. (2001) *The Invisible Heart: Economics and Family Values*, New Press: distributed by W.W. Norton, New York.

Fraser, N. (1989) *Unruly Practices: Power, Discourse, and Gender in Contemporary Social Theory*, University of Minnesota Press, Minneapolis.

Goodin, R. E. (1985) *Protecting the Vulnerable: A Reanalysis of Our Social Responsibilities*, University of Chicago Press, Chicago.

Gornick, J. C. & Meyers, M. K. (2005) *Families that Work: Policies for Reconciling Parenthood and Employment*, Russell Sage, New York.

Hankivsky, O. (2004) *Social Policy and the Ethic of Care*, University of British Columbia Press, Vancouver.

Hays, S. (1996) *The Cultural Contradictions of Motherhood*, Yale University Press, New Haven.

Held, V. (2006) *The Ethics of Care: Personal, Political, and Global*, Oxford University Press, New York.

Heymann, J. (2000) *The Widening Gap: Why America's Working Families Are in Jeopardy and What Can Be Done About It*, Basic, New York.

Ignatieff, M. (1984) *The Needs of Strangers*, Penguin, New York.

Kittay, E. F. (1999) *Love's Labor: Essays on Women, Equality and Dependency*, Routledge, New York.

Knijn, T. & Kremer, M. (1997) 'Gender and the Caring Dimension of Welfare States: Toward Inclusive Citizenship', *Social Politics*, Vol. 4, no. 3, pp. 328–61.

Koggel, C. M. (1998) *Perspectives on Equality: Constructing a Relational Theory*, Rowman & Littlefield, Lanham, MD.

Lewis, J. (1997) 'Gender and Welfare Regimes: Further Thoughts', *Social Politics*, Vol. 4, no. 2, pp. 160–77.

Machiavelli, N. (1979) *The Portable Machiavelli*, Penguin, Harmondsworth.

Nedelsky, J. (2008) 'Reconceiving Rights and Constitutionalism', *Journal of Human Rights*, Vol. 7, no. 2, pp. 139–73.

Noddings, N. (1984) *Caring, a Feminine Approach to Ethics & Moral Education*, University of California Press, Berkeley.

Noddings, N. (2002) *Starting at Home: Caring and Social Policy*, University of California Press, Berkeley.

Nussbaum, M. C. & World Institute for Development Economics Research (1987) *Nature, Function, and Capability: Aristotle on Political Distribution*, World Institute for Development Economics Research of the United Nations University, Helsinki, Finland.

Page, S. (2005) 'What's New about the New Public Management? Administrative Change in the Human Services', *Public Administration Review*, Vol. 65, no. 6, pp. 713–27.

Piercy, M. (1976) *Woman on the Edge of Time*, Knopf, New York.

Preskill, H. S. & Russ-Eft, D. F. (2005) *Building Evaluation Capacity: 72 Activities for Teaching and Training*, Sage, Thousand Oaks, CA.

Razavi, S. (2007) 'The Political and Social Economy of Care in a Development Context: Conceptual Issues, Research Questions and Policy Options', in *Gender and Development Programme*, United Nations Research Institute for Social Development, Geneva.

Ruddick, S. (1989) *Maternal Thinking: Toward a Politics of Peace*, Beacon, Boston.

Ruddick, S. (1995) *Maternal Thinking: Toward a Politics of Peace*, Beacon, Boston.

Schorr, L. (1997) *Common Purpose: Strengthening Families and Neighborhoods to Rebuild America*, Anchor Books, New York.

Scully, J. L. (2008) *Disability Bioethics: Moral Bodies, Moral Difference*, Rowman & Littlefield, Lanham, MD.

Sevenhuijsen, S. (1998) *Citizenship and the Ethics of Care: Feminist Considerations on Justice, Morality, and Politics*, Routledge, London and New York.

Silvers, A. (1995) 'Reconciling Equality to Difference: Caring (F)or Justice for People with Disabilities', *Hypatia*, Vol. 10, no. 1, pp. 30–55.

Tronto, J. C. (1993) *Moral Boundaries: A Political Argument for an Ethic of Care*, Routledge, New York.

Ungerson, C. (1997) 'Social Politics and the Commodification of Care', *Social Politics*, Vol. 4, no. 3, pp. 362–81.

Waerness, K. (1984a) 'Caring as Women's Work in the Welfare State', in *Patriarchy in a Welfare Society*, ed. K. Waerness, Universitetsforlaget, Oslo, pp. 67–87.

Waerness, K. (1984b) 'The Rationality of Caring', *Economic and Industrial Democracy*, Vol. 5, no. 2, pp. 185–211.

Waerness, K. (1990) 'Informal and Formal Care in Old Age: What is Wrong with the New Ideology in Scandinavia Today?', in *Gender and Caring: Work and Welfare in Britain and Scandinavia*, ed. K. Waerness, Harvester Wheatsheaf, London, pp. 110–32.

Wagner, D. & Bear, M. (2009) 'Patient Satisfaction with Nursing Care: A Concept Analysis within a Nursing Framework', *Journal of Advanced Nursing*, Vol. 65, no. 3, pp. 692–701.

Walker, M. U. (1998) *Moral Understandings: A Feminist Study of Ethics*, Routledge, New York.

Walker, M. U. (1999) 'Getting Out of Line: Alternatives to Life as a Career', in *Mother Time: Women, Aging and Ethics*, ed. M. U. Walker, Rowman & Littlefield, Lanham, MD, pp. 97–112.

Williams, F. (1999) 'Good-enough Principles for Welfare', *Journal of Social Policy*, Vol. 28, no. 4, pp. 667–88.

Williams, F. (2001) 'In and Beyond New Labour: Towards a New Political Ethics of Care', *Critical Social Policy*, Vol. 21, no. 4, pp. 467–93.

Xenos, N. (1989) *Scarcity and Modernity*, Routledge, Chapman & Hall, London.

Interweaving Caring and Economics in the Context of Place: Experiences of Northern and Rural Women Caregivers

Heather Peters, Jo-Anne Fiske,
Dawn Hemingway, Anita Vaillancourt,
Christina McLennan, Barb Keith and
Anne Burrill

While caregiving in northern, rural and remote communities takes place in the context of conditions unique to smaller communities, caregivers live with social policies that are shaped by urban norms rather than rural realities. In times of economic decline and government cuts rural issues of limited services and infrastructure as well as dependency on a single industry can lead to unemployment, community and family instability, and a decline in health and well-being. During these times caregivers face increased pressure to voluntarily fill the gaps left by service cuts. Research with women caregivers in four communities in northern British Columbia (BC), Canada explores the experiences of caring and the social, geographic, economic and political contexts within which the caregiving occurs. The discourse of economic efficiencies that speaks solely to the monetary value of care is contrasted with the human condition of connectedness and relationships. These two contradictory perspectives are uncovered during interviews with women caregivers and analyzed in the framework of Olena Hankivsky's discussion of an ethic of care.

Heather Peters is an associate professor in the School of Social Work, University of Northern British Columbia, Canada. Jo-Anne Fiske is Professor of Women's Studies and Dean of the School of Graduate Studies at the University of Lethbridge. Dawn Hemingway is Associate Professor and Chair of the University of Northern BC School of Social Work and an adjunct professor in Community Health Sciences and Gender Studies. Anita Vaillancourt is a PhD candidate in the Factor-Inwentash Faculty of Social Work at the University of Toronto. Christina McLennan is a Continuing Sessional Instructor in the Thompson Rivers University School of Social Work and Human Services in Kamloops BC. Barb Keith is the Clinical Supervisor at Evergreen Addiction Services for Vancouver Coastal Health, as well as a part-time instructor at the University of Northern British Columbia. Anne Burrill is a Social Planner with the City of Williams Lake and a Sessional Instructor with the School of Social Work at UNBC.

Introduction

While caregiving in northern, rural and remote communities takes place in the context of conditions unique to smaller communities, caregivers live with social policies that are shaped by urban norms rather than rural realities. Interviews were conducted with women caregivers in four communities in northern British Columbia (BC), Canada. These four communities were facing economic decline combined with service cuts, which affected caregiving experiences. This article begins by describing the ways in which northern, rural and remote places are relevant to understanding care and caregiving. The relationships between gender, caregiving and service cuts are also discussed. Neo-liberal governments and economists explain current service cuts and restructuring via the concept of economic efficiencies. Economic efficiencies which speak solely to the monetary value of care are contrasted with the human condition of connectedness and relationships. These two contradictory perspectives are uncovered during interviews with women caregivers and analyzed in the framework of Olena Hankivsky's discussion of an ethic of care.

Northern, Rural and Remote Contexts

Northern, rural and remote contexts serve as the locale within which caregiving, an ethic of care, and economic efficiencies of service provision are explored in this research. While they are not homogeneous, small and northern communities have commonalities which result in complex conditions distinct from more populated regions. Northern or small community realities include limited infrastructure and services, large geographic areas, social and physical isolation, poor transportation, harsh winter climates and high travel costs, among others (Schmidt 2005). Services are typically concentrated in larger centres and people in smaller communities are forced to travel long distances often in poor conditions, or go without necessary services (Schmidt 2005; Self & Peters 2005). The lack of rural services and infrastructure for people in need of care places multiple and conflicting demands on women who are expected to fill the service gaps.

Service inadequacies in resource-based communities are exacerbated by economic changes including boom to bust economic cycles, shifts in international trade relations, and globalization. Small, northern communities tend to be resource dependent, often with only a single industry to power their economy (Collier 2006). Collier describes the relationship between northern and southern communities as a hinterland metropolis relationship where northern communities are economically dependent on raw resources that are shipped to metropolises in the south for processing and exporting. Thus northern communities have limited economic diversification and are dependent on southern urban communities and international demand for natural resources. The single-industry reality leaves these communities more susceptible than urban areas to the swings of boom and bust economies (Collier 2006; Schmidt 2000). During difficult economic times, these factors can undermine the quality of life in rural and northern communities by leading to unemployment, decline in personal wealth, negative impacts on health and well-being, and dislocation of individuals and families (Hanlon *et al.* 2007).

At the time of the research (2004–08) the four communities being studied were experiencing economic decline, with some movement toward economic growth near the end of the research period, although the growth proved to be short lived given the international economic crisis that followed in 2008 and 2009 (Fiske *et al.* in press). Globalization combined with natural resource issues results in negative repercussions for families and communities (Ewart & Hemingway 2008). The depletion of fish stocks affected one community (Prince Rupert) with the others (Quesnel, Fraser Lake and Prince George) being hit by difficulties within the forestry industry. Disputes between Canada and the United States over softwood lumber agreements, stalled housing starts in the United States, and the pine beetle epidemic that destroyed significant stands of trees in northern BC resulted in the forestry industry experiencing slowdowns or closures of mills and a significant decrease in lumber exports (Ministry of Forests 2004).

In spite of economic difficulties, the provincial neo-liberal government made the decision to decrease spending. Cuts were made across the public sector including to health care, income assistance, and public-sector employment (Hanlon *et al.* 2007; Lee *et al.* 2005; Wallace *et al.* 2006). According to Lee *et al.* (2005) these changes disproportionately hit resource-dependent communities in BC's northern and rural regions. Results included a loss of jobs, loss of care and other government services, and tightening of eligibility requirements for some programs. Thus in the four research communities issues of already limited infrastructure and services were exacerbated by economic decline and government cuts.

Caregiving: Gender and Service Cuts

Women have traditionally carried the burden of caring for children and family members in addition to being more likely to hold paid positions in government social and healthcare sectors (Hanlon *et al.* 2007; Luxton & Reiter 1997). Care is not only gendered but is also related to race and class where minorities, immigrants and people with lower incomes, typically still women, carry the burden of care work (Lawson 2007; Tronto 2005b). Women who are active in the paid labour force also do the majority of work in the home (Luxton & Reiter 1997). As well as providing care, women are more likely than men to be the recipients of government services (Luxton & Reiter 1997; Neysmith 1997). In addition, caring work is more likely to be devalued:

> 'Care' proves to be an undervalued and highly gendered activity assumed largely by families, and when publicly undertaken, underfunded and limited to the

maintenance of basic functioning rather than to enabling autonomy and participation. (Aronson & Neysmith 2001, p. 153)

It is therefore necessary to understand that gender is intricately woven through all aspects of care.

Gender and caregiving are fundamentally connected to service decline and need to be understood in the context of national and provincial neo-liberal responses to global economic change. Canadian governments have adopted an agenda of downsizing and downloading social programs as a central strategy to manage challenges of global and national economic pressures (Yalnizyan 2005). Cuts to services in rural and small communities have been occurring in Canada for the last two decades (Hanlon & Halseth 2005). Provincial and federal govern-ments have initiated cuts in order to save money: 'Increasingly, urban-based models of efficiencies and market parameters have been applied to welfare service evaluation, funding and provision ... A repeated result has been the closure of rural and small town services' (Hanlon & Halseth 2005, p. 7). Closures and cuts affect not only health and social services but also other public-sector offerings such as post offices, employment centres and government agencies. The effects include a loss or decline of the services, jobs and income tax base vital for providing the necessary infrastructure to support economic and social development. One consistent finding in the literature is that cuts to care services move care work from the realm of paid work to unpaid work, which is downloaded onto women (Armstrong 1996; Hanlon et al. 2007; Hemingway & MacLeod 2004). Women are expected to take on more work on a volunteer basis at the same time that their paid positions are being cut.

Caregiving: An Ethic of Care and Economic Efficiencies

Care can be described as having two components: 'a mental disposition of concern' and the 'actual practices we engage in as a result of that concern' (Tronto 1998, p. 1). In Tronto's definition of care, the practices of care include 'everything that we do to maintain, continue, and repair our "world" so that we can live in it as well as possible' (p. 2). An ethic of care begins with the notion of the irrefutability of human interdependence and the centrality of relationships and care in human existence. If relationships and caring for each other are central to life, then an understanding of these dynamics must also be central to the way society is structured, particularly in the development of policies and services related to the provision of care (Lawson 2007).

Hankivsky argues that a social justice perspective provides an important but incomplete start to social policy knowledge, and that an ethic of care needs to be added to this framework to provide a complete foundation for policy analysis and development (Hankivsky 2004). She outlines three principles of an ethic of care that are applicable to social policy. The first is contextual sensitivity that moves beyond universality to incorporating a nuanced understanding of diversity consistent with postmodern insights. As with a postmodern perspective, contextual sensitivity pays attention to the fluidity and multiplicity of individuals, relationships and contexts. Rather than applying policies in a uniform way to all people and situations, contextual sensitivity seeks to acknowledge and respect difference in its development and implementation of policy. The second principle is one of being responsive to, and in a dialectical relationship with, others while keeping in mind the complex diversities of people's lives. Hankivsky's third principle is that policy development and analysis needs to move beyond the level of the hypothetical to understanding, in a concrete way, how policy does and will affect people. The goals of policy implementation should be to alleviate suffering and improve people's lives.

Over the last three decades many developed nations including Canada have moved to a neo-liberal paradigm that has led to the restructuring and retrenchment of care service provision in the context of cost–benefit and cost–effectiveness analyses (Hankivsky 2004; Smith 2005). The neo-liberal starting point for these changes is based on an economic context which is presumed to be 'given, not made' (Smith 2005, p. 1). This discussion has resulted in a tug of war between those arguing for economic efficiencies and those lobbying for needed services; this has perhaps been most apparent in Canada and BC in the debates over healthcare restructuring.

According to the neo-liberal paradigm, individuals seek to maximize their profits and come together for this purpose: 'Interactions are focused on an ideal market in which prices form the only necessary form of communication. Thus, the relationship between buyer and seller is assumed to be the model of all human interactions' (Hankivsky 2004, p. 83). Values of selflessness, caring and sacrificing for the good of others are not understood to be a part of the public sphere and a liberal ideology 'is unable to ... separate between what aspects of our lives should and should not be commodified' (Hankivsky 2004, p. 84). However, to apply only an economic approach to public policy is to deny that there are social consequences to those decisions (Hankivsky 2004). Economics is neither neutral nor value free. When economic reasoning and advice is applied to public policies, the repercussions reverberate through people's lives, often with unacceptable consequences. An understanding of potential social consequences must, therefore, be a part of the analyses in the first place. Hankivsky argues that traditional economic analyses result in relationships and care being made invisible. She suggests that it is necessary to utilize economic analyses cautiously, in appropriate situations and in the context of an ethic of care that prioritizes individual and societal well-being over profit. A discussion of the connections and contradictions between economics and care proved to be central for caregivers in this research.

The unique conditions of small and rural communities provide an important research opportunity to better understand ways in which place and caregiving interact (Hanlon & Halseth 2005; Hanlon et al. 2007). Place informs how care is carried out and how policy is interpreted (Poland et al. 2005). Thus the interaction of place and caregiving is dynamic and changing; place informs the activities of caring and in turn caregivers and their work shape place. 'The suggestion here is that for rural places in particular, care [...] is configured in specific ways as a result of the particular economic, political and social geographies of such locations' (Parr & Philo 2003, p. 472). The purpose of this research is to explore women's experiences and understandings of caregiving in the context of northern, rural and remote realities of limited service access, economic decline and care policy and service restructuring in northern BC.

Description of the Research

Data collection and analysis involved three stages conducted over four years. Based on an initial literature review, proposed research themes were taken to four community meetings, one in each of the identified communities, for the first step of data collection. Local women from a variety of backgrounds were invited to collaborate with researchers to further develop the research questions, to discuss caregiving in the framework of local conditions, and to describe the current economic, political and social contexts for their community. Information from these meetings informed the interview questions.

The second stage of data collection consisted of interviews with women caregivers in each of the four communities. The initial community meeting and literature review suggested three areas of caregiving, and researchers recruited women caregivers from all three fields. The definition of paid caregiving, the first field, was left open and caregivers worked in various areas including social services such as child protection or women's centres, as well as health care, long-term care, and others. Familial or domestic caregiving involves care activities with or for family members, friends or neighbours who may be living in the caregiver's home or elsewhere. Third is unpaid or volunteer labour connected to a formal organizational setting. Women from across the lifespan and from a variety of ethnic, cultural and socio-economic backgrounds were recruited and efforts were made to reflect local community diversity. Recruitment strategies included purposive and snowball sampling through a variety of organizations in each community, researchers' local connections, and participants at the initial research meetings. Approximately 15 interviews were held in each community for a total of 58 interviews across all four communities. Women were asked about their activities in the three fields of caregiving. Research questions examined women's understandings of their caregiving responsibilities in light of personal circumstances and geographic, social and political contexts.

The third stage of data collection revolved around the return of preliminary results to women in each of the four communities at another public meeting. Women present were involved in a community analysis and discussion of the data. The presentations of preliminary results utilized a variety of methods such as verbal sharing, visual displays and interactive opportunities. Information and data from these community meetings were then included in the final analysis.

Data analysis methods started with a thematic and content analysis of the transcripts and occurred across a variety of groupings, with the first level of analysis being by community. Findings for each community were then examined together to determine whether themes were specific to a particular community or were common to all communities. The next step was to review the transcripts and themes with the lens of critical discourse analysis with the goal of uncovering deeper, or more layering of, themes or patterns. Finally, all themes and data were analyzed in the context of community histories and current political, economic and social circumstances and shifts. Critical theory, structural social work theory, political economy and socialist feminist theories all formed the basis of the research from proposal writing and data collection to analysis.

Results

Two interconnected layers of findings were uncovered through the analytic process. The first layer of findings was of themes and patterns found in the data for at least three and usually all four of the communities (see Table 1). The second layer of findings offered more than themes: these findings were more like threads that were consistently woven across and throughout the themes in the first layer (see Table 2). In many ways these threads tie the themes together in a deeper and more meaningful way. The threads across the findings are particularly relevant to this article, although these threads must be examined within the framework of the first layer of themes.

Table 1 First layer of research findings: care and caregiving themes across the four research communities

---

- Multiple caregiving roles were the norm and all women do multiple types of caregiving over their lifespan, with many doing multiple types simultaneously
- Participants did not describe their work as 'caregiving' but rather discussed it as: activities inherent in relationships; a responsibility, duty or obligation; and a part of one's identity
- The effects of caregiving: positive rewards (e.g. feeling good about helping others); negative experiences (e.g. stress, health issues, isolation, exhaustion, etc.); increased utilization of support networks
- Caregiving was often connected to finances as it was one's employment or it cost money to access additional care services
- Policies affected women caregivers and had specific repercussions for caring work and accessing care services in rural and small communities
- In the face of hardship, people in northern regions came together as a community to support each other
- Where participants lived, including choice of housing and the community, was related to relationships, caregiving and economics

---

Table 2 Second layer of research findings: threads woven throughout and across research themes and communities

---

- Caregiving is more about relationships than it is about work or activities, and relationships are woven through women's lives at work, at home and in the community
- Economics at personal, regional and global levels is inextricably linked to all aspects of caregiving
- The threads of relationships and economics are intertwined

Research Themes

The first theme is that the three types of caregiving (familial/domestic, unpaid volunteer, and paid) overlapped in women's lives with all women engaged in more than one of these over their lifespan: many women were multiple caregivers, that is, they did two or more of these types of caregiving simultaneously:

> women are socialized ... to do this double juggling ... I think that it's ... our life. (Jean)

When women were overwhelmed by their work they had to prioritize their caregiving roles or try to 'do it all'; both of these options created difficulties and stress for participants.

The second theme is that the women for the most part rejected the use of the terms caregiver, caregiving, or care work to describe themselves or their work. Caring for others was described as being about relationships and 'caregiving' as being about activities rather than being about the entire relationship. In speaking about her paid care work, one participant said of a client:

> 'They become a member of your family' and 'this is what home care is supposed to be'. (Polly Anna)

In addition, caring was described as a necessary responsibility, not usually a choice, and that it is a part of how the women described themselves and their identity:

> And uh, when I moved back, I had to take care of all of them. I had to cook for them and clean for them and everything else, so it's just normal now. (Dawn)

When caregiving is both an obligation and one's identity, the description of it as 'care work' does not adequately describe it, and thus for some women the term demeaned their caring.

The third theme is the effects of caregiving on women. These effects could be affirmative in that the women felt a sense of reward or accomplishment for their efforts. Negative experiences included exhaustion, stress, developing health problems, no time to care for one's self, isolation, among others. In describing their experiences of caregiving women made a diverse range of comments:

> rewarding. (Joy and Anne)
> I like the fulfillment of helping people. (Cindy)
> 'feeling good' and 'achieving something'. (Daffy)
> 'incredibly hard' and 'I feel spiritually drained'. (Lane)
> 'an extra load' and 'non particular worry, stress'. (Jean)
> it's really affected my health ... there's just been massive problems with my
> body, headaches and just everything else all of a sudden this year. (Dawn)

These potentially contradictory descriptions occurred not only between women but within individual women. Caregivers also experienced the need for assistance in dealing with daily living activities and many relied on their support networks to assist them in their caregiving roles.

A fourth theme is that caregiving is connected in various ways to finances or economics. Some women were engaged in paid care work because they needed the money. In addition, they talked about family members or others who needed care beyond public services and whether or not they could afford the care. Women also described how personal financial pressures, which were related to regional and global economic conditions, could force them to prioritize their paid caregiving over their familial obligations:

> You go to work instead of care for your kids. You love your work and not your kids.
> (PR-A)

The result was often one of stress and feelings of guilt:

> I haven't been able to do that caregiving and the guilt that, you know, comes with
> it. (Abby)

Women were also very clear about the ways in which social and health policies affected their caregiving and how these policies could be especially problematic for rural communities. This is the fifth theme. They talked about the lack of infrastructure and resources in small communities, as has been identified in the literature review, and they outlined the various cuts to health and social services and the ways in which their caregiving became increasingly difficult as services were reduced or eliminated. One woman talked about how the move to discharge her husband from hospital placed increased pressure on her and the family to provide the care he still needed:

> it's 'good to be at home and not in hospital ... but responsibility falls on family'.
> (Jean)

Caregivers in paid positions also commented on the cuts, saying:

> it's resulted in 'very, very limited services'. (Lane)
> what they [clients] really need is things that aren't really offered in our system.
> (Jean)

Comments also indicated that service cuts were exacerbated in small, rural and remote communities where services were limited to begin with and where accessing services meant time-consuming and expensive trips to larger centres.

In spite of the difficulties with living in small northern communities, the sixth theme is the way in which women spoke highly of the northern community spirit. They identified that in the face of hardships, people would come together to support each other:

> I think there is still some of that frontier spirit of community and working together and, for the good of all ... that's one of the wonderful things I think about living here. (PG-A)

The last theme is that the choice of where one lived, from housing to the larger community, was related to their care work, their relationships and economic realities. Women most often said that they moved to their current community because of employment opportunities for themselves or their spouse. The move to their current housing was related to what they could financially afford, but their decision to stay or move to another house or community was discussed in terms of their relationships. People talked about the importance of a sense of community and connections to neighbours as factors in a decision to stay in their neighbourhood or town. Small communities were often seen as more affordable as well as more community minded. Housing was also connected to care work, with one participant saying that she could not do her paid caregiving work (taking clients into her home) in a smaller house, while simultaneously being unable to afford her home unless she took in clients. Another woman described leaving her paid care position to stay at home to care for her own children and consequently the loss of her income resulted in the loss of the family home and the need to move to a more affordable house.

Threads across Research Themes

Additional research analysis identified threads woven throughout all of the themes. The most prominent thread is that of relationships. This was the most apparent in the second theme where women did not identify their work as caregiving but rather identified it as a responsibility of being in relationships. In this sense relationships were about caring for one another and so they were not telling researchers about their caring work, they were telling researchers about their relationships. One caregiver said:

> Yeah, it's a connection. It's almost like, yeah. Having some kind of connection with people and you know you get to know them after awhile. It's almost like family. (Daffy)

For multiple caregivers, the overwhelming sense of being unable to do everything meant that they were prioritizing relationships, not activities. This was extremely difficult for women to do: the repercussions of prioritizing were not about tasks left undone but about relationships being abandoned or damaged:

> My 'biggest fear in that is that sometimes you can go to a certain point that you just keep, to try and keep up with the economy ... That you lose family values, the family time, the quality time ... And, and lose that whole kinship thing because you're so busy doing this, doing this.' (Tess)

The thread of relationships was also woven through their choice of housing and their feelings about the community in which they lived. Several participants said we have 'good neighbours' (Alfie & Anne) and I 'love our neighbours', the neighbourhood is 'good for kids' (Lane). Women's appreciation for their communities was also expressed in terms of relationships: 'communities are only as nice as the people' (Alfie); I have a 'strong belief in relationship & community' (Lane); and I stay in this community because 'people are friendly' (Polly Anna). One woman said she wanted to stay in her community because the relationships and sense of community resulted in 'the personal level at which you can live your life' (Jean).

The second thread is that of economics, both a personal financial situation as well as larger market forces. Paid care work was taken up for a variety of reasons, including the need for money for daily living. Flexibility in paid positions was seen as important as it allowed women to engage in familial care work: 'if we have the expectation that we will provide care [to family members] ... I think our workplaces need to support that' (Jean). Yet for most women this was not a reality. Women in multiple caregiving roles who became overwhelmed by their responsibilities sometimes resorted to hiring someone else, usually another woman, to take on some of their care work in the home. Accessing care above what government provides was also about whether or not one could afford those 'extra' services. Economic decline combined with cuts to government spending in care services downloaded caregiving to women who tried to increase their unpaid care activities, within limited available time, while struggling to meet the financial and emotional needs of their families. Global economies were also relevant. As industries expand or decline, entire families, or the primary wage earner, must move to follow the jobs which strains or eliminates long-established relationships.

Most importantly, the threads of relationships and economics are intertwined. Paid work was an opportunity to develop friendships: 'Every new job your network of people opens' (Daffy). Work can also be problematic for relationships. One woman described financial need leading her to take on paid care work in the home, but that this was difficult for her husband: 'I think at first he [my husband] ... may have resented it' (Polly Anna). One woman talked about shopping locally as a way to develop relationships with people in her community, suggesting that an adequate income is about more than survival; it is also about one's ability to participate in community and develop support networks, friendships and relationships.

Although the concept of economic efficiencies is contrasted with an ethic of care, economics in a broader sense is contradictory for the participants. On the one hand, economic decline and cuts to services in the name of economic efficiencies were clearly damaging for women in many ways, such as: loss of care services increased pressure on women to take on escalating unpaid care duties; it put women in a position of having to prioritize work over relationships; and it forced people to move which destabilized relationships and support networks and separated people from their caregivers. On the other hand, participation in the economic market, whether through paid work, shopping or purchasing a home of one's choice, provided an opportunity for women to develop relationships and a sense of belonging in one's community. Personal income also allowed women to purchase care services that they needed but were not provided through the public system, or hire someone to do in-home care work that they were unable to do themselves. The key to the positive benefits of the economic system is *access to an adequate income*. One participant summed it up this way:

> Really the only time people ... say, 'Oh well money isn't everything,' is if you've got enough to live on ... I mean money ... unfortunately it *can* buy you better health. (PG-B)

Discussion

The research results and themes echo many of the findings in the literature. Northern, rural and remote communities have fewer services and more limited infrastructure than urban areas. In times of economic difficulties rural communities often face the loss of their primary industry, which increases stress on families. When economic decline is combined with service cuts there is increased pressure on women to take on more care work in unpaid roles. Because northern, rural and remote communities have decreased access to government health and social care services they experience an increased reliance on familial and volunteer care. These findings are consistent with results from other studies (Hanlon & Halseth 2005; Hanlon *et al.* 2007; Parr & Philo 2003; Schmidt 2000, 2005).

In addition, what caring looks like and how it is experienced by women is influenced by northern, rural and remote realities. Parr and Philo describe one way in which rural communities are distinctly different from urban areas:

> In some rural places, exactly the opposite social-geographical relationships to those in urban locations can arguably be found in that people are *physically distant* from neighbours ... but more *socially proximate*. (Parr & Philo 2003, p. 475; emphasis in original)

This is important in understanding caregiving; greater distances often decrease access to formal services, but social proximity can contribute to a more complex network of informal care. While the women in this research talked about the rewards of informal care, they also described the ways in which the increased pressure on women takes its toll emotionally, physically and spiritually. Social familiarity can also decrease access to privacy because people in small communities share information about what is going on in the lives of others (Parr & Philo 2003). Women in this research also commented on the ways in which familiarity 'has its downsides as well' (Jean) and that they wanted a balance between privacy and a caring community; something that is not easy to achieve. Caring activities are dynamic and change over time and as environments change. Women talked about the ways in which service cuts increased their responsibilities and forced them not only to take on more unpaid care work but also to prioritize not just care tasks but their relationships, creating stress and feelings of guilt. This is consistent with Hanlon *et al.*'s work:

> We assert that economic restructuring, welfare retrenchment and population aging are important triggers in the reconfiguration of social care networks, and that closer attention to these catalysts for change will contribute to a more nuanced understanding of the relation between social care and place. (Hanlon *et al.* 2007, p. 479)

The threads across the research themes provide new insights into discussions of an ethic of care and economic efficiencies. The two threads are simplistically aligned with each aspect of this discussion: the thread of relationships is intrinsic to an ethic of care and the thread of economics is aligned with discussions of economic efficiencies. The discourse of caregivers describing their work as being about a relationship rather than as care work is also reflected in other research with rural caregivers: 'it's very difficult to call yourself a carer—I'm just somebody's mother' (Parr & Philo 2003, p. 481). The discourse of caregiving being about relationships, obligations and a part of one's identity at first glance seems to corroborate neo-liberal ideologies that separate the public and private, and identify caregiving as more properly within the realm of private family life. This superficial interpretation of the data seems to suggest that government efficiencies that cut public services and move care to unpaid realms of women's labour are supported by research participants. However, the women's discussions of government policy and service cuts strongly dispute this interpretation as they are clear that the loss of these services is damaging to women, families and communities.

> We've experienced huge change, um, since the election in terms of the lack of services available and the dynamics that, the lack of options that our women have. And so you're seeing a lot more ... women coming through the system. (Abby)

Some participants participated in organizing to oppose government decisions that they saw as negatively affecting their families and their communities:

> I'm not afraid to advocate ... to talk to um the MPs or the Minister of anything. (Tess)
> ... there are a lot of progressive people here and they're kind of forced to be active ... it's kind of a scrappy community I find. (Kate)

In the lives of women caregivers, there was no separation of public and private.

77

CARE ETHICS

It is Hankivsky's discussion of an ethic of care that provides a bridge to understanding the women's seemingly disparate stances on care as being about relationships while also disagreeing with service restructuring that moves care work back onto the unpaid shoulders of women. Hankivsky argues that an ethic of care is premised on an understanding that 'human interdependence' is central to the concept of care and thus should be central to social policy (Hankivsky 2004, pp. 2, 127). This is what the women in this research are also saying: that economics, relationships and caregiving are intertwined, and a separation of public and private with the resulting focus on economics alone to address social issues results in a disruption of social life that is damaging to people's health, to relationships and to community:

> An ethic of care reveals that care and human connectedness are key aspects of the human condition and, at the same time, that traditional economics renders them invisible. (Hankivsky 2004, p. 93)

Hankivsky states that in a focus on economic efficiencies, 'market forces are increasingly shaping our values and our lives' when it should be our values of interdependence that instead shape policy and services (Hankivsky 2004, p. 103). The women in this research agree. Throughout the research they demonstrated that an understanding of their care work as being grounded in relationships is the key to shifting social policy analysis and development from a focus on economics to an analysis that incorporates the realities of their lives. One woman described it this way:

> I just don't understand society's, you know, money-saving measures when we look at the long term cost ... They've burnt out family members so there's nobody left. (Lindy)

Women doing paid and unpaid caregiving are very aware of the impact of policies on their work and their lives. Lindy went on to say:

> Why can't we support families, women in particular, because that's who's doing the bulk of the, the unpaid caregiving. Why women aren't being supported through policies that, you know, allow flexibility in the workplace and policies that allow access to services or um, money for services. (Lindy)

Hankivsky argues that social policy analysis and development need to go beyond the 'use of a one-dimensional economics measure' (Hankivsky 2004, p. 104) to incorporate an ethic of care that brings with it the principles of contextual sensitivity, responsiveness to others and to diversity, and an understanding of the social consequences of decisions. A key element of the principle of contextual sensitivity is understanding the diversity and plurality of human life and experiences and then incorporating these diverse voices into policy discussions and analysis. In this perspective social policy analysis and restructuring would take into account human relationships at the intersection of place in the context of northern, rural and remote communities in service delivery and care provision.

An ethic of care applied to policy analysis and service provision would ask the people most affected by the provision of care services about the potential repercussions of policy changes on their lives. It would seek to understand the consequences of policy shifts in the context of location and the differences between urban and rural. It would create policy that was flexible and could reflect different needs in different communities. It would understand that an adequate income at an individual level is necessary for quality of life and also for a healthy national and global economy. Policy analysis in the context of an ethic of care would understand that outcomes are about more than cost savings, but also about the communities, relationships, and societies we seek to develop and build.

Acknowledgements

The authors wish to acknowledge and thank the Social Sciences and Humanities Research Council for funding the research from which this information is drawn (Grant # 410-2004-1646). Thanks are also due to the women we interviewed for their time and knowledge which were graciously shared with us, and to the communities including many organizations which assisted with the facilitation of the research process.

References

Armstrong, P. (1996) 'Unraveling the Safety Net: Transformations in Health Care and their Impact on Women', in *Women and Canadian Public Policy*, ed. J. Brodie, Harcourt Brace, Toronto, pp. 129–49.

Aronson, J. & Neysmith, S. M. (2001) 'Manufacturing Social Exclusion in the Home Care Market', *Canadian Public Policy*, Vol. 27, no. 2, pp. 151–65.

Collier, K. (2006) *Social Work with Rural Peoples*, 2nd edn, New Star Books, Vancouver.

Ewart, P. & Hemingway, D. (2008) 'Devastating Mill Shutdowns: What Can Towns Like Mackenzie Do?, 12 June, available at: <www.opinion250.com> (accessed 7 March 2010).

Fiske, J., Hemingway, D., Vallaincourt, A., Peters, H., McLennan, C., Keith, B. & Burrill, A. (in press) 'Health Policy and the Politics of Citizenship: Northern Women's Care Giving in Rural British Columbia', in *Rural Women's Health in Canada*, eds B. D. Leipert, B. Leach & W. Thurston, University of Toronto Press, Toronto, ON.

Hankivsky, O. (2004) *Social Policy and the Ethic of Care*, UBC Press, Vancouver.

Hanlon, N. & Halseth, G. (2005) 'The Greying of Resource Communities in Northern British Columbia: Implications for Health Care Delivery in Already-underserviced Communities', *Canadian Geographer*, Vol. 49, no. 1, pp. 1–24.

Hanlon, N., Halseth, G., Clasby, R. & Pow, V. (2007) 'The Place Embeddedness of Social Care: Restructuring Work and Welfare in Mackenzie, BC', *Health & Place*, Vol. 13, no. 2, pp. 466–81.

Hemingway, D. & MacLeod, T. (2004) 'Living North of 65: A Community Process to Hear the Voices of the Northern Seniors', *Rural Social Work*, Vol. 9, pp. 137–46.

Lawson, V. (2007) 'Geographies of Care and Responsibility', *Annals of the Association of American Geographers*, Vol. 97, no. 1, pp. 1–11.

CARE ETHICS

Lee, M., Murray, S. & Parfitt, B. (2005) *BC's Regional Divide: How Tax and Spending Policies Affect BC Communities*, Canadian Centre for Policy Alternatives, Vancouver.

Luxton, M. & Reiter, E. (1997) 'Double, Double, Toil and Trouble. Women's Experiences of Work and Family in Canada, 1980–1995', in *Women and the Canadian Welfare State: Challenges and Change*, eds P. M. Evans & G. R. Wekerle, University of Toronto Press, Toronto.

Ministry of Forests, G.o.B.C. (2004) 'Resolving the Softwood Lumber Dispute', available at: <http://www.for.gov.bc.ca/HET/Softwood/index.htm> (accessed 26 August 2004).

Neysmith, S. M. (1997) 'Towards a Woman-friendly Long-term Care Policy', in *Women and the Canadian Welfare State: Challenges and Change*, eds P. M. Evans & G. R. Wekerle, University of Toronto Press, Toronto, pp. 222–45.

Parr, H. & Philo, C. (2003) 'Rural Mental Health and Social Geographies of Caring', *Social & Cultural Geography*, Vol. 4, no. 4, pp. 471–88.

Poland, B., Lehoux, P., Holmes, D. & Andrews, G. (2005) 'How Place Matters: Unpacking Technology and Power in Health and Social Care', *Health and Social Care in the Community*, Vol. 13, no. 2, pp. 170–80.

Schmidt, G. (2000) 'Remote, Northern Communities: Implications for Social Work Practice', *International Social Work*, Vol. 43, no. 3, pp. 337–49.

Schmidt, G. (2005) 'Geographic Context and Northern Child Welfare Practice', in *Violence in the Family*, eds K. Brownlee & J. R. Graham, Canadian Scholars' Press, Toronto, pp. 16–29.

Self, B. & Peters, H. I. (2005) 'Street Outreach with No Streets: A Rural Nursing Initiative in the British Columbia Interior', *Canadian Nurse*, Vol. 101, no. 1, pp. 20–24.

Smith, S. J. (2005) 'States, Markets and an Ethic of Care', *Political Geography*, Vol. 24, pp. 1–20.

Tronto, J. (1998) 'An Ethic of Care', *Generations*, Vol. 22, no. 3, pp. 15–20.

Tronto, J. (2005a) 'Care as the Work of Citizens: A Modest Proposal', in *Women and Citizenship*, ed. M. Friedman, Oxford University Press, New York, pp. 130–45.

Tronto, J. (2005b) 'The Value of Care', *Boston Review*, available at: <http://boston review.net/BR27.1/tronto.html> (accessed 27 February 2010).

Wallace, B., Klein, S. & Reitsma-Street, M. (2006) *Denied Assistance: Closing the Front Door on Welfare in BC*, Vancouver Island Public Interest Research Group and Canadian Centre for Policy Alternatives, Vancouver.

Yalnizyan, A. (2005) 'Divided and Distracted: Regionalism as an Obstacle to Reducing Poverty and Inequality', available at: <www.policyalternatives.ca> (accessed 8 March 2010).

Gratitude and Caring Labor

Amy Mullin

I argue that it is appropriate for adult recipients of personal care to feel and express gratitude whenever care providers are inspired partly by benevolence, and deliver a real benefit in a manner that conveys respect for the recipient. My focus on gratitude is consistent with important aspects of feminist ethics of care, including its attention to the particularities and vulnerabilities of caregivers and care recipients, and its concern with how relations of care are shaped by social hierarchies and public institutions. In addition, it goes beyond the current preoccupations of care ethicists both by introducing gratitude as an important aspect of morally valuable relations of care and by stressing the significance of attending not only to the needs but also the capacities of recipients of care.

I offer a general account of interpersonal gratitude and argue that it is important to think about gratitude in the context of caring labor. My approach is based on a feminist ethics of care, and my focus is on caring labor in which the recipients are adults and the care they receive meets needs they would find it difficult or impossible to meet on their own. The care involved might include assistance with showering, eating, or getting in and out of a wheelchair or walker. Because my topic is gratitude, I consider only those recipients who are capable of recognizing and appreciating the benevolent efforts of others.

When we think about gratitude in the context of caring labor, we need to contest the idea that gratitude is owed whenever the recipient has received a benefit and the idea that those who are paid to care are not appropriate targets of gratitude. I am therefore especially interested in paid caring labor. I hope to

Amy Mullin is Professor of Philosophy at the University of Toronto. Her research interests include social philosophy, aesthetics, and feminist philosophy, with a focus on questions about relationships involving the provision of care. She is the author of *Reconceiving Pregnancy and Childcare: Ethics, Experience and Reproductive Labor* (Cambridge) as well as journal articles and book chapters on the subjects mentioned above.

show that gratitude has an important role to play in generating respect for care providers and care receivers alike. In addition, I will argue that when we develop policies and practices around the provision of caring labor, we need to leave room for the development of relationships where gratitude will be both merited and expressed.

I first explain my methodological approach, by indicating what I consider the most important features of a feminist ethics of care. I then move to a discussion of gratitude, generally, and gratitude for personal care more specifically. An ethics of care emphasizes the importance of thinking about and seeking to meet the particular needs of particular people. Early versions of the ethics of care emphasized the needs of recipients of care in close personal relationships, and urged caregivers not only to consider the point of view of a care recipient but also to take it on (Noddings 1984). Responses to feminist critiques led to the following important characteristics of a feminist ethics of care. Such a feminist ethics of care asks who cares and who receives care, and attends to how sex, class and ethnicity, other dimensions of social difference, and public institutions shape the allocation and delivery of care (Bubeck 1995; Tronto 1993). A feminist ethics of care does not assume that all relationships should be maintained, and worries about the exploitation of caregivers and the danger of self-abnegation in caregiving (Hoagland 1991). A feminist ethics of care attends to the vulner-abilities and needs of caregivers and care recipients alike (Kittay 1999). It recognizes the separate nature and needs of the care recipient and does not assume that the caregiver will find it easy to understand what the care recipient needs (Tronto 1993; White 2000). Its mandate is an investigation of care both locally and globally, and it is concerned with both the private and the public provision of care (Noddings 2002; Robinson 1999; Tronto 1993; White 2000).

To this list of criteria I add two of my own. First, a feminist ethics of care must attend not only to the vulnerabilities of both caregivers and care recipients but also to their capacities. It must recognize recipients of care as more than bearers of need. To date, feminist care ethics has focused more on caregivers and what is needed to care well, while also meeting caregivers' needs, than on questions about the responsibilities and capacities of recipients of care. Given its concern to distinguish the perspectives of caregiver and care recipient (Bubeck 1995; Card 1990; Hoagland 1991), attention has been paid to the autonomy of both parties (Clement 1996), but the autonomy of recipients has been investigated mainly in terms of care-recipients' determination of their own needs (White 2000). Although the capacities and responsibilities of those who need care have not been sufficiently addressed or thematized in feminist care ethics thus far, my first additional criterion is consistent with important feminist commitments. These are commitments to recognize capacities for agency and responsibility even in those who have limited access to resources and power, and to promote agency in all subjects.

Second, a feminist ethics of care should aim not only at avoiding unhealthy relationships (involving exploitation or inappropriate paternalism) but also at achieving healthy ones. Healthy relationships, characterized by deserved trust and mutual respect, are widely sought and morally valuable. Healthy relationships are nurtured when we attend as much to the capacities and responsibilities of recipients of care as those of caregivers. In my focus on gratitude, I aim to contribute to an ongoing project of recognizing the importance of attending to the capacities of recipients of care, and their ability to contribute to healthy relationships with their caregivers. Gratitude is one such contribution.

What is gratitude? Interpersonal gratitude, or gratitude *to* a person, as opposed to being grateful *that* some particular thing has occurred, involves appreciative attitudes towards both a benefit and a benefactor (Walker 1988). Patrick Fitzgerald notes that standard philosophical analyses of gratitude require benevolence from the benefactor and receipt of a benefit on the part of the grateful party. He goes on to criticize this standard account for neglecting to find gratitude appropriate towards those who harmed us or indirectly and unintentionally benefited us (Fitzgerald 1998). I find his account implausible.

We may be appropriately grateful to those who help us transform past harms into sources of strength, but we are not appropriately grateful *to* those who harm us. Moreover, since expressions of gratitude tend to reinforce the behavior for which we are grateful, it seems misguided to show appreciation for harmful behavior. When others unintentionally benefit us, we might be grateful that their behavior has positive unintended consequences, but we should not be grateful to them. I therefore reject Fitzgerald's argument. Instead, I concur with the view that gratitude requires that a benefit is received, and the benefit is seen as given out of benevolence. However, I will argue below that benevolence is insufficient and needs to be accompanied by respect to merit gratitude. The standard conception of gratitude is shared by psychological studies of gratitude (see, for instance, Tsang 2006a). Therefore, when those studies discuss gender differences in gratitude, or the positive effects of gratitude, they will be applicable to my analysis.

Gratitude is sometimes confused with indebtedness. However, it is distinguished from indebtedness both by the motivation imputed to the benefactor and the attitude of the recipient. When we are grateful, we impute motives of goodwill and caring on the part of the benefactor and not expectations of equivalent payback as is associated with indebtedness. Those who feel gratitude typically feel positively valenced emotions as opposed to the discomfort and uneasiness associated with indebtedness (Tsang 2006b; Watkins *et al.* 2006).

It is inappropriate to feel either gratitude or indebtedness in the absence of any benefit. It is also inappropriate to feel gratitude towards a person we believe has accidentally benefited us, or benefited us without concern for whether we would regard the good or service as a benefit, or towards someone who conveyed a benefit with a malevolent ulterior purpose (for instance so as to cause suffering when the benefit is withdrawn). Gratitude is merited only when the provider of a benefit has done so at least in part out of goodwill towards us. In addition, gratitude is appropriate only when a benefactor expresses not only goodwill but also respect for the recipient.

This last point is typically omitted, perhaps because it is assumed that respect invariably accompanies goodwill, but we are capable of feeling goodwill without respect. For instance, someone may genuinely desire to benefit someone who is regarded as a kind of favored pet, or as a needy and infantilized object of pity. In such cases, I cannot see how gratitude towards the benefactor would be merited or associated, as it generally is, with good feelings towards the benefactor. The recipient might still be grateful *that* his or her needs were met in some part, but respectful appreciation of the patronizing or demeaning bene-factor cannot be appropriate. As Card argues: 'one's gratitude is a response to another's benevolence, more specifically, to the valuing of oneself presupposed in another's benevolence: gratitude acknowledges and reciprocates that valuing, thereby demonstrating that one does not value others merely as useful for one's own ends' (Card 1988, p. 117). Interpersonal gratitude would demonstrate severely damaged self-respect if it did not require that the benefactor demonstrate not only goodwill but also respect for the one benefited.

I mentioned above that gratitude is merited only when the giver of a benefit does so at least in part out of goodwill towards the recipient. It is important to note that motives for giving, as with motives for pretty much anything we do, are generally mixed, and gratitude would rarely be merited if only called for when the benefactor provides the benefit at enormous sacrifice, due solely to goodwill for the beneficiary. As Walker argues:

> while I may be under no obligation to the person who benefits me inadvertently or entirely out of self-interest, we must not inflate this point and claim that only benefits motivated purely by goodwill require gratitude. We should allow that obligations of gratitude are generated when benefits are the result of mixed motives and conferred from a mixture of self-interest and goodwill. (1988, p. 208)

The important point is that if the benefit is conveyed purely out of self-interest, with expectation of equivalent payback, then gratitude is not called for, but instead the beneficiary may be expected to feel indebted.

When we feel grateful, we have goodwill towards our beneficiary, and desire to manifest our appreciation and respect. While we may wish to benefit our benefactor in turn, we do not feel indebted or constrained to provide any specific type of benefit in return. Instead, we are often creative in our expressions of appreciation, expressions that at a minimum are intended to demonstrate respect for the benefactor. Studies show that women are generally more comfortable feeling and expressing gratitude than are men, and get more rewards from doing so. Older men, particularly those who identify with a masculine identity, tend to feel some discomfort if they feel expected to be grateful (especially to other men), and studies suggest that they may conflate gratitude and indebtedness, or associate gratitude with unwanted dependency (Kashdan *et al.* 2009, p. 709).

This association between gratitude and dependency is in keeping with Aristotle's claim in the *Nicomachean Ethics* that the great-souled man will not feel gratitude because he would be ashamed to be in a position to receive benefits from another. His claim is that the superior person gives benefits and the inferior person receives them (1980, p. 92). If we reject this picture of human interdependency as a sign of weakness, and remember that gratitude is merited only when the benefactor has respect for the beneficiary, then we must reject Aristotle's view, and celebrate the declining tendency to associate gratitude and unwanted dependency in more recent generations of men.

As mentioned above, fewer women have problems with notions of human interdependence than do men, some of whom view gratitude as an acknowl-edgment of a power differential between the one who gives and the one who receives a benefit. Interestingly, far from viewing gratitude as a threat to autonomy, women who regularly feel and express gratitude experience more well-being and feel more autonomous than those who do not. In experimental studies of the effects of gratitude, as compared to men, 'women derived greater benefits from gratitude, including (1) greater satisfaction of the need to feel connected to and cared for by others (belongingness) and (2) increased feelings of freedom to act in ways that are consistent with core values (autonomy)' (Kashdan et al. 2009, p. 720). This is interestingly consistent with feminist work on relational autonomy, often taken up in the ethics of care (Sherwin 2000). Women who do not regard interdependence as a threat to autonomy find that gratitude enhances their feeling of control over their lives and their ability to act freely. The first benefit is consistent with psychological research showing that gratitude has a key role to play in relationship building overall (Bartlett & DeSteno 2006).

Having given a basic account of the nature of interpersonal gratitude and discussed when it is merited, I turn now to my second aim: to discuss interpersonal gratitude in the context of caring labor, specifically caring labor provided to adult recipients capable of acknowledging and appreciating others' efforts on their behalf. Here I contend that, in contexts of caring labor, paid and unpaid, gratitude is the morally appropriate response not to care provided in an impersonal or disrespectful manner but to care provided in a manner that recognizes and respects the humanity of the recipient.

What kinds of respect are relevant in relationships of care? Stephen Darwall and Robin Dillon provide helpful accounts distinguishing between respect owed someone as a person with inherent dignity, whatever she may have done and whatever she may be like, and respect based on an assessment of her particular characteristics. For Darwall, the former is a variety of recognition respect, which requires us to regulate our conduct towards an object in virtue of its nature. When what we respect is another person's dignity, then we respect their ability to make a claim on us, and to demand respect from us, in virtue of being a free and rational agent (2004, p. 44). For him, recognition respect contrasts with appraisal respect, or esteem, which is based on an assessment of someone's character, conduct, or both. Since we address demands to respect our dignity only to other people, recognition of dignity is inherently reciprocal (2004, p. 43). To demand that others respect our dignity while failing to respect their dignity is hence a contradiction. This will be important in our discussion of gratitude for caring labor.

Dillon accepts Darwall's distinction between recognition respect and appraisal (or evaluative) respect, and elaborates on care respect as a variety of the former. For Dillon, and for care ethicists more generally, care respect is due all people, but is based not on our being free and rational, or autonomous agents, but on our being particular people, with our own self-conceptions, perspectives, and needs. She writes: 'The object of care respect is the whole, specific individual human "me" as such ... the core of an appropriate response is paying attention to and valuing the person in her particularity' (2009, p. 32). In addition, care respect involves trying to understand another 'in her own terms; and second, it includes seeking to promote the other's well-being' (2009, p. 36). Dillon recognizes that the other may have a deeply flawed self-conception (perhaps because of a history of exploitation, perhaps for more idiosyncratic reasons), and may fail to recognize some of what he or she needs. Nonetheless, in our attempts to care for others, we are always to consider their perspectives, and be humble in recognition of our limited ability to accurately assess what another person needs (2009, pp. 38–40). Dillon recognizes that there is a tension between 'regarding each person as just as valuable as every other and regarding this individual as special' but she sees the tension as constructive and akin to what we manage to do when we see our various friends or children as equally and yet uniquely valuable (2009, p. 35). I am less sanguine that our ability to treat our friends or children this way suggests that we can or should regard everyone as simultaneously equally valuable and special. Especially when it comes to our friends, we interact with them because of features that we admire in them, the value of our history together, and our appreciation of their contributions to our relationship. There is less cause to think we will find all others we encounter to be equally valuable, or that we should do so.

In addition, there is an important role to be played by evaluative respect once we actually enter into any kind of close personal relationship with another, such as is required to meet their needs for care. Instead of Dillon's view that care respect should lead us to find everyone equally and uniquely valuable, I argue that care respect is the attitude we should bring to our encounters with others who need care, as a starting point. We should regard others whose needs we aim to meet as concrete people with perspectives, needs and capacities we should strive to discover and take into account in our dealings with them. Feminist care ethicists often contrast this with responding to a generalized other (Benhabib 1985). We should also, as Dillon urges, be slow and cautious in making evaluative judgments (2009, p. 36). However, respect for particularity demands that we take it seriously, and respond to what we discover. Once we have engaged enough with recipients of our care (and their other caregivers and intimates, and others from their cultural group, if the culture is unfamiliar) to get a good sense of their particular characters and the meaning of their conduct, it is incumbent on us then to evaluate those characters and conduct, particularly with regard to how they relate to us. We should not meet or deny care-recipients' basic needs in response to our judgments. Instead, how we relate to care recipients, what we expect of them, and the relationships that we build with them should respond to our assessment.

How does this understanding of care respect as a kind of recognition respect, and evaluative respect as something that may or may not follow from care respect, shape our understanding of when gratitude is called for in response to caring labor? It suggests that even benevolent caregivers who fail to manifest care respect in their dealings with recipients of care do not merit gratitude. If a caregiver does not treat a recipient of care as a particular person whose perspective needs to be sought and taken into account, then he or she is not treating the recipient as someone with dignity. This does not mean that a care recipient should treat the caregiver in turn as someone without dignity, but it does mean there is no reason to feel or express gratitude towards the caregiver.

What if a caregiver treats a recipient of care as someone with dignity, but, after seeking to understand the care-recipient's perspective and while taking it into account in caregiving, nonetheless fails to find much in the recipient to esteem? Or what if the caregiver esteems certain character traits and aspects of conduct, but clearly abhors others or finds them understandable but regrettable (the impatience and swearing is due to pain, the anger is due to embarrassment, the prejudice is due to an inability to rise above a racist upbringing)? When someone fails to find another person to be particularly estimable, this does not manifest a lack of basic recognition respect, and so it should not negate a responsibility to respond to the benevolent and respectful provision of a real service with gratitude.

We have a responsibility to be grateful only when another has treated us with the kind of recognition respect that is consonant with our dignity. In situations involving caregiving (contra Dillon, I think not necessarily in all situations), we are treated with dignity only if we are treated as particular people whose well-being matters, whose needs must be discovered rather than assumed, and whose perspective needs to be acknowledged and taken into account, even if our perspective does not alone determine how care is provided. Since a claim to dignity is a claim we address to other people, gratitude towards a caregiver who has treated us with dignity is a matter of reciprocal recognition of our mutual personhood. The expression of merited gratitude therefore simultaneously recognizes the caregiver's humanity and asserts the humanity of the recipient. Since our being treated with respect by others is important for our self-respect (Honneth 1992), merited gratitude can enhance the self-respect of each party and enable the development of a positive relationship. It is therefore unsurprising that, in Moskos and Martin's survey and analysis of over 1,000 Australian direct care workers who care for elderly people, those care workers frequently mentioned the gratitude they received, and the caring relationships they formed, as two of the most rewarding aspects of their work (2005).

Although it can be tempting for care recipients who resent or feel shamed by their dependency to depersonalize the caregiver, and treat him or her as a mere instrument, this is unfair to the caregiver and expresses alienation from the care-receiver's vulnerability, rather than asserting the consonance of dignity and vulnerability. It would be easier to gain social recognition of this consonance if we focused not only on the needs but also the capacities of recipients of care. The direct care workers discussed above repeatedly mentioned the extent to which they appreciated and learned from the elderly people they cared for, often mentioning the wisdom of care recipients, the stories that recipients told, and how recipients make workers feel valued and appreciated. For instance, one worker said that the best thing about direct care work is 'being able to make the residents feel they are still human beings and have a lot to offer', while another wrote that the best thing about the job is 'to personally be able to care for elderly residents, treating them with respect, encouraging independence where possible, and developing a trusting friendship' (Moskos & Martin 2005, p. 10). Many of the workers, who range from nurses and physiotherapists to personal care workers, mention listening to the elderly residents who have 'a great wealth of knowledge to impart' (2005, p. 10). The workers respond to the recipients of their care as particular people with both needs and capacities to give.

Until we have greater social recognition of the co-existence of important capacities with significant need, whether in elderly people or younger adults with disabilities, it can be difficult for individuals to accept that needs they associate with childhood (like assistance with toileting and bathing) do not demean them. There has been some mockery of and discomfort with the development of 'robocarers' to assist the elderly, and fear that care is becoming explicitly depersonalized when a robot assists with their care. Nonetheless, innovations to assist with tasks such as bathing, if expenses could be brought down, might be genuinely helpful given the current lack of such social recognition. Of course, socially isolated elders (or people with disabilities who require such forms of intimate care) also need social contact and caring relationships (to have the opportunity to be recognized as people with dignity, among other things, something that can only come from other people). However, so long as innovations such as robotic baths (that close around a person in a wheelchair and wash and rinse the person's body) are a supplement to, and not a replacement for, contact with a caring person, they can not only spare caregivers some physically demanding work but also enable recipients to avoid shame still often associated with bodily need (Robichon 2004).

To summarize this section of my essay, gratitude is merited only when a benefit is conveyed in a manner that makes the recipient feel its giver has both goodwill towards and respect for the beneficiary. The kind of respect at issue is a form of recognition respect, or respect for dignity. Dillon's conception of care respect as requiring us to attend to the particularity of the recipient of care is an important elaboration of how we can respect dignity in providing care. When caregivers attend to the particularities of a recipient of care, it is important that they seek not only to recognize the particular needs of the person and that person's understanding of her needs and how they should be met but also to recognize the particular capacities of the person needing care. It is important for caregivers, therefore, not only to feel and express care respect but also to be open to feeling and expressing evaluative respect when it is merited by recipients' character and conduct, including conduct within the caring relationship. One example of conduct deserving evaluative respect is a care recipient's expression of merited gratitude.

Even unpaid volunteer care laborers will not merit gratitude if they do not manifest both goodwill and recognition respect, and paid care laborers may well merit gratitude. For example, if recipients have reason to believe that care labor directed at them is intended not only to make ends meet for the laborer but also that the care laborer has also chosen a field of work in which he (or more likely she) can meet real needs in a respectful manner, then the paid laborers merit gratitude. In the survey of direct care workers discussed above, many of the care workers report that they stick with their work, despite its low pay and low social status, precisely because they feel it allows them to meet real needs and develop rewarding relationships with the people they care for (Moskos & Martin 2005, pp. 10–13). It is important to stress that feeling gratitude towards someone engaging in care labor is not at odds with the recipient feeling that his or her basic needs should be met as a matter of justice, since the recipient can still be grateful to the care laborer for why and how she seeks to meet the recipient's needs.

I now consider a challenge to my claim that gratitude has an important place in caring labor. Galvin argues that some people with disabilities are disturbed by expectations of gratitude and experience them as a significant burden. First, it is important to remember that gratitude is merited only when someone acts towards us with both goodwill and respect. Galvin's stories of people who receive inadequate care, delivered without care and consideration, are not stories where gratitude is merited but are examples of situations when it is wrong to expect gratitude. Thus, for instance, one woman insists that her caregivers need to remember that they are acting as her hands and feet and not as her head. She says: 'This is the way I see it. They are paid to do a job. What's their job? It's being my hands and feet but not my head' (Galvin 2004, p. 142). Her caregivers treat her as incompetent to decide for herself about her needs. While her caregivers expect gratitude, they are wrong to do so, since gratitude is not merited when recognition respect is absent.

Second, it is important to stress that gratitude differs from indebtedness. When someone acts towards us in a way that suggests they expect a return equal to their investment, then it is not gratitude that is called for, but, supposing we have requested or accepted the benefit given on those terms, indebtedness. What is called for is repayment rather than broadly based goodwill towards and respect for the provider of the benefit.

Gratitude may still be expressed in either of these situations (when care is inadequate or presented with the expectation of tit–for-tat reciprocity), but this would be either out of fear or out of hope—fear that the needs one has barely had met will be neglected altogether, or hope that the expression of gratitude will help shift the relationship into one based on a new foundation of mutual respect. Expression of gratitude in such circumstances may be strategic but is not merited. As Galvin writes, 'people who were reliant on informal assistance could not afford to appear ungrateful, because gratitude was seen to be the only currency available with which to secure support' (2004, p. 145). This kind of strategic gratitude is more likely to be expressed in societies where people's basic needs are not met by public institutions or through public provision of funds, so that people with significant dependency needs are forced to rely upon informally provided care.

Third, Galvin gives an account of people with disabilities who have had bad experiences of inappropriately demanded gratitude, understandably resent this, and delight in paying care providers in cash rather than gratitude. It is nonetheless wrong for a care receiver to insist that people she acknowledges to act respectfully and out of goodwill do not merit gratitude. Galvin quotes another woman as saying: 'Nowadays I have my own funding and my own carers and they've mostly been with me for a long, long time. And it's just a very good relationship. They do things for me and they'll even go the extra mile and I pay them and I don't have to be grateful for it' (2004, p. 145). It is understandable this woman is happy not to have to express gratitude given her bad past experiences, but to fail to express gratitude is to wrong care laborers who act out of goodwill and respect (in addition to the desire to be paid for their labor).

As stressed above, a feminist ethics of care attends to the vulnerabilities of both caregivers and care recipients, and often explores the manner in which public institutions can mitigate or exacerbate these vulnerabilities; for instance, when care is publicly funded. Kirstein Rummery does both. She reminds us that care laborers are often from lower socio-economic classes and disadvantaged ethnic groups, and are caught up in the same struggle for autonomy that Galvin described in the case of care recipients (Rummery 2007). Both care laborers and those adult recipients who need assistance in meeting needs for bodily care are often treated in ways that disrespect them and therefore risk damaging their self-respect. Both should be treated in ways consonant with at least recognition respect as well as evaluative respect for those who act in ways that respect others. Moreover, both groups are disproportionately female, with care laborers, both paid and unpaid, especially likely to be women.

Galvin's main point in her article is that people who are forced to rely upon informal and typically unpaid care to meet their basic needs are also often forced to express gratitude whether they feel it or not, adding one more social burden to their lives. I share her opposition to forced gratitude. She notes that the disabled people she studied who were happiest with their care arrangements were those who were able to pay for their own care, either from their own resources or because they received government funds to do so. Rummery stresses that state provision of care often benefits care laborers as well as care receivers (particularly when there is some oversight of the conditions of their labor), even though it has not had any effect on the gendered provision of care labor (Rummery 2008). I strongly support the call to recognize that meeting the basic needs of people with disabilities is a matter of justice, rather than a matter solely of compassion (Becker 2005 makes just this case). My point is merely that our rejection of misplaced or forced gratitude should not carry over to a rejection of the appropriateness and benefits of expressing gratitude to those care laborers who deserve it.

Above, I discussed men who confuse gratitude and indebtedness and view receiving a benefit (especially from another man) as a sign of their weakness and dependence. Those people with disabilities who were resentful of expectations of gratitude similarly saw gratitude as confirmation of their dependence upon others. Many of the women studied by psychologists, by contrast, saw gratitude as an expression of their interconnection with others and as enabling them to live autonomously and interdependently (Kashdan *et al.* 2009). We need greater social recognition, among men and women alike, of the compatibility of need and autonomy, and more just distribution of social resources so that no one needs to express gratitude simply for having their basic needs met, no matter how inadequately or callously.

That we have needs does not take away from our possession of traits that demand evaluative respect, or the importance that recognition respect for our values and perspective has for us. When adults have needs that are shared by vulnerable and dependent children, such as the need for assistance with bathing or eating, this does not mean the adults are now childlike. Greater recognition of the widespread nature of human vulnerability and dependency and the compatibility of dignity and need should make the positive role of gratitude easier to acknowledge. It is a hopeful sign that women rarely conflate interdependency and immaturity, and that men are decreasing the extent that they do so. The kinds of changes I am calling for may be facilitated by increasing recognition of the contributions that people with dependency needs can make to others and the larger society, including but by no means limited to their demonstrations of respect and value for others in expressions of gratitude.

When we acknowledge the compatibility of gratitude with self-respect and respect for caring others, we can start to learn about the many positive aspects of feeling and expressing gratitude, and the contributions that gratitude can make to well-being, autonomy, pro-social behavior and relationship building. Given the vulnerability of both the recipients and the providers of caring labor, these are groups of people who need support. It is therefore very important that, when caring labor is funded through public or private means, there is time left for care laborers to demonstrate their goodwill and respect for care recipients, and time as well for care receivers to express, and care laborers to acknowledge, gratitude for benefits conveyed in a way that demonstrates both goodwill and respect.

A main complaint of direct care workers (raised nearly as often as complaints about low social status and pay) is the time constraints on their work, especially insofar as those time constraints limit the time they can spend attending to and interacting with those they care for (Moskos & Martin 2005, statistical summaries on p. 26). Care laborers who barely have time to assist their clients with bathing will not have time to listen to and learn from their clients about how they may best meet not only their physical needs but also their need to maintain their dignity and privacy in the midst of their vulnerability. It is therefore vital that those who oversee the provision of care, those who fund it and those who train and supervise caregivers recognize the importance of giving enough time for caregivers to learn about and demonstrate recognition respect for the recipients of their care. People who need extensive personal care are often socially isolated, and interactions with their caregivers may be one of the few opportunities they have to interact with others in a manner than demonstrates mutual respect. Care laborers who have time to listen and learn and demonstrate respect for care recipients will not only do a better job of meeting their clients' needs but are also more likely to find their work rewarding, and to experience gratitude from others that recognizes not only the value of their work but also their value as people. Care recipients gain from receiving care that not only meets bodily needs but also recognizes their value and demonstrates recognition respect for them as individuals, and they are likely to gain as well, in many ways, from their own expressions of the gratitude such care merits.

In conclusion, a focus on gratitude is consistent with important aspects of feminist ethics of care, including its attention to the particularities and vulnerabilities of caregivers and care recipients alike, and its concern with how relations of care are shaped by social hierarchies and public institutions. In addition, it goes beyond current preoccupations of care ethicists both by introducing gratitude as an important aspect of morally valuable relations of care and by stressing the significance of attending not only to the needs but also the capacities of recipients of care.

References

Aristotle (1980) *Nicomachean Ethics*, trans. D. Ross, revised by J. L. Ackrill & J. O. Urmson, Oxford University Press, Oxford.

Bartlett, M. Y. & DeSteno, D. (2006) 'Gratitude and Prosocial Behavior: Helping When it Costs You', *Psychological Science*, Vol. 17, no. 4, pp. 319–25.

Becker, L. C. (2005) 'Reciprocity, Justice and Disability', *Ethics*, Vol. 116, pp. 9–39.

Benhabib, S. (1985) 'The Generalized and the Concrete Other: The Kohlberg–Gilligan Controversy', *Praxis International*, Vol. 4, pp. 402–24.

Bubeck, D. (1995) *Care, Gender and Justice*, Clarendon Press, Oxford.

Card, C. (1988) 'Gratitude and Obligation', *American Philosophical Quarterly*, Vol. 25, pp. 115–27.

Card, C. (1990) 'Caring and Evil', *Hypatia*, Vol. 5, pp. 101–8.

Clement, G. (1996) *Care, Autonomy and Justice*, Westview Press, Boulder.

Darwall, S. (2004) 'Respect and the Second-person Standpoint', *Proceedings and Addresses of the American Philosophical Association*, Vol. 78, no. 2, pp. 43–59.

Dillon, R. (2009) 'Respect and Care: Toward Moral Integration', in *Respect for the Elderly: Implications for Human Service Providers*, eds K.-t. Sung & B. J. Kim, University Press of America, Lanham, MD, pp. 23–44.

Fitzgerald, P. (1998) 'Gratitude and Justice', *Ethics*, Vol. 109, pp. 119–53.

Galvin, R. (2004) 'Challenging the Need for Gratitude: Comparisons between Paid and Unpaid Care for Disabled People', *Journal of Sociology*, Vol. 40, no. 2, pp. 137–55.

Hoagland, S. (1991) 'Some Thoughts about Caring', in *Feminist Ethics*, ed. C. Card, University Press of Kansas, Lawrence, pp. 246–63.

Honneth, A. (1992) 'Integrity and Disrespect: Principles of a Conception of Morality Based on the Theory of Recognition', *Political Theory*, Vol. 20, pp. 187–201.

Kashdan, T. B., Mishra, A., Breen, W. E. & Froh, J. J. (2009) 'Gender Differences in Gratitude: Examining Appraisals, Narratives, the Willingness to Express Emotions, and Changes in Psychological Needs', *Journal of Personality*, Vol. 77, no. 3, pp. 691–729.

Kittay, E. F. (1999) *'Love's Labor: Essays on Women, Equality, and Dependency'*, Routledge, New York.

Moskos, M. & Martin, B. (2005) *What's Best? What's Worst? Direct Carers' Work in their Own Words*, National Institute of Labour Studies, Flinders University, Adelaide, Australia, available at: <http://nils.flinders.edu.au/> (accessed 23 October 2009).

Noddings, N. (1984) *Caring: A Feminine Approach to Ethics and Moral Education*, University of California Press, Berkeley.

Noddings, N. (2002) *Starting at Home: Caring and Social Policy*, University of California Press, Berkeley.

Robichon, F. (2004) 'Robots Help Japan Care for its Elderly', *Popular Mechanics*, available at: <http://www.popularmechanics.com/technology/industry/1288241.html> (accessed 29 October 2009).

Robinson, F. (1999) *'Globalizing Care: Ethics, Feminist Theory and International Relations'*, Westview Press, Boulder.

Rummery, K. (2007) 'Caring, Citizenship and New Labour: Dilemmas and Contradictions for Disabled and Older Women', in *Women and New Labor*, eds C. Annesley, F. Gains & K. Rummery, Policy Press, Bristol, pp. 175–92.

Rummery, K. (2008) 'The Role of Cash-for-care in Supporting Disabled People's Citizenship: Gendered Conflicts and Dilemmas in Social Citizenship', unpublished MS, available at: <http://www2.sofi.su.se/RC19/pdfpapers/Rummery_RC19_2008.pdf> (accessed 19 July 2009).

Sherwin, S. (2000) 'A Relational Approach to Autonomy in Health Care', in *Readings in Health Care Ethics*, Broadview Press, Peterborough, Ontario.

Tronto, J. (1993) *'Moral Boundaries: A Political Argument for an Ethic of Care'*, Routledge, New York.

Tsang, J.-A. (2006a) 'Gratitude and Prosocial Behavior: An Experimental Test of Gratitude', *Cognition and Emotion*, Vol. 20, pp. 138–48.

Tsang, J.-A. (2006b) 'The Effects of Helper Intention on Gratitude and Indebtedness', *Motivation and Emotion*, Vol. 30, pp. 199–205.

Walker, A. D. M. (1988) 'Political Obligation and the Argument from Gratitude', *Philosophy and Public Affairs*, Vol. 17, no. 3, pp. 191–211.

Watkins, P. C., Scheer, J., Ovnicek, M. & Kolts, R. (2006) 'The Debt of Gratitude: Dissociating Gratitude and Indebtedness', *Cognition and Emotion*, Vol. 20, no. 2, pp. 217–41.

White, J. A. (2000) *Democracy, Justice, and the Welfare State: Reconstructing Public Care*, Pennsylvania State University Press, University Park.

The Productivity of Care: Contextualizing Care in Situated Interaction and Shedding Light on its Latent Purposes

Alessandro Pratesi

Care work may be connected with emotional and psychological exhaustion but also gratification, reward, and self-empowerment. Caregivers experience both positive and negative emotional states in caring situations, and further studies on the rewarding and energizing aspects of care may help us to broaden our understanding of how we can reduce the degree of burden while increasing the sense of satisfaction. This article shows how the focus on emotion is a necessary step to show the ambivalences and the grey areas connected with the concept of care as well as to challenge the not fully explored assumption that care is often associated with burden and stress and viewed as a result of circumstances. It reports the findings of a micro-situated study of daily care activities among 80 caregivers. Care is seen as a strategic site to grasp deeper insights into the interactional mechanisms through which the emotional dynamics revolving around care produce unanticipated outcomes in terms of symbolic and practical productivity.

The study of emotions in everyday life helps remedy the failure of the social and psychological sciences to appreciate the hidden sensual and aesthetic foundations of the self. (Katz 1999)

Introduction

Care is a complex phenomenon and is becoming all the more so due to the ongoing demographic trends and cultural transformations involving family, parenthood, marriage, cohabitation, and an increasingly ageing population.

Alessandro Pratesi is Research Associate at the Research Institute for Health and Social Change, Manchester Metropolitan University, UK.

The flexible character of its definition, at the intersection between informal communities and formal organizations, makes the phenomenon of care quite problematic and in need of further specification. This is because care transcends typical distinctions between work and leisure, public and private, and productive and reproductive relations. The complex nature of care leaves open several unsolved contradictions, notably those connected with the gendered definition of private and public spheres.

What exactly are individuals doing when they engage in care work? What are its symbolic and social implications? How are symbols of care created and how do they circulate differently for different caregivers? How does care work intertwine emotional/inner processes and public/outer processes involving power and status dimensions? Starting from these central questions, I present here a close scrutiny of *informal care*, which I define as *unpaid and non-professional care of a physical, emotional, and social nature that is provided by partners, relatives, or friends*. I discuss the emotional implications of care by focusing on different kinds of care arrangements, as they emerge in different kinds of family contexts and other forms of intimate relationships. The interactional dynamics of unpaid care relationships have been central to an ethic of care as developed by many care theorists in the last 25 years (Gilligan 1982; Noddings 1984; Tronto 1994; Held 2006). The focus in this article is on the role of *emotion* in unpaid care relationships.

Emotion is a fundamental component in showing the ambivalences and the grey areas connected with the concept of care and challenging the assumption that care work is associated with burden and stress and a result of circumstances or default. Informal care may be connected with emotional and psychological exhaustion, but also with emotional and psychological gratification, reward, self-empowerment, and energizing processes. Nonetheless, there has been considerably less published on the positive aspects of care. By shedding light on the less visible and less investigated nature of care and its deep connections with emotions, I will shed light on the *latent purposes of care*, purposes that diverge substantially from the manifest purposes of tending to and looking after someone. In doing this, I aim to contribute to the project of a general theory of care, which has been pursued by a range of scholars (Tronto 1994; Thomas 1993; Leira 1994; Graham 1991; Bubeck 1995; Fisher & Tronto 1990; Ruddick 1995; Noddings 2003; Kittay & Feder 2002).

The analysis is carried out in light of approaches to the sociology of emotions that have already inspired a rich research agenda: addressing the emotional mechanisms through which social structures are interactionally and situationally reproduced (Kemper 1990; Gordon 1990; Collins 1990, 1993, 2004; Katz 1999; Barbalet 2001; Scheff 1990; Turner 1999, 2000; Hammond 1990). More specifically, I describe how the emotional dynamics revolving around care can challenge our conventional view of care-related inequality and produce unexpected outcomes in terms of symbolic and practical *productivity*. In what follows, I briefly review current theoretical perspectives on care and illustrate how emotions can help us to unpack and highlight its less visible rationales.

What do we Know about Care?

Recent feminist research suggests that both the conceptual and empirical boundaries between formal and informal care are dissolving in ways that have gendered impacts. Yet the theoretical dispute on the dissolving boundaries between the two kinds of care still seems to be open (Graham 1991; Thomas 1993; Ungerson 1995, 1997; Himmelweit 1999). In addition, care theorists have argued that care activities are different from, but need to be integrated with, other activities in both the economic and political spheres (Hochschild 1983; Zelizer 2005; Folbre & Nelson 2000).

Some early care theorists emphasized the emotional components of care, describing care as meaningful and fulfilling to many women and viewing care as a model to be extended to the larger social arena (Gilligan 1982; Ruddick 1998). Others emphasized the practical/material components of care, describing care as oppressive to women, who are compelled to provide care by a variety of material and ideological forces (Finch & Groves 1983).

As a concept, 'care' encompasses both instrumental tasks and affective relations, ranging from *activity* to *ethics*, that is, from '*taking charge*' of others' physical well-being to '*feeling concern*' for others' physical and psychological well-being (Graham 1983; Noddings 1984; Ruddick 1998; Thomas 1993; Leira 1994; Kittay 1999; Kittay & Feder 2002). It defines a particular kind of work, an activity directed to identify and meet the needs or well-being of certain others, and it challenges dichotomous thinking opposing *head* with *heart* and *rationality* with *emotion* (Waerness 1984).

The composite nature of informal care has been central to an ethic of care as developed by many care theorists in the last 25 years, notably in the contributions of Gilligan (1982), Noddings (1984), Tronto (1994) and Held (2006). However, much can still be learned from the sociological literature on the *positive role of emotion* in unpaid care. We can expand on these contributions by referring to Randall Collins' theory of *Interaction Ritual Chains* (2004), according to which the essential mechanism holding society together is *emotional* rather than cognitive.

Highlighting the Role of Emotions in Unpaid Care

Collins suggests that emotions are the *common denominator of rational action* because rationality depends on assessing the utility (the capacity to confer positive affect) of alternatives lines of conduct (Collins 1993, 2004). The rational actor perspective, he says, collides with a number of problems: first, there are a whole series of behaviours that do not fit with cost/benefit analysis; second, it lacks a *common metric* that allows actors to compare costs and benefits across whatever range of situations they may encounter; and third, is the simple evidence that people are not always compulsively obsessed calculators.

The centre of Collins' micro-sociological explanation is not the individual but the situation. Interactions, not individuals, are ontologically basic, and the search for successful interactions is the basic human engine. Every interaction generates status and power effects, and one of the primary goods of a successful interaction is the feeling of solidarity with a group: a sense of status membership or status inclusion. Collins describes this sense of status member-ship in terms of *emotional energy*, which is similar to the psychological concept of 'drive' but with a specific social orientation: it is a long-lasting emotion that builds up across situations and makes individuals initiate or fail to instigate interactions. It is a feeling of confidence and enthusiasm for social interaction (2004, p. 108).

Emotional energy is thus both the ingredient and the outcome of the interaction. People's choices, behaviours, and decisions regarding daily-life issues are in fact based on the emotional outcomes and inputs, and people's chance to gain or lose emotional energy is affected strongly by their perceived sense of status membership. In other words, within such a model, people's choices circuit in the loop of emotional energy production and we can think about *social stratification* as an *unequal distribution of emotional energy* rather than an unequal distribution of material resources or social positions. Moreover, we can empirically visualize social stratification through a careful analysis of how emotional stratification is enacted in micro-situations.

The Subjects of Care—Sample and Methods

My critical interpretive inquiry[1] draws on a multi-method approach: semi-structured in-depth interviews, weekly diaries, participant observation, online discussion forums between members of parents' associations, ongoing conversa-tions with the respondents beyond the interview context, key-informants interviews, secondary sources on informal care and parenthood collected from adoption agencies and local associations, journal and newspaper articles, and the web. Between winter 2005 and summer 2007, I interviewed 80 caregivers, mostly living in the Philadelphia urban and suburban areas.[2] The respondents were different in terms of gender, sexual orientation, and marital status. Both child care and elderly care were included in my study, although parental care is the main kind of informal care I explored. The sample included gay/lesbian caregivers not only because they have been thus far excluded from the conceptual category of 'normal' caregivers and from 'normal' research on informal care, but also because they represented a key-subject to visualize the less explored rationales of care and the crucial role of emotion in the

---

1. The analysis was guided mostly by what Denzin (2001) calls *interpretive interactionism* and other scholars have called *interpretive phenomenological analysis* (Smith 2004; Smith *et al.* 1999).
2. Broadly definable as belonging to the middle class and upper middle class.

reproduction of social inequality.[3] The goal of the empirical part of the research was to gain insights into how emotional stratification is reproduced in specific kinds of *interaction ritual chains*.

Internal Conversations and Permanent Visitors

My argument is that we can look at care activities as chains of micro-interactions.[4] The specific kind of interaction on which I focus is the ongoing internal dialogue between the subject caregiver and a whole network of generalized others, or what Norbert Wiley (1994) calls 'permanent visitors', that is, all those people who are variably present in our thoughts and with whom we are in a constant inner conversation (also McMahon 1996; Archer 2003, 2007; Doucet 2008). Within the context of care, the acknowledgement of the relation as a caring relation from both the subject caregiver and these generalized others is an essential condition to give *visibility, entitlement* and *legitimacy* to the status of caregiver and to confer on the latter a sense of belonging to what I shall call here *the intangible community of fully entitled and successful caregivers*.

During her permanent internal dialogue with all these visitors, the caregiver is constantly verifying or disconfirming her status membership. 'Am I acknowledged, and therefore, do I feel entitled as a legitimate and successful caregiver?'—the caregiver constantly asks herself. In Collins' model, status membership (or status inclusion) is the criterion that defines whether an interaction is successful and, therefore, whether there is an increase or decrease in the supplies of emotional energy.

Care, especially in parenthood, can be lived as a site of status inclusion or exclusion, independent of people's sex, marital status, or sexual orientation. One belongs to the community of 'parents' and consequently feels excluded from other groups or communities, such as, for instance, the groups of single friends with different lifestyles, or the community of successful colleagues with more impressive résumés or qualifications, and so on. However, single parents and gay parents can experience care activities as sites of status exclusion in a more prescriptive and rigid way than their heterosexual counterparts. In fact, the image of the nuclear family still provides a powerful interpretive template to cast in people's minds a series of generalized others with whom people engage in internal conversations. For both single and gay parents, the sense of status

3. Research on gay/lesbian parenthood has concerned mainly the different styles of parenting, the different networks of resources, and the different developmental outcomes between children raised by lesbian and gay parents and those raised by heterosexual parents. No studies have considered how and under what conditions the caregiver's sexual orientation can enhance or hinder feelings of well-being, self-confidence, enthusiasm, support, and trust during the care episode or 'souvenir', intended here as a form of *third-order circulation of symbols* in Collins' terms (2004, p. 99).

4. Within the continuum which in Collins' Interaction Ritual model goes from formalized and strongly focused to informal and relatively unfocused interactions, I am referring here mostly to the informal and less focused interactions, which nonetheless define clearly structured *individual reputations*, increasingly more important than categorical identities (2004, pp. 272, 291, 295).

membership in the community of *fully entitled parents* is affected by the normativity of the nuclear family; for gay/lesbian caregivers, it is also affected by heteronormativity. What does that mean in terms of feeling like *fully entitled parents*? Does it require a different kind of effort, for a single or a gay parent, to handle the issue of 'belonging' by constantly trying to attain good 'individual reputations' as a parent? Yes and no. Yes, it does require a different effort. Yet such a different effort does not automatically relocate single parents and gay parents in a subordinate position in terms of emotional stratification.

The fast-growing phenomenon of lesbian motherhood and the remarkable number of single women who opt for motherhood outside of marriage[5] provide us with additional insights on how the self-empowering effects of the *pursuit of motherhood* can compensate for the sacrifices preceding, accompanying, and following their care choice. While they are tossing out conventional definitions of motherhood and family, these mothers nonetheless embrace quite conventional roles concerning child-rearing. By the same token, the new generations of gay men are more likely than their straight brothers to look for alternative and less conventional routes to personal affirmation and social success, and more likely to embrace nurturing, care-taking, and domestic activities without feeling that their masculine identity is threatened or their emotional energy drained (Stacey 2005, 2006). What accounts for these growing phenomena? How is difference (and inequality) actually reproduced through care? Is the activity of care in itself—with its unequal distribution of tasks—what makes a difference or is it rather *the ways people live, reflect on*, and *feel* the care experience that account for differences and inequalities between the different kinds of caregivers?

The Latent Purposes of Care

The internal processes of *thinking* and *feeling* care, I claim, are what mostly makes the difference and thus produces inequality: an inequality based on the long-term effects of the emotional stratification, which ultimately stems from the ongoing process of reflexivity. I, therefore, hypothesize that care is not only about tending to or caring for someone but also about *status inclusion* and *emotional energy production*, which I suggest are its latent purposes. Without necessarily being aware of it, all caregivers participate in this invisible process of self-induced internalized stratification. Indeed, a not-so-latent purpose of care as a fundamental source of emotional energy production is explicitly admitted by Kendrick, who candidly confesses that his decision to become a father responded to a pretty much 'selfish' fundamental desire. Caring for somebody and 'being able to love somebody' makes him feel good, fulfilling one of the basic human emotional needs:

---

5. See Rosanna Hertz (2006); Frank Furstenberg (2002, 2005).

> Yeah, I think in the broad sense is that it's a very selfish thing, I mean I have children because it makes me feel good, you know [...] People always say, oh, that's such a noble thing you're doing, what a wonderful thing you're doing. No, it's all selfish, I did it for me. The benefit is, I think, he is a good kid and we have a great relationship, I think I'm raising him well; but let's be honest about it, I mean, that was kind of a fundamental desire, I had this need and there he was.

We have seen that emotional energy is the long-lasting sense of self-confidence, enthusiasm, and initiative that is produced by and instigates a successful interaction. A successful interaction generates a sense of status membership or inclusion which increases the supply of emotional energy and fosters the loop of emotional energy production. Care activities and responsibilities generate forms of group membership or *status enhancement* and consequent outcomes in terms of emotional energy that alter people's emotional stratification. This in turn affects people's ability to successfully manage future interactions. Reflexivity is the essential condition by which caregivers judge their care experiences as successful or unsuccessful. Without denying the weight of structural and cultural factors in the reproduction of inequality, I claim that these factors need active mediation—the capacity and the willpower of individuals to act independently and to make their own choices—in order to be effective and productive. Through their internal conversations, individuals reflect upon and mould their social situation in light of care-related tasks and concerns (Wiley 1994; Archer 2003, 2007). These inner dialogues govern caregivers' responses to social forces, their actual and potential patterns of social interaction, and whether they contribute to social inequality; an inequality that is based on the *felt experience* of care.

The missing link between society and the individual, I suggest, is to be found in the production of emotional energy which occurs during the constant interaction of *Self* with a whole set of generalized others with whom the individual is in constant conversation, be it actual or virtual. I consider the care experience as a crucial site to observe the ongoing processes of reproduction of emotional stratification that is the basis of social inequality. These unexplored aspects of care also allow us to reframe current discourse on care and to challenge the assumption that care is routinely associated with burden and stress and viewed as a result of circumstances. In the following section, I will navigate through some of these astonishing and overlooked aspects of the phenomenology of care that I claim constitute its core nature.

The Productivity of Care

Contrary to common belief, care does not necessarily produce stress or make people less productive—at least not always and not under all circumstances. Even in its most draining aspects, care seems to make people find their 'second wind', as William James used to call it: an unexpected strength and energy allowing them to overcome challenges and difficulties that stem from their *caring about* their beloved ones.[6] Far more than we are willing to admit, *being caring* also means *being productive*. For some, this might mean giving more attention to quality than to quantity; for others, it might mean keeping the same standards in terms of quantity and paying less attention to the quality of the end products. What emerges as quite evident from all the interview accounts is that caring activities, under certain conditions, make people more efficient and increase their capacities to get more things done in a more focused way.

It is also evident that one of the latent purposes of care is the production of emotional states that go in the direction of what Hammond (1990) calls 'affective maximization', a more or less conscious strategy to maximize the supply of positive emotions. It does not matter, for our purposes, whether this unantici-pated outcome of care is conscious or unconscious, whether it is planned or unintended. The point is that the search for the 'meanings of care' in the entire ecology of people's lives brings to the surface important and understudied elements, perhaps a blend of new and old elements, which acquire a completely new sense in light of the Interaction Ritual model and with the inclusion of gay and single parents. One of these elements concerns precisely the energizing and empowering effects of care responsibilities that clearly help people not only to overcome the exhaustion connected with multi-task operations but also to balance their perceived status exclusion from other settings.

Parenting Gives me Energy

The energizing nature of care is illustrated by Jason's case. In the following passage, Jason underlines the self-empowering effects of care responsibility, when he recalls the challenging period during which he was finishing his dissertation, teaching full-time, and being a dad:

> R: It was a hellish couple of years. But at the same time I think being a dad helped me to balance out some of that. I mean I think if I would not have been a dad and would have just been trying to finish the dissertation while teaching full-time, I think I would have driven myself crazy [...] Because for me parenting really gives me energy.

On the other hand, Sarah, a single mother, highlights how inhabiting all at once the statuses of single mother, part-time student, and full-time worker can create a sense of 'non-fitting' or status exclusion:

> R: Yeah, like I don't know, it makes me feel like I don't fit in very well at school.
> I: You don't fit in?
> R: Well, because nobody in my department really has children [...] and so I don't know, the people are like at a different stage in their life because, even though they're around the same age as me, they don't have like a lot of responsibilities in life so they can go out and socialize and do whatever. And me, I don't get to go

6. James (1913).

out and socialize ever, and if I do, I have to take her with me. So it's a different kind of social life.

She also provides a description of the labelling process connected to the categorical identity of a single mother when she expresses other people's negative prejudice toward her being a full-time working mother and a student:

> R: I feel like a lot of times when people find out that I'm a single parent they always have all these stereotypes of what I am and [...] you know what I mean, stereotypes of what I'm supposed to be like [...] People just have stereotypes of what single parents are like, you know, that I don't spend time with her and stuff like that. And I spend more time with her than most married moms do [...] People just have these stereotypes about ... like that whole unwed mother kind of thing and me be a kind of stereotype [...] Yeah, like a married couple where the mother is like a homemaker and all that crap.

However, neither the non-fitting feeling nor the stereotypes connected to her status of single mother seem to affect her sense of self-confidence, energy, and motivation for action, in short, her level of emotional energy, when she concludes:

> R: I am [energetic]. I manage my time extremely well because I know [...] other people, who have a lot less on their plate, who struggle to get all their work done; and I always get everything I need done, always.

The Busier I Am, the More Effective I Am

In the same regard, Roger, father of three children, underscores an interesting paradox of care when he realizes how the challenges connected to the difficult balance between work, a master's program, his wife's pregnancy, and other family care related issues pushed him to become more effective and productive:

> R: [...] My son was born in January of 2002 and the following August I started a master's program at night. And those two things forced me to become a much better manager of time, to really allocate, you know, this much time for this, this much time for this [...] When I have a little bit less requirements to get done, fewer requirements, I've gotten lazy about being careful [...] Well, there's an expression that if you want something to get done, ask a busy person to do it. And I think that definitely holds true for me. The busier I am, the more effective I am.

Several other interviewees confirm the idea of the increased efficiency connected to the massive workload quite clearly. Byron, a wealthy financial advisor who, at the age of 52, decided to have a child with a close lesbian friend of his, is one of them. Byron and his friend live in separate homes and worlds, but they share childcare responsibilities:

> R: I became extremely efficient after the baby was born in doing the work with 30 or 40 percent less time and I still managed to do it all.

I: Really?

R: Absolutely, mm, hmm. Because time had many more things packed into it so I had to become more efficient—a rather easy thing to do. If you want someone to do something, you pick someone who is busy to make sure it gets done.

Energy Begets Energy

Not only can care responsibilities produce an extra layer of energy, inducing people to become more efficient and more focused in achieving their goals and getting things done; they also possess an emotion-enhancing effect which creates positive loops of emotional energy production. Roger raises quite spontaneously the theme of the 'energizing power' of care, stressing how the emotional energy deriving from his caring activities not only compensates for the physical exhaustion but is also positively reflected on his job. Referring to his three children, he says:

> It's unbelievable, they just have two speeds it seems, fast forward and stop. And that has to carry over to some degree. On the one hand it makes you exhausted because you have to keep up with them all the time, but on the other hand energy sort of begets more energy. So the kids go to bed and I'm tired, but at the same time I'm energized and I have the energy and the strength to keep working later at night that I might not have if they weren't there.

Several examples follow a similar wavelength. Julia, a single mother who happened to be delivering her daughter at the same time she lost her job, attributes the merits of her further education to the birth of her daughter, explaining how the energetic loop in which she was involved pushed her to think that it would 'be best to nip it in the bud' and get through an additional temporary strain in order to reach a better social and economic position:

> R: [...] And in fact I probably wouldn't have pursued education, the truth be known, had Sarah not been born. I made that decision based on her. I would have continued in the mental health field and not thinking about summers off or the hours I'm working or the breaks I have off.
> I: So you improved your education because you had a kid.
> R: Right, I went back to school.
> I: It sounds like a paradox.
> R: Right, and I decided it would be best to nip it in the bud, get it over with when she was young, go full force, gung-ho, get through it and then I can relax and I'd have a career. And my income doubled, that was another good part of going back to school.

The word 'energy' is constantly and spontaneously raised by all interviewees, and the energy loops that childcare 'brings in' seem to be something that not only drive people to accomplish ordinary tasks but also to explore completely new details of their life experience, details they probably would never have explored otherwise.

'Good Stress' and 'Bad Stress'

An interesting distinction between 'good stress' (which is not resented or is even experienced as a 'good thing') and 'bad stress' is made in the following:

> There's good stress and there's bad stress, but the stress that causes the feeling of responsibility in care giving, in a way, that's not resented. I like the opportunity to have the pressure and the stress of caring for this child, so it's a good thing.

Most respondents define the stress associated with their care activities as 'good stress'; and even when it is 'bad stress' it can be transformed. An example of *bad stress* transformed into *good stress* is offered by Jean, a single caregiver who looked after her dying father for a long period. Critical care can activate a loop of automatisms by which people just keep on getting things done or developing new habits which are all focused on taking care of the emergency while at the same time upholding working routines and preserving a psychological equilibrium. Even in the worse and most critical circumstances, care seems to become at the same time the cause of the distress and its remedy that is the emotional energy with which to handle it:

> It was hard. I did not go on vacation for the last two years; I did not do anything but work, play some sports locally and take care of my family. And, you know, I had a drink every night when I got home, I had a glass of wine as soon as I got home because that was the only thing that I could, like I needed to decompress for a half an hour by myself. Every day was a fight, was a struggle. I got up because, and I got out of bed and I went to work because I knew that I might have to take care of my father for the rest of his natural life, however long that was [...] I got up in the morning because my dad was around. That was what I did.

A serious illness cannot but be a traumatic event with severe repercussions on the caregiver's psychological, emotional, and physical health. Jean's story assumes dramatic tones during the interview because she was particularly affectionate to her father and looked at him as a unique model of reference. Nevertheless, beyond the unquestionably draining aspects of her care experience, she eventually finds her way to give it a totally different meaning. At the end of her exhausting, draining, and solitary journey through her father's illness and death, Jean recuperates a new sense of her personal identity and self-worth.

> He was my guy and I miss him. [Crying] I cry daily for my dad. I mean he's been gone for six months—he was the best guy in the world.

Jean does not seem to realize that what she probably misses now is not only her father but also *her taking care of him*—that chaotic, critical, and distressful period itself that produced so much pressure on her. One of the common characteristics about critical care is forgetting soon about its negative or more problematic aspects and not viewing even the most difficult times as unbearable anymore. Eventually, people rediscover new balances and existential priorities, which are often characterized not only by higher levels of emotional maturity but also by a sharper awareness of their trajectory as caregivers. The 'activating' or motivating power of care seems to drive people not only to get things done but also to find a correct and effective balance between different needs. What Jean is still mourning is not just the absence of her father but also the *absence of care*, the sudden vacuum created after such a dense and intense emotional period, for better or for worse.

Concluding Remarks

Most of the scholarship on care typically focuses on the gendered costs of care and on its draining aspects. Less attention is paid to the consequences of *being excluded from care* or not being acknowledged as an entitled and legitimate caregiver. Even less attention is paid to the inherently rewarding aspects of care and to its positive consequences in terms of status membership, increased productivity, and emotional energy production.

Emotions constitute the link between *doing care* at the micro level of interactions and *doing* or *undoing difference* at the macro level of social structures. Different ways *to do care* and *to do gender* must be taken into account if we want to grasp a truly comprehensive picture of the phenomenon of care. It is important, therefore, to add a focus on different kinds of carers, not only theoretically—to fill the gaps—but also strategically—to increase equality. By focusing on the interactional processes that reproduce inequality, the phenomenological approach I propose here helps us to shed light on both the conservative forces reproducing inequality and the potential for cultural change. Since social categorizations (such as gender or sexual orientation) are not likely to disappear, we can at least reduce the cultural beliefs attached to them that reproduce inequality. Thus, for example, if sex categorization is so embedded in social relations that it is most likely to persist, the interactional processes can change or cancel cultural beliefs about male rationality or female emotionality (Ridgeway & Correll 2000). Similarly, if the labelling process by which we reproduce a difference between gay parents (or single parents) and heterosexual parents (between 'atypical families' and 'traditional families') is likely to remain in the near future, the interactional processes can challenge and erode cultural beliefs about heterosexual parenthood and families as 'natural' and gay or single parenthood and families as unusual and/or 'odd'. Repositioning care in situated interaction, while shedding light on its latent purposes and clarifying the central role that emotions play in the reproduction of inequality, allows us to address many of the theoretical problems connected to reification and to transform them into empirical ones, analysed in specific contexts.

Caregivers experience both positive and negative emotional states in caregiving situations. They can perceive both moderate burden and great satisfaction at the same time. Further studies on the rewarding and energizing aspects of care may help to broaden our understanding of how we can reduce the degree of burden while increasing the sense of satisfaction. Acknowledging the intrinsic value of care and highlighting its *productivity* and self-empowering consequences does not mean giving voice to a romanticized view of the world or failing to recognize the draining aspects of care, but rather *capitalizing* on care as a long-term investment and a resource. Such capitalization can be accomplished by facilitating conditions under which care is self-empowering and productive and by reducing those under which it is constraining or emotional-energy draining. In doing that, we can also reduce the inequality connected to this fundamental activity.

Acknowledgements

This research was funded with a five-year William Penn Fellowship at the University of Pennsylvania (USA) and three summer fellowships ('Gertrude and Otto Pollak' summer research fellowship, University of Pennsylvania, 2005–2007). The author would like to thank Professor Randall Collins, Professor Robin Leidner and Professor Frank Furstenberg for their comments and advice on this research.

References

Archer, M. (2003) *Structure, Agency, and the Internal Conversation*, Cambridge University Press, New York.

Archer, M. (2007) *Making Our Way through the World: Human Reflexivity and Social Mobility*, Cambridge University Press, Cambridge.

Barbalet, J. M. (2001) *Emotion, Social Theory, and Social Structure: A Macrosociological Approach*, Cambridge University Press, Cambridge.

Bubeck, D. E. (1995) *Care, Gender, and Justice*, Clarendon Press, Oxford.

Collins, R. (1990) 'Stratification, Emotional Energy, and the Transient Emotions', in *Research Agenda in the Sociology of Emotions*, ed. T. D. Kemper, SUNY Press, New York, pp. 27–57.

Collins, R. (1993) 'Emotional Energy and the Common Denominator of Rational Action', *Rationality and Society*, Vol. 5, pp. 203–30.

Collins, R. (2004) *Interaction Ritual Chains*, Princeton University Press, Princeton and Oxford.

Denzin, N. K. (2001) *Interpretive Interactionism*, 2nd edn, Sage, Thousand Oaks, CA.

Doucet, A. (2008) 'From her Side of the Gossamer Wall(s): Reflexivity and Relational Knowing', *Qualitative Sociology*, Vol. 31, pp. 73–87.

Finch, J. & Groves, D. (eds) (1983) *A Labor of Love: Women, Work and Caring*, Routledge & Kegan Paul, London.

Fisher, B. & Tronto, J. (1990) 'Toward a Feminist Theory of Caring', in *Circles of Care: Work and Identity in Women's Lives*, eds E. Abel & M. Nelson, SUNY Press, New York, pp. 35–62.

Folbre, N. & Nelson, J. A. (2000) 'For Love or Money—Or Both?', *Journal of Economic Perspectives*, Vol. 14, no. 4, pp. 123–40.

Furstenberg, F. F. (2002) 'What a Good Marriage Can't Do', Editorial, *New York Times*, 13 August 2002, available at: <http://www.nytimes.com/2002/08/13/opinion/13FURS.html>.

Furstenberg, F. F. (2005) 'The Future of Marriage', in *Family in Transition*, 13th edn, eds A. S. Skolnick & J. H. Skolnick, Pearson/Allyn & Bacon, Boston, MA, pp. 190–96.

Gilligan, C. (1982) *In a Different Voice: Psychological Theory and Women's Development*, Harvard University Press, Cambridge, MA.

Gordon, S. L. (1990) 'Social Structural Effects on Emotion', in *Research Agenda in the Sociology of Emotions*, ed. T. D. Kemper, SUNY Press, Albany, pp. 145–79.

Graham, H. (1983) 'Caring: a Labour of Love', in *A Labour of Love: Women, Work and Caring*, eds J. Finch & D. Groves, Routledge and Kegan Paul, London, pp. 13–30.

Graham, H. (1991) 'The Concept of Caring in Feminist Research: The Case of Domestic Service', *Sociology*, Vol. 25, pp. 61–78.

Hammond, M. (1990) 'Affective Maximization: A New Macro-theory in the Sociology of Emotions', in *Research Agendas in the Sociology of Emotions*, ed. T. D. Kemper, SUNY Press, Albany, pp. 58–81.

Held, V. (2006) *The Ethics of Care: Personal, Political, and Global*, Oxford University Press, Oxford.

Hertz, R. (2006) *Single by Chance, Mothers by Choice: How Women are Choosing Parenthood without Marriage and Creating the New American Family*, Oxford University Press, Oxford and New York.

Himmelweit, S. (1999) 'Caring Labor', *Annals, AAPPS*, Vol. 561 (January), pp. 27–38.

Hochschild, A. (1983) *The Managed Heart: Commercialization of Human Feeling*, University of California Press, Berkeley.

James, W. (1913) *The Energies of Men*, Moffat, Yard, New York.

Katz, J. (1999) *How Emotions Work*, University of Chicago Press, Chicago.

Kemper, T. D. (1990) 'Social Relations and Emotions: A Structural Approach', in *Research Agendas in the Sociology of Emotions*, ed. T. D. Kemper, SUNY Press, Albany, pp. 207–37.

Kittay, E. (1999) *Love's Labor: Essays on Women, Equality, and Dependency*, Routledge, New York.

Kittay, E. & Feder, E. (2002) *The Subject of Care: Feminist Perspectives on Dependency*, Rowman & Littlefield, Lanham, MD.

Leira, A. (1994) 'Concepts of Caring: Loving, Thinking, and Doing', *Social Service Review*, Vol. 68, pp. 185–201.

McMahon, M. (1996) 'Significant Absences', *Qualitative Inquiry*, Vol. 2, pp. 320–36.

Noddings, N. (1984) *Caring: A Feminist Approach to Ethics and Moral Education*, 2nd edn (2003), University of California Press, Berkeley.

Ridgeway, C. L. & Correll, S. J. (2000) 'Limiting Inequality through Interaction: The End(s) of Gender', *Contemporary Sociology*, Vol. 29, pp. 110–20.

Ruddick, S. (1995) *Maternal Thinking: Towards a Politics of Peace* (1989), 2nd edn, Beacon Press, Boston.

Ruddick, S. (1998) 'Care as Labor and Relationship', in *Norms and Values: Essays on the Work of Virginia Held*, eds J. G. Haber & M. S. Halfon, Rowman & Littlefield, Lanham, MD, pp. 3–25.

Scheff, T. J. (1990) *Microsociology Discourse, Emotion, and Social Structure*, University of Chicago Press, Chicago.

Smith, J. A. (2004) 'Reflecting on the Development of Interpretative Phenomenological Analysis and its Contribution to Qualitative Research in Psychology', *Qualitative Research in Psychology*, Vol. 1, pp. 39–54.

Smith, J. A., Jarman, M. & Osborn, M. (1999) 'Doing Interpretative Phenomenological Analysis', in *Qualitative Health Psychology: Theories and Methods*, eds M. Murray & K. Chamberlain, Sage, London, pp. 218–40.

Stacey, J. (2005) 'The Families of Man: Gay Male Intimacy and Kinship in a Global Metropolis', *Signs: Journal of Women in Culture and Society*, Vol. 30, no. 3, pp. 1911–35.

Stacey, J. (2006) 'Gay Parenthood and the Decline of Paternity as We Knew It', *Sexualities*, Vol. 9, pp. 27–55.

Thomas, C. (1993) 'De-constructing Concepts of Care', *Sociology*, Vol. 27, pp. 649–69.

Tronto, J. (1987) 'Beyond Gender Difference to a Theory of Care', *Signs*, Vol. 12, pp. 644–63.

Tronto, J. (1994) *Moral Boundaries: A Political Argument for an Ethic of Care*, Routledge, New York.

Turner, J. H. (1999) 'Toward a General Sociological Theory of Emotions', *Journal for the Theory of Social Behavior*, Vol. 29, pp. 133–62.

Turner, J. H. (2000) *On the Origins of Human Emotions: A Sociological Inquiry into the Evolution of Human Affect*, Stanford University Press, Stanford.

Ungerson, C. (1995) 'Gender, Cash, and Informal Care: European Perspectives and Dilemmas', *Journal of Social Politics*, Vol. 24, no. 1, pp. 31–52.

Ungerson, C. (1997) 'Social Politics and the Commodification of Care', *Social Politics*, Vol. 4, no. 3, pp. 362–81.

Waerness, K. (1984) 'The Rationality of Care', *Economic and Industrial Democracy*, Vol. 5, pp. 185–211.

Wiley, N. (1994) *The Semiotic Self*, University of Chicago Press, Chicago.

Zelizer, V. A. (2005) *The Purchase of Intimacy*, Princeton University Press, Princeton.

The Individual in Social Care: The Ethics of Care and the 'Personalisation Agenda' in Services for Older People in England

Liz Lloyd

The ethic of care provides not only a basis for understanding relationships of care at the micro level but also a potent form of political ethics, relevant to the development of welfare services. Williams (2001), for example, argues that the concept of care has the capacity to be a central referent in social policy—a point at which social and cultural transformations meet with the changing relations of welfare (Williams 2001, p. 470). English social care services are currently in another period of change precipitated by the 'personalisation agenda'. This agenda is seen as having the potential to revolutionise social care, to create the conditions needed to tailor services to individual needs, and to give service users greater choice and control, including, where possible, control over their own service budgets or direct possession and management of care funds. These developments are inextricably linked to broader economic and social trends, key amongst which are the ageing of the population and changing economic conditions affecting both the labour market and the market for care services. This article applies the feminist ethic of care to an analysis of the personalisation agenda in the context of care for dependent older people. It highlights fundamental political questions posed concerning the nature and extent of older people's need for care, responsibility for meeting these needs and the associated costs. It questions whether the personalisation agenda could potentially offer a more responsive form of care, by placing more power and control in older people's hands. Key points considered are the individualisation of care and the ways in which control is conceptualised. The article concludes with an assessment of the feminist ethic of care as a basis for policy evaluation.

Introduction

The term 'personalisation' has become something of a catch-all phrase in English social policy but is nonetheless contentious. Boxall *et al.* (2009) distinguish

Liz Lloyd is a senior lecturer in the School for Policy Studies, University of Bristol, UK.

between *personalisation*, which focuses on the particular needs of individuals in preference to a one-size-fits-all approach to services, and *self-directed support*, which is about the control that service users can exert over the definition of their needs and the ways in which these should be met. In broad policy terms, personalisation is both '*The way in which services are tailored to the needs and preferences of citizens*' and the means by which the state empowers citizens '*to shape their own lives and the services they receive*' (DH 2008a, p. 4).

The need to personalise services arises because, its proponents argue, services remain institutionalised and driven by professional and managerial agendas, rather than those of service users. A key characteristic of the personalisation agenda in social care specifically is that an individual's interpretation of her/his needs and the ways in which these should be met must be at the heart of any intervention.

The process for the transformation of social care policy involving personalisation is regarded as requiring far-reaching effects:

> Reforming social care to achieve personalisation for all will require a huge cultural, transformational and transactional change in all parts of the system, not just in social care but also for services across the whole of local government and the wider public sector. (DH 2008a, p. 5)

The required cultural transformations include shaping and building the market for care (DH 2008a). Quoting Williams (1975), Ferguson argues that the term personalisation is in danger of becoming a 'warmly persuasive word' (2007, p. 389), which is hard to be against but which, because of its association with individualisation and market-based approaches, should be viewed critically by social workers. The ethic of care provides a valuable basis for such a critical analysis because its attention to the intrinsic rather than instrumental value of caring activities highlights the problems associated with the extension of markets into areas of social life that have been traditionally outside this realm (Held 2006). Indeed, Held argues that the market value of caring is one of the least appropriate ways in which to think of its value.

Personalisation as envisaged in contemporary policies in England entails the delegation of service procurement and management to the level of the individual in need of help. This might be in the substitution of cash for services, as in the provision of Direct Payments, or through Individual Budgets, in which the individual's needs are assessed and the cost of meeting these identified so that the service user can negotiate with a professional service provider how to obtain the optimum level of support within the overall resources available to them. Individual Budgets represent an attempt to capture the personalised aspects of services (tailor-made rather than standardised) whilst demanding less of service users than would be the case if they had responsibility for managing a budget.

In their evaluation of the pilot scheme of Individual Budgets Glendinning *et al.* (2008) identified lower levels of satisfaction amongst older people than other service users. Reasons for this include:

- older people often approach social care services for the first time when they are at a point of crisis and not in a good position to make decisions about how a budget for care should be spent;
- inflexible organisational arrangements and a lack of alternatives to already existing services hampered the implementation of new forms of support for older people through Individual Budgets;
- service providers identified a narrower range of needs amongst older people and allocated less money to their individual budgets than to those of other age groups.

There are, therefore particular age-related concerns to consider in this critique of personalisation, including the nature of older people's needs, how these are perceived by service providers and the kind of help perceived as appropriate. Such perceptions are powerfully influenced by demographic trends, given by policy makers as a fundamental rationale for change to the social care system. Demographic trends have generated a sense of urgency for policy makers and strategic managers as they seek solutions to predicted pressures on the social care system. Personalisation is expected therefore not only to offer more responsive, individualised support but also to provide a system that is *sustainable* over the long term and capable of meeting the increased demands of an ageing population and proving value for money for taxpayers.

The implementation of the personalisation agenda in services for older people might therefore be regarded as something of as a litmus test of its efficacy, since it is the ageing of the population that presents the greatest challenge to future service provision whilst older people appear to be the least enthusiastic of service user groups about the proposed solution.

The Ethic of Care Perspective

The following discussion considers how an ethic of care approach contributes to an understanding of the issues raised concerning the need for care in old age and the personalisation agenda. Feminist ethicists (e.g. Held 2006; Kittay 2002; Sevenhuijsen 2000; Williams 2001; Tronto 1993) argue that it is because dependency and vulnerability are inherent within the human condition that the need for care arises. Kittay (2002), for example, refers to 'inevitable dependencies', which are a facet of human life and give rise to a need for care but which remain largely unacknowledged. Because this need for care is antithetical to the political aim of fostering independence and self-reliance as essential qualities of full citizenship, modern Western societies have devalued care and confined it to the private sphere. Feminist ethicists argue that the need *to* care is also inherent within the human condition. However, the interests of those who need and those who provide care are not always congruent and may in fact be in conflict. It is necessary therefore to give due consideration to the needs of all involved in caring relationships—either as care giver or receiver. Kittay's (2002) concept of *'nested dependencies'* describes how care is also required by those who provide care.

Tronto's model for an ethic of care (1993) has influenced a number of subsequent critical analyses of social policies (see, for example, Sevenhuijsen 2000; Williams 2001). She conceptualises care as a process with four 'phases': attentiveness (caring about), responsibility (taking care of), competence (care giving) and responsiveness (care receiving). These are not to be regarded as neatly sequential, and Tronto argues that for an ethic of care to be realised, *all* of the above four stages must be integrated. Tronto's model has been criticised for being somewhat abstract (Fine 2007) and more relevant to micro-level caring relationships than to broader societal-level concerns about the politics of care (O'Neill 1996). However, it is arguably directly relevant to this discussion of personalisation. For example, responsibility is a fundamental element of the debate on social care set out in the British government's discussion document *Shaping the Future of Care Together* (DH 2009), which poses the question: what constitutes a fair balance of responsibility between the individual and the state for taking care of social care needs? Moreover, Tronto's concept of responsiveness is at the heart of the personalisation agenda, since enabling those using services to define their needs and how these should be met is, ostensibly, what personalisation is all about. The profound dissatisfaction expressed by many within the social care system is irrefutable, particularly the sense of being subjected to institutionalised regimes and unable to exercise choice and control. It is largely due to the advocacy work of service user groups that attention has been drawn to the need for system change.

The ethic of care is political (Sevenhuijsen 1998, 2000). If care is placed at the centre of public political discourses, Sevenhuijsen argues, it becomes possible to develop a clearer understanding of different interpretations of need and of conflicts of interest that exist between those in need of care and those who provide it. She defines care as a 'social practice', a human activity that is 'underpinned by formal or informal institutions, usually a combination of these' (Sevenhuijsen 1998, p. 21). Social and organisational contexts shape interpretations of need and actions taken to meet these. For Sevenhuijsen, universal ethical principles are required, not just as a framework for micro-level caring relationships but more broadly in public life. Once the principle is established that everybody needs care it follows that, in a democratic society, citizens should be enabled to both give and receive care. This means that the right to care and be cared for should be enshrined within the constitutional rights of citizens, which Sevenhuijsen argues could be achieved through a 'life-plan' approach that guarantees the right to take time for unpaid caring activities (see also Williams 2001).

In the context of social care, Tronto's (1993) observation that the moral agenda of rights and justice is usually conceptualised quite separately from the political agenda of resources also has particular resonance. Issues on the moral agenda, such as the promotion of service-user choice and control, frequently remain as unfulfilled aspirations because in the day-to-day reality of service organisation and provision the political agenda of resources always takes precedence. In many ways the personalisation agenda reasserts the aims of the community care reforms of the 1990s, when 'tailor-made' services were envisaged but never implemented in full because of a consistent shortage of resources (Means *et al.* 2003). With a projected 1.7 million more adults needing social care services by 2026 it is perhaps not surprising that the British government's concerns about resources and future funding options are dominant but they jeopardise the aims of service users for greater choice and control over services.

The Ageing Population and the Personalisation Agenda

The next part of the discussion will focus on the context of an ageing society, how demographic trends are understood and how this understanding is applied to the personalisation agenda. Particular attention is given to key themes within the personalisation agenda: the individualisation of care and the focus on service-user control.

Demographic Trends and Needs Over the Life Course

Reference has already been made to the way in which the ageing of the population has generated a sense of urgency for policy makers. Currently, the emphasis is on finding ways to reduce the cost of providing care, with a number of strategies being followed including increasing preventive and re-ablement services and technological support that helps to maintain people in their own homes for as long as possible, as well as Direct Payments and Individual Budgets (DH 2008a).

However, demographic trends have another implication which is rarely considered in policies but which is highly relevant to a discussion of social care for older people. This concerns the connection between improved life expectancy and the concentration of death in old age. When the welfare of older people was being debated at the turn of the twentieth century just 24 per cent of deaths in the UK population were of people aged over 65. By the turn of the twenty-first century this had grown to 84 per cent. The evidence demonstrates clearly that at whatever age we die, it is in the period prior to our deaths that our claims on health and care services are the greatest. Premature deaths are equally demanding on resources and the costs associated with old age might therefore be more accurately understood as the costs associated with dying (Lloyd 2010). Increased life expectancy is also related to changes in the circumstances of dying and the increase in chronic illnesses as causes of death. From an ethic of care perspective chronic illness can be understood as increasing the intensity of dependency in the period prior to death. Looked at from this perspective care must necessarily encompass more than the restoration of independence. Ultimately, what feminist ethicists refer to as inherent human vulnerability is inextricably linked with mortality, and while restoring or maintaining independence is crucially important for some older people, the needs of others for whom this is no longer a possibility should also be acknowledged in social care policies.

Age-related Needs for Care

The discussion document *Shaping the Future of Care Together* (DH 2009) sets out the kinds of support that could be provided through personal budgets. These include further or higher education, training to prepare for a job, employment, bringing up children, caring for other family members, volunteering, involvement in sport, leisure and social activities. There is clearly little evidence here of *attentiveness* to older people's needs that arise from events, such as a fall or stroke, or from growing frailty, degenerative illness or cognitive impairment. On the contrary, policy aims such as these represent a highly instrumental view of social care, portraying services as a means of restoring people to their functions as active citizens.

Waerness (2001) comments that there are separate and parallel discourses on care for older people: the public management perspective of care and the 'real world' practices of care. She argues that these two parallel discourses should be brought together and that feminist ethicists should seek to do this through the production of knowledge that is relevant to policy makers (see also Twigg 2002). When policy makers speak of social care for older people their focus is not on the daily activities of helping them to wash and dress or to prepare and eat their meals but on the economic challenge this need generates. Service providers conceptualise care as a commodity and focus on its procurement, funding and management. By contrast, an ethic of care would entail attentiveness to the practicalities associated with dependencies that arise from frailty and ill-health in old age. With its emphasis on human relationships and connectedness, an ethic of care perspective would also consider how responsibility for taking care of older people's needs should be shared and would regard the question of resources not only terms of how the costs of care should be managed and controlled but how they should be allocated to meet needs in a competent and responsive manner that does not exploit those who provide care.

Being 'in Control'

In contemporary social care policies, placing service users in control is regarded as an unquestionable benefit for service users, ensuring that care is provided in a way that reflects their particular preferences and requirements. An ethic of care perspective raises a more complex picture by highlighting differences in needs and priorities between care providers and receivers.

Waerness (2001) distinguishes three basic forms of care: caring for dependants (where because of illness or disability one individual is dependent on another person to help them); caring for superiors (such as in employer/assistant relationships); and caring in symmetrical relationships in which balanced reciprocity is evident and the individuals involved in the relationship 'care for' each other. This last form reflects the experiences of many older people, whose giving and receiving of care reflects symmetry in the relationship and means it can be difficult to distinguish the carer from the cared for.

Waerness's typology is useful in demonstrating how in caring relationships power is not always in the hands of the carer but it is essential not to make assumptions about the quality of a relationship or to determine how control is exercised simply by looking at its form. For example, the provision of cash in lieu of services places service users in the position of employer, shifting them from the first to the second type, but the degree to which they are able to exercise control will vary significantly according to a wide range of factors. For example, the implementation of personalised budgets is a top-down process at the local level, with service providers determining the rates at which budgets are set. This will affect the rates at which care workers are paid and the local supply of care worker, thus impacting on the extent to which choice and control can be exercised. In addition, service users have widely differing capacities, which will impact on their caring relationships and their ability to exert control and manage their own care arrangements.

Kittay *et al.* (2005) argue that from an ethical standpoint independent living schemes should also be viewed from the perspective of the personal assistant, who is often invisible in debates concerning the provision of cash in lieu of services. They point out how in the North American context the supply of personal assistants depends on the migration of women from developing nations whose pay and conditions of work are extremely poor. From a UK context a related point is made by Yeandle and Steill (2007) who identify both positive and negative experiences amongst personal assistants employed through Direct Payments who found that their work could be more satisfying because of the friendships that developed between them and the people they supported but that these friendships could also make it difficult to assert their rights as workers, for example, in keeping to their contracted hours of work.

Control over caring arrangements also needs to be understood within the wider power dynamics of the relationships. Kittay (2002) draws attention to the relationship between dependency and power and the potential for domination of vulnerable people by those with responsibility for their care. This is a highly pertinent point to consider in relation to the vulnerability of older people. Maintaining people in their own homes can be a way of avoiding institutionalisation and can enhance reciprocal or symmetrical family caring relationships However, evidence on the nature and extent of abuse of older people points to greater risks associated with dependency for care on family, friends or neighbours (Manthorpe *et al.* 2008). According to a recent survey by the organisation Action on Elder Abuse, 66 per cent of abusers were either family members or neighbours and acquaintances. Arguably, safeguarding older people from abuse should be at the heart of the implementation of the personalisation agenda, yet a report by the Commission for Social Care Inspection in 2008 identified a lack of awareness of the links between the two areas of practice and a lack of involvement in the personalisation agenda by managers responsible for safeguarding adults (CSCI 2008). An ethic of care would be attentive to the potential for abuse within families and would minimise isolation in caring relationships through appropriate support for both carer and cared for.

Individualism

With its focus on the individual, the personalisation agenda represents a point around which different approaches to social care coalesce. Social work traditions, consumerist values of individual choice and control and the political aims of disabled people for non-institutionalised forms of care all share an emphasis on individual self-determination and are open to criticism from the perspective of the ethic of care. In social work, the personalisation agenda is perceived to offer an opportunity to re-establish core social work values by shedding the heavily bureaucratic administrative approach that has dominated community care services. Carr and Dittrich (2008), for example, argue that personalisation originated at least in part from social work values, which have always stressed respect for the individual and self-determination:

> Good social work practice has always involved putting the individual first; values such as respect for the individual and self-determination have long been at the heart of social work. In this sense the underlying philosophy of personalisation is familiar. (p. 8)

Carr and Dittrich's comments overlook long-standing debates in social work concerning its individualistic values. Jordan (2004), for example, argues that its individualistic focus allies social work with consumerist agendas of choice and independence and that this alliance runs the risk of creating an enforced form of independence for those who are poor and have little choice. Newman *et al.* (2008) make a similar point that the ideal of the consumer citizen within the personalisation agenda is vulnerable to neo-liberal political agendas in which the individual is expected to take greater responsibility for self-care, thus subverting the aims of enhanced choice and control.

A related point is made by Roulstone and Morgan (2009), who argue that personalisation runs the risk that enforced individualism and isolation will replace the enforced collectivities of old-style institutionalised services. This point calls into question the claims concerning the capacity of personalisation to enhance choice, since the chances of making a positive choice to move to a care home would be reduced, but it also directs attention to the conditions in which older people live in their own homes when they become more dependent. For example, the emphasis on maintaining people in their own homes has driven the development of telecare, which enables remote surveillance of older people's movements around their home and triggers rapid responses to unusual activities or alarms. From an ethic of care perspective, telecare is not undesirable if it is used in the context of supportive caring relationships, but it undoubtedly has significant potential to exacerbate isolation and loneliness. Where the aim is simply to enable an individual older person to remain in their own home, using telecare misses the point about the fundamental human need for social relationships.

From an ethic of care perspective, individuals are not already formed prior to engaging in relationships but it is through relationships with each other that individual identity is forged. Thus the older person should be seen in the context of their relationships, including those with carers. This perspective generates a different set of concerns. For those older people who lack supportive and caring relationships the aim of maintaining them in their own homes would need to be balanced against their need for social contact. Another concern is that older people's health status frequently fluctuates and changes and this poses a challenge to their identity as they experience a loss of self-reliance and growing dependency on others for help with everyday activities. In the context of a society that characterises them as a burden such challenges can be experienced in highly negative and damaging ways.

There are implications also for those who take on the identity of 'carer'. Kittay's concept of nested dependencies provides a constructive model for understanding the impact of caring on the identities of both carer and cared for, as it draws attention to the influence of wider relationships, including with health and social care professionals (Kittay 2002). In the UK context a question arises concerning the adequacy of support for carers in the context of increasing levels of care at home. The British government claims that the personalisation agenda will address pressures on family carers (DH 2008b) but the campaigning group Carers UK argues for a more holistic approach that understands carers not only within their caring role but in their lives more generally (Carers UK 2009).

Ageing, Dependency and the Ethic of Care

A focus on issues related to individualism and service-user control pinpoints the tensions within contemporary social care services and the impact of these on older people. The ethic of care provides a relevant and useful framework through which to analyse the current personalisation agenda in England. In terms of attentiveness, it is evident that the personalisation agenda fails to take account of the diversity of older people's needs and in particular neglects the needs of many who turn to social care services when their health is declining in the period before their deaths. Socio-economic inequalities across the life course are frequently exacerbated in old age and those who are least able to provide for their own care in old age are likely to have the greatest need for care. There are also important gender considerations in that women are most likely to be widowed and live alone but also least likely to have accrued resources to fall back on in old age because of their disadvantaged position in the labour market.

Such inequalities highlight the dangers associated with the individualism of the personalisation agenda in allocating responsibility for care. From an ethic of care perspective, responsibility for care needs to be shared and, in Kittay's terms, spread to the outer reaches of the nested dependencies (Kittay 1999). The question of the adequacy of resources for social care, including resources to support family carers and to provide good conditions of work for paid care workers can be examined by reference to Tronto's (1993) concept of competence.

Responsiveness—seeing things from the perspective of the one receiving care—is fundamental to personalisation. However, as argued, although greater choice and control for service users is promised there is no guarantee that a market for care will generate this and the personalisation agenda is not responsive to the diversity of support needed by older people. It also remains unclear how the personalisation agenda will promote the well-being of older people who do not gain access to the social care system, particularly in a climate where cutbacks in services have become the norm. Pressure by service users has undoubtedly influenced policy and a stronger political movement of disabled people exists now in comparison to the period when community care was introduced, but limited resources for care in a more economically challenging climate coupled with demographic trends mean that the implementation of personalisation in social care will face similar challenges.

There are also questions to consider concerning the value of the ethic of care both as an explanatory model and as a way of identifying how social care for dependent older people should be developed. Meyers (1998) argues that care should be understood as primarily a political rather than an ethical issue and in his view this entails drawing a distinction between the *context* and the *activities* of care. Thus, at the societal level solidarity between people rather than individualistic accounts of responsive care comes to the forefront of analysis. However, a separation of context and activities misses the point raised above concerning the need to make connections between policy making and the practicalities and daily experiences of receiving and providing care (Waerness 2001). There are particular political and ethical issues to consider in relation to old age. For example, whilst there are successful campaigns on issues relating to retirement and to age discrimination it is less likely that people's experience of frailty and dependency in the last stage of their life course would provide a basis of solidarity on which to build a political campaign. Ensuring that people's needs are met in these circumstances is therefore an *ethical* agenda because it addresses moral concerns about ensuring that those who are dependent on others are treated well. It is also political in nature because it concerns the rights of individuals to receive and to give care. Importantly, this agenda is not limited to those with an aged or service-user identity but is of general concern. The right to care in old age concerns us all at whatever stage of the life course we happen to be.

Conclusion

Older people in need of social care are in an invidious position. The current policy debate on the future of social care is framed almost entirely within a perspective of their burdensomeness, which is exacerbated by demographic trends. The ethic of care perspective provides a sound and logical explanation for the inattentiveness of the policy-makers' agenda: dependent older people are regarded as 'the other' and the priorities of the working-age public are presented as separate from and antagonistic to those of dependent older people, as though ageing was not a shared experience.

The campaigning agenda of disabled service users for control over care provision has coincided with policy-makers' agenda of delegating responsibility for care but arguably is equally inattentive to the needs of people who become old and frail. The ethic of care approach is regarded by some as antithetical to disabled people's campaigns for full citizen rights. For Beresford the concept of care frames disabled people as dependent and is 'inherently unequal and controlling' (2008, p. 13). As argued, the personalisation agenda stresses the importance of service-user control as part of a wider campaign for citizen rights by disabled people. But from an ethic of care perspective the counter analysis is not that the concept of care frames disabled people as dependent but that vulnerability and dependency are inherent in the human condition, meaning that we all have a need for care and, as Sevenhuijsen (1998) argues, that citizenship must be understood differently.

However, the persistence of this viewpoint means that it is all the more important for an ethic of care perspective to place the perspectives of those who are in need of care centre-stage, and to emphasise responsiveness. A focus on the need for care in circumstances of frailty and ill-health in old age is a valuable way of developing understanding of the dependencies that human beings share in common. How people live towards the end of their lives in old age is currently poorly understood by researchers, policy makers and service providers alike. The ethic of care is an effective framework for developing knowledge concerning the giving and receiving of care that has the potential to influence not only the ways in which social care services are provided but also the ways in which dependency is experienced at this stage of the life course.

References

Beresford, P. (2008) *What Future for Care?*, Joseph Rowntree Foundation, York.
Boxall, K., Dowson, S. & Beresford, P. (2009) 'Selling Individual Budgets, Choice and Control: Local and Global Influences on UK Social Care Policy for People with Learning Difficulties', *Policy and Politics*, Vol. 37, no. 4, pp. 499–515.
Carers, UK (2009) *Policy Briefing: The National Strategy for Carers*, Carers UK, London.
Carr, S. & Dittrich, R. (2008) *Personalisation: A Rough Guide*, Social Care Institute for Excellence, London.

Commission for Social Care Inspection (CSCI) (2008) *Raising Voices: Views on Safeguarding Adults*, Commission for Social Care Inspection, London.

Department of Health (DH) (2008a) *Transforming Social Care*, Local Authority Circular DH (2008)1, Department of Health, London.

Department of Health (DH) (2008b) *Carers at the Heart of 21st Century Families and Communities: A Caring System on Your Side, a Life of Your Own*, Department of Health, London.

Department of Health (DH) (2009) *Shaping the Future of Care Together*, Cm7673, The Stationery Office, London.

Ferguson, I. (2007) 'Increasing User Choice or Privatizing Risk? The Antinomies of Personalization', *British Journal of Social Work*, Vol. 37, no. 3, pp. 387–403.

Fine, M. (2007) *A Caring Society? Care and the Dilemmas of Human Service in the 21st Century*, Palgrave Macmillan, Basingstoke.

Glendinning, C. *et al.* (2008) *Evaluation of the Individual Budgets Pilot Programme: Final Report*, Social Policy Research Unit, University of York.

Held, V. (2006) *The Ethics of Care: Personal, Political, and Global*, Oxford University press, Oxford.

Jordan, B. (2004) 'Emancipatory social work? Opportunity or oxymoron', *British Journal of Social Work*, Vol. 34, no. 1, pp. 5–19.

Kittay, E. F. (1999) *Love's Labor: Essays on Women, Equality and Dependency*, Routledge, New York and London.

Kittay, E. F. (2002) 'When Caring is Just and Justice is Caring: Caring and Mental Retardation', in *The Subject of Care: Feminist Perspectives on Dependency*, eds E. F. Kittay & E. K. Feder, Rowman & Littlefield, Lanham, MD, pp. 257–76.

Kittay, E. F., Jennings, B. & Wasunna, A. A. (2005) 'Dependency, Difference and the Global Ethic of Long-term Care', *Journal of Political Philosophy*, Vol. 13, no. 4, pp. 443–69.

Lloyd, L. (2010) 'End of Life Issues', in *The Sage International Handbook of Ageing*, eds D. Dannefer & C. Phillipson, Sage, London and New York, pp. 618–29.

Manthorpe, J., Stevens, M., Rapaport, J., Harris, J., Jacobs, S., Challis, D., Netten, A., Knapp, M., Wilberforce, M. & Glendinning, C. (2008) 'Safeguarding and System Change: Early Perceptions of the Implications for Adult Protection Services of the English Individual Budgets Pilots—A Qualitative Study', *British Journal of Social Work*, Vol. 39, no. 8, pp. 1465–80.

Means, R., Richards, S. & Smith, R. (2003) *Community Care: Policy and Practice*, 3rd edn, Palgrave Macmillan, Basingstoke.

Meyers, P. A. (1998) 'The "Ethic of Care" and the Problem of Power', *Journal of Political Philosophy*, Vol. 6, no. 2, pp. 142–70.

Newman, J., Glendinning, C. & Hughes, M. (2008) 'Beyond Modernisation? Social Care and the Transformation of Welfare Governance', *Journal of Social Policy*, Vol. 37, no. 4, pp. 531–57.

O'Neill, O. (1996) *Towards Justice and Virtue: A Constructive Account of Practical Reasoning*, Cambridge University Press, Cambridge.

Roulstone, A. & Morgan, H. (2009) 'Neo-liberal Individualism or Self-directed Support: Are We All Speaking the Same Language on Modernization?', *Social Policy and Society*, Vol. 8, no. 3, pp. 333–45.

Sevenhuijsen, S. (1998) *Citizenship and the Ethics of Care: Feminist Considerations on Justice, Morality and Politics*, Routledge, London.

Sevenhuijsen, S. (2000) 'Caring in the Third Way: The Relation between Obligation, Responsibility and Care in Third Way Discourse', *Critical Social Policy*, Vol. 20, no. 1, pp. 73–80.

Tronto, J. (1993) *Moral Boundaries: A Political Argument for an Ethic of Care*, Routledge, London.

Twigg, J. (2002) 'The Body in Social Policy: Mapping a Territory', *Journal of Social Policy,* Vol. 31, no. 3, pp. 421–39.

Waerness, K. (2001) 'Social Research, Political Theory and the Ethics of Care', *Research Review,* Vol. NS 17, no. 1, pp. 5–16.

Williams, F. (2001) 'In and beyond New Labour: Towards a New Political Ethics of Care', *Critical Social Policy,* Vol. 21, no. 4, pp. 467–93.

Williams, R. (1975) *Keywords: A Vocabulary of Culture and Society,* Fontana, Glasgow.

Yeandle, S. & Steill, B. (2007) 'Issues in the Development of the Direct Payments Scheme for Older People in England', in *Cash for Care in Developed Welfare States,* eds C. Ungerson & S. Yeandle, Palgrave Macmillan, Basingstoke.

A Comparative Analysis of Personalisation: Balancing an Ethic of Care with User Empowerment

Kirstein Rummery

Developments in the provision of care and support services for disabled and older people across developed welfare states have led to the expansion of personalisation (sometimes called cash-for-care, direct payments, care payments, etc.) schemes, whereby cash is paid in substitute for care services and support. Although these schemes vary considerably in their scope and operation (sometimes paying carers directly, sometimes enabling disabled and older people to act as direct employers, sometimes mixing paid and unpaid care), they share the characteristics of commodifying care and support services and will have a potentially profound impact on the relationship between individuals, families, communities and the welfare state. Although the schemes have been evaluated within their own national contexts, little work has been done so far to explore the theoretical implications of their development and extension, particularly from an ethics of care perspective. This paper intends to fill that theoretical gap by drawing on comparative evidence from several schemes across different national contexts to develop an analysis which draws on feminist theory and an ethics of care approach to examine (a) the gendered policy outcomes and impact of such schemes; (b) a feminist analysis of the governance implications of personalisation; (c) the implications for the gendered division of work, particularly between paid and unpaid care work and between different groups of paid and unpaid carers; (d) an ethics of care analysis of the impact of personalisation over the lifecourse of disabled and older people, and carers; and (e) a discussion of the relationship between commodification, empowerment, citizenship and choice drawing on the work of care ethicists. It will draw conclusions about the outcomes of a range of types of personalisation schemes and thus have implications for theory, policy and practice.

Kirstein Rummery is Professor of Social Policy in the School of Applied Social Science, University of Stirling.

Introduction

Social, demographic and political changes have led to a rising demand for 'care' and support, particularly for disabled and older adults, across developed welfare states (Pierson 2001). On a positive note, these demands can be seen as a reflection of the success of welfare states in promoting longevity, well-being and reduced morbidity, as health and social services have made a significant contribution to the welfare of citizens. Indeed, Walker and Lowenstein (2009) and others have referred to the so-called 'demographic timebomb' (i.e. the rise in demand for welfare services due to an ageing population) as one of the most significant 'successes' of twentieth-century social policy in developed welfare states. One response to these changes has been the development of 'personalisation' services: formal, or semi-formal payments for care services designed to replace either formal state care services or to support informal family- or community-based care. Although there are substantial variations in the form and function of these services, they are essentially a way of routing cash directly to disabled or older people to purchase care and support.

The social, demographic and political changes referred to above do not just affect the state and the way in which it provides for the needs of its citizens. Feminist analysts, particularly those basing their analysis on Gilligan's (1982) and Sevenhuijsens' 'ethic of care' (2000) have pointed out that no matter what form the welfare state takes, welfare, care and support are provided by a mix of families, communities and (sometimes) the state. State policies regarding care (and related areas), even though often not overtly concerning gender equality or gender issues, nevertheless have a gendered impact (as well as a differential impact regarding other social divisions, such as class and age). Understanding who undertakes, pays for, and receives care is a crucial part of understanding both the form and practice of gender-related oppression (Lewis 2002). Moreover, even policies which are not overtly gendered in their normative framing will have normative cores which are implicitly gendered, resting on sometimes very powerful assumptions about the role and value of care work as 'feminised' (Lewis 2002). Most theoretical developments concerning the role that these different constituent parts play in the 'welfare mix' which draw on feminist theory have focused on the gendered roles associated with *providing* care. Whilst this has led to a rich empirical and theoretical tradition informed by feminist analysis, the perspectives of those *receiving* care, with a few notable exceptions (e.g. Morris 1996; Kroger 2009; Lloyd 2000), have not necessarily been viewed through a theoretical lens informed by this perspective.

This paper will therefore discuss comparative developments in personalisation and care services from a feminist perspective, examining the gendered outcomes for both carers and the cared-for. It will then use feminist ethic of care theoretical perspectives to discuss the governance implications of these developments. It will examine the implications from these developments for the gendered division of labour (both paid and unpaid), the gendered impact of personalisation across the lifecourse of disabled and older people and carers, and a discussion of what the evidence so far from these developments means in terms of the relationship between commodification, choice and empowerment.

Personalisation and the Ethic of Care

Recent years have seen several important changes in policy direction in the development of health and social care services across developed welfare states. Firstly, in response to increasing life expectancy and reduced morbidity there is a growing concern amongst developed welfare states to cap the perceived rising demand for resources, particularly from disabled and older adults. This has led to a shifting of responsibilities across different parts of the public sector (e.g. from health to social services, or from centralised to localised provision) and across sectors (e.g. from state to private or third sector, or state to family provision). Secondly, there have been changes in the governance of welfare across different sectors, including the increasing commodification of services and the associated de-professionalisation of health and social care practitioners (Newman 2005). Thirdly, there has been a growing politicisation of disability rights organisations, and in some cases older people's organisations, who have responded to what they have seen as the increased fragmentation and unresponsiveness of services resulting from poor-quality state provision by demanding more choice and control over care and support services.

This combination of factors has led to the development of what is known as 'personalised', or cash-for-care, services. These vary considerably in terms of their design, scope and function: however, there are certain factors which unite them. They are ways in which the state pays disabled and older people cash benefits in order to enable them to directly purchase their care or support: either from formal service providers, or informal carers, or a mixture of both. In some cases this payment replaces services directly provided by the state, and in other it acts as a commodified form of supporting informal care, usually from family members.

The role that a reliance on family-based care plays in creating and reinforcing inequalities has long been understood (Lewis 2002). On the one hand, care policies that rely on family care are based on the assumption that care work is legitimately seen as both 'private' and 'feminised', with the result that it is undervalued, in market terms, and seen as not subject to scrutiny by the state, unless it fails and the state needs to replace it (Lewis 2002). Welfare states, particularly those that rely on engagement in paid work as a mark of citizenship, have often accorded carers a second-class status because of this assumption: whilst at the same time the working of a capitalist economy relies on care work being provided 'free' or being undervalued, which serves to legitimise the lower levels of participation in market-valued work by carers (Fraser 1994).

Ever since Gilligan (1982) took issue with what she perceived as a male-dominated view of 'justice' which did not allow for the true value of women's caring to be articulated, feminist analysts have sought to re-value care work, pointing to its legitimacy and necessity as well as its value (Tronto 1994; Sevenhuijsen 2000). Articulating the different components of caring, particularly the link between the pragmatic and the emotional aspects of care (e.g. taking responsibility for, and caring about, as well as the actual hands-on delivery of physical care) does serve the purpose of making care work visible and allows for an understanding regarding the meeting of welfare need that is not simply about individuals and the state allocating resources (Ellis 2004). It also serves the valuable purpose of exposing the neo-liberal myth that engagement in the fulfilment of citizenship duties is possible only through participation in paid work—i.e. work that is valued by the market: indeed, it highlights the distortion of the market through the undervaluing of unpaid, or low-paid care work. Fisher and Tronto (1991) have developed a four-point schema for a political ethic of care that incorporates a moral precept: attentiveness (caring about), responsi-bility (taking care of), competence (care giving), and responsiveness (responding to the needs of the cared-for).

However, this reframing of care work from the perspective of those who *provide* care leaves underdeveloped the role of those who *receive* care. Ungerson (1987) and others have developed a feminist framework of social policy analysis that points out that policy is personal, and that reliance upon unpaid or undervalued care is a way of legitimating gender inequalities: however, they have been taken to task by feminist disability rights authors for undertheorising the power differentials experienced by those receiving care (Morris 2004), who point out that reliance on unpaid family care creates a 'burden of gratitude' that is intrinsically disempowering and exploitative (Galvin 1994; Brisenden 1986). Moreover, Ellis and Morris have pointed out that the development of care policies which privilege the attainment of 'independence' do so in a neo-liberal and patriarchal way, by normatively framing 'independence' in a way which does not allow for reliance on others. Both feminists and disability rights analysts have highlighted the way in which this 'myth' of independence does not allow for the complex reality of interdependence, and reciprocity of care and support, that make up the lives of everyone, not just those who are deemed to be 'disabled', or 'carers'. As Oliver (2009) point outs, no one who uses an aeroplane to travel from the United Kingdom to Australia is considered to be 'dependent' on the plane: but someone who uses a wheelchair is often seen as 'dependent' on it by non-disabled carers. A tension exists, therefore, between two ostensibly opposing sets of theories. On the one hand, care ethicists would like to see both the emotional and practical aspect of caring properly legitimated and valued. On the other, disability activists would like to see 'care' removed altogether and replaced with a notion of independence that involves being in control of the type of support individuals receive.

Personalisation schemes sit uneasily in between these two theoretical perspectives. As discussed above, they have been developed to meet a variety of sometimes conflicting policy objectives, and these in themselves have their origins in different theoretical underpinnings. Different models have emerged, depending in part on the different aims and normative frameworks: they include care allowances paid directly to disabled and older people, personal care budgets allowing the direct employment of care workers, allowances paid directly to informal carers—sometimes as part of income-replacement schemes which compensate informal carers for lost paid employment. They have been criticised for commodifying and re-familiasing care (Ungerson 1997; Spandler 2004), for devolving responsibility and risk onto vulnerable people and for de-professionalising social care (Ferguson 2007). However, they have been shown to be valued by both carers and the cared-for, and Kroger (2009), Rummery (2006, 2009) and others have discussed the way in which they might bring a kind of synthesis to these ostensibly opposing worlds by introducing elements of *choice* and *control* to both parties. The remainder of this paper will use both an ethic of care and disability rights framework to draw on comparative international evidence from different types of personalisation schemes, examining the potential for improved outcomes in terms of care, choice and empowerment for carers and the cared-for.

Examples of Personalisation Schemes

United Kingdom

Prior to 1996 it was illegal for statutory social services departments to give cash directly to service users to enable them to purchase their own services; however, several ad hoc and quasi-legitimate schemes showed that this was preferred by some users to receiving state-funded services. Following various schemes all disabled and older people who are deemed eligible for state-funded support services are entitled to apply for cash payments (sometimes called direct payments, self-directed care, personalised care or individual budgets). England has piloted the combining of various health and social care funding streams which enable users to purchase a fairly wide range of services—payments are usually used to directly employ formal carers, or to purchase services from not-for-profit care agencies. It is not possible to directly employ family members: this scheme is intended to replace formal, not informal care. There is little formal protection for workers employed under this scheme, and there is little assistance with the recruitment of care workers. It is implemented by local authorities and based on locally determined eligibility criteria and needs assessments; there is therefore considerable local variation in how schemes operate and on their take-up (Rummery 2006). Users are also eligible for a fairly complex range of means-tested care allowances which are under review.

The Netherlands

The year 1991 saw the introduction of a personal care allowance scheme that in 1995 became part of the national long-term care insurance scheme. This allows recipients to choose to receive cash payments instead of state-provided care and support services; like the UK scheme, it replaces formal care provision. However, unlike the UK scheme, it is possible to pay family members, which enables users to combine formal and informal care provision much more flexibly. The scheme is fairly strictly regulated and provides a degree of protection for directly employed carers which makes it impossible either to employ illegal workers or for the money to be used on general family expenditure rather than care and support. Compared to the other schemes in this paper, it is relatively generously funded, although recent concerns about rising demands and costs have led to some political pressure to limit its expansion. In common with other schemes, it has proved more cost effective than directly providing state-funded services, and is therefore likely to continue to be popular (Weekers & Pijl 1998).

Italy

Unlike the United Kingdom and the Netherlands, Italy has seen very little development of formal care and support services for disabled and older people. A high reliance on family and informal care (supported by comparatively low levels of full-time female workforce participation) has been matched by a very decentralised state system which has shown resistance to the development of formalised, centralised state-funded support. A national non-means-tested care allowance is paid directly to disabled and older people who are deemed to be 'dependent', and it is not graduated according to need. Its use is not restricted or policed, with the result that it is often used to employ illegal workers, or becomes part of the general family finances (particularly in low-income house-holds). It is supplemented by locally provided means-tested care allowances (which vary according to their eligibility criteria and therefore access and take-up also vary considerably). The lack of formalised provision or the development of a not-for-profit care market means that payments are most often used to employ individual care workers (with very little employment protection), paid directly to informal carers or become part of general family finances (Gori & Da Roit 2007; Pavolini & Ranci 2008).

Austria

Like Italy, Austria has historically had relatively low levels of formal care service provision, relying heavily on informal family provision and emphasising a 'male breadwinner' model of welfare (Bettio & Platenga 2004). However, unlike Italy, Austria is a strongly social-democratic state and in 1993 it introduced a long-term care allowance system whereby a non-means-tested benefit is paid directly to disabled and older people who qualify (Oesterle 2001). Like the Dutch system it can be used to purchase formal care services from individuals and organisations, and to reimburse family carers, thus giving a high degree of flexibility. However, more in line with the Italian than the Dutch system, there are very low levels of regulation associated with what the payment can be used for, with the result that it is often used to employ illegal labour with very low levels of employment protection, or to reimburse family carers: both options have the result of supporting a gendered division of labour within the family (Kreimer & Schiffbaenker 2005).

France

France is often portrayed as a combination of high levels of insurance-based welfare provision coupled with high reliance on family for care and support (Le Bihan & Martin 2006). Care allowances were introduced in 1997, which were replaced by a more formalised system in 2002. These are paid directly to older people who qualify, and can be supplemented by related means-tested benefits. They can be used to purchase care services from professionals or relatives (but not spouses) and are most often used to purchase services from formal, not-for-profit care organisations rather than directly employing individual carers. Care workers thus have relatively high levels of employment protection: indeed, some commentators have argued that these payments were introduced primarily to protect the employment of formal care workers rather than to 'personalise' care services (Bresse 2004). There is little evidence that the balance between formal and informal care has altered substantially, nor that the gendered division of labour in care work has been affected (Le Bihan & Martin 2006).

Sweden

Sweden has a long social-democratic history of welfare provision, with long-term state-funded care provision being established in the 1950s. Reforms to the system in 1992 shifted responsibility for care provision to a more localised level, tightening the criteria for accessing services and expanding reliance on family-based informal care, in line with developments across other welfare states facing similar demographic pressures. Cash payments are beginning to be developed—for example, an attendance allowance scheme for older people was extended in 1994 to cover disabled people and enables users to purchase their own care and support, including employing relatives, and some commentators argue that this marks the end of universal state-funded care support (Le Bihan & Martin 2006)—although, in comparison to other schemes under discussion, the Swedish scheme remains relatively marginal to mainstream care provision, and, unlike other schemes, social workers manage the care payment on behalf of users.

United States

Of all the countries discussed in this paper, the United States probably has the highest degree of policy decentralisation: there is a considerable amount of variation in care policies at federal level. The national Medicaid programme has allowed the development of different 'consumer-choice' schemes which enable disabled and older people to directly hire their own care workers (Mahoney *et al*. 2000). Care workers are usually employed with whom users have an ongoing relationship—formal, or through kinship networks. Such schemes have proved popular and are becoming an increasingly mainstream feature of care provision across several states (Keigher 2007), commodifying informal care. Like the Italian case, often such schemes are not replacing state-provided care but are instead seeking to underwrite family-based care.

Personalisation Policies and an Ethic of Care

There are several normative cores underpinning the development of personalisation schemes. The more overt consist of a push towards cost containment, neo-liberal support for individualisation in welfare, and the increased commodification of care and support services. However, there are more covert but nonetheless powerful normative cores that concern expectations of care giving that are being played out in the design and implementation of personalisation schemes. Where schemes are explicitly about the state reducing its role in the direct provision of support (particularly in cases with previously high levels of state support, such as the Netherlands, Sweden and France) there seems to be a push towards a (re)familiasation of care: and when the state expects family to step in, this usually (but not always) means a feminisation and undervaluing of care work (Pateman 1988). Whilst in some respects this fits with an ethic of care thesis (because the state is recognising and recompensing carers for the care work that they undertake), nevertheless the way in which the levels of payment have been set low to make savings indicates that the state values the care provided by family less than the care provided by the state (although state-provided carers are also underpaid and undervalued, in market terms).

However, personalisation schemes in all seven countries chosen as examples have been developed at least in part as a response to users' concerns about having more control over the kind of care and support they receive, rather than as part of a campaign to address the undervaluation of care. For example, politicised user movements in the United Kingdom, the Netherlands and the United States have been directly involved in the development of personalisation schemes (Donellan 1991), and have argued that unpaid care is potentially exploitative and damaging for both carers and the cared-for because of the way in which it reinforces dependency and powerlessness on both sides (Morris 2004). Commodifying care by introducing cash payments recognises carers' work by compensating them (Lister 2002) and can be seen as an important achievement for the support of an ethic of care perspective and carer parity in welfare (Fraser 1994). This is a particularly powerful argument where personalisation schemes are recompensing carers who would previously have been unpaid (such as in Austria, the United States and Italy) rather than where personalisation schemes are replacing care and support previously provided by the state (such as the Netherlands, the United Kingdom, Sweden and France).

Whether personalisation schemes address the undervaluing of care depends largely on how the payments are used. Where schemes free up previously 'unpaid' carers to participate in the labour market they will also have the effect of recompensing previously 'unpaid' carers for their work: in both cases, carers will benefit financially from such schemes. Where personalisation schemes are used to protect the employment of carers who were previously paid by the state (France and, to a lesser extent, the Netherlands), there is the potential for the state to maintain the value it places on care work, even if that is not substantially increased. In both cases, public policy legitimises and values care work, whilst freeing carers to chose whether, and how, to provide care.

Governance, Personalisation and the Ethic of Care

Some of the schemes under discussion in this paper have been designed explicitly to allow a considerable degree of localised variation in their design and implementation (particularly the United Kingdom, Italy, Austria and the United States). They can be understood as falling within a policy objective of shifting services from centralised to localised provision—often legitimated ostensibly to allow for greater *responsiveness* to need, which fits with an ethic of care framework (Fisher & Tronto 1991). However, such localisation means that there is considerable scope for inequalities and inequities in the system to be magnified. For example, the different type of employment protection available to paid care workers and the differential impact that introducing payments for care can have on previously unpaid carers (see below) can lead to situations where carers who are already marginalised and vulnerable (e.g. through low income, poor employment prospects and poor access to resources and support) can be made even more marginalised by low levels of state governance over the operation of the schemes. Failure to protect the status of carers can be seen as undervaluing care, as well as running the risk of exploiting the emotional aspect of caring, particularly the attentiveness and responsibility aspects.

The different ways in which the schemes are governed has an impact on how far an ethic of care can be operationalised. How the schemes are run, including the different ways in which users are held to account for the way in which they spend the money, gives rise to different levels of policing and surveillance over people's lives and care relationships. Some personalisation schemes are highly regulated (e.g. France and the Netherlands), which gives a very high level of protection to potentially vulnerable users and carers. This is particularly the case for France, where the scheme is designed specifically to protect the employment rights of care workers (Le Bihan & Martin 2006). This gives the state an important role in policing and surveilling intimate caring relationships: it undertakes to ensure that two dimensions of Fisher and Tronto's ethic of care, namely *competence* (care giving) and *responsiveness* (responding to the needs of the cared-for), are accounted for. However, an ethic of care framework argues that the other two precepts, *attentiveness* (caring about) and *responsibility* (taking care of), are intrinsically linked with the others. Levels of state policing which seek to regulate the emotional aspects of caring have the potential to exert considerable power and influence over carers' lives, whilst limiting the choice and control that users have over the type and quality of care and support they receive. Caring relationships are often complex, involving reciprocal ties and obligations which are linked to both the emotional and physical aspects of providing and receiving care. Formalising and policing such arrangements run the risk of pulling apart the interlinked components of an ethic of care.

However, the risks of *under*governance of personalisation schemes are also worrying. In schemes such as those in Austria and Italy, which are deliberately unregulated, there is evidence that the state's role in regulating users' and carers' lives is reduced, which enables a high degree of personal flexibility concerning the way in which care needs and relationships are negotiated. To a certain extent this allows for the complexity of interpersonal giving and receiving of care to be recognised, and for users to receive care from a mix of paid and unpaid carers, thereby relieving some of the burden on family. Nevertheless, these schemes allow for the proliferation of an unregulated and unprotected employment market for paid carers. This has the potential for the exploitation and abuse of vulnerable workers—particularly illegal and migrant workers, and reinforces the under-valuation of care work which serves to support and exacerbate divisions of labour along lines of gender, ethnicity and poverty/class. Commodifying care by introducing cash into relationships without governing the quality of care does not allow for the protection of either the physical or emotional aspects of caring. By reneging on its responsibility to ensure that it takes responsibility for and is attentive to care needs, the state is running the danger that care could in these situations be incompetent and unresponsive, thus failing to meet the moral, physical and emotional precepts of an ethic of care. Moreover, the danger that money is not used for care at all (particularly in the Italian case) places users in a potentially vulnerable position: the state has ostensibly discharged its responsibilities to citizens without actually meeting care needs.

Empowerment and Choice

Notwithstanding the many concerns discussed above, the evidence across all the schemes suggests their growing popularity; particularly where they replace state-provided care and services their uptake is increasing and qualitative evidence suggests they appeal to users and carers (both formal and informal). Personalisation schemes are successful at recognising the complexity of caring relationships: they can encompass the interconnected moral, emotional and physical dimensions of an ethic of care by introducing an element of *choice* into care. The social identities of citizens are often not easily divided into carers and cared-for. Many disabled and older people can simultaneously be receiving and giving care and support in formal and informal ways: for example, a disabled mother can be an employer (of a carer, or child carer), a carer (mother), and worker (paid and/or unpaid) as well as being a 'citizen' in many other ways (Rummery 2007; Lloyd 2000). Personalisation schemes can recognise these complex social identities in a way that state-provided, and family-provided, care alone cannot. Enabling disabled and older people to exercise choice over who provides care, and the level and type of care they provide, lets them control the care and support they receive, and combine formal and informal networks. It also enables them to carry out their own caring duties and participate more fully in society as competent citizens (Rummery 2006).

Fisher and Tronto (1991) indicate that all four moral precepts must be present for an ethic of care to have relevance: *attentiveness* (caring about), *responsibility* (taking care of), *competence* (care giving), and *responsiveness* (responding to the needs of the cared-for). The experiences of both carers and the cared-for indicate that whilst these elements are valued by both sides, a crucial consideration for whether care is exploitative or empowering lies in whether carers and the cared-for feel *in control* of their lives and choices. If carers feel 'trapped' into providing care then both the practical and emotional aspects of care giving will feel exploitative and abusive. If those who are cared-for feel 'trapped' into receiving care that they are not in control of, they will feel exploited and abused. Personalisation schemes therefore offer an opportunity for both carers and the cared-for to avoid the exploitation and abuse that is entailed in being trapped into unwanted caring relationships. Carers are in a much stronger position to be able to be attentive, competent, responsive and take responsibility for people if they entered into caring relationships on a basis which enables them to exercise choice over which elements of care they provide, and how. Disabled and older people are in a much stronger position to ensure that the care they receive is attentive, competent and responsive if they can exercise choice and control through paying for it directly.

Personalisation schemes also enable users to purchase care which is not easily provided through inflexible state services: for example, care which crosses sectoral divides (such as health and social care, or social care and education). It can enable users and carers to exercise choice about which caring tasks they undertake (or want unpaid carers to undertake) and which they 'outsource' to formal carers. This has the effect of decoupling relationships from care: allowing intimate relationships to be characterised by being spouses, or parents, or children first and foremost, rather than carers. An ethic of care approach to analysing personalisation schemes would indicate that the value of care work should be understood and articulated. Enabling carers to engage in work which is valued by themselves, those they care for and the state opens up new ways of participating in society and exercising citizenship rights and duties. However, a disability rights approach to understanding the strength of personalisation schemes rests on the acceptance that those *receiving* care should be the ones in control of how that care is delivered. How can these perspectives be reconciled?

Conclusions: Reconciling Personalisation, Empowerment and an Ethic of Care

In attempting to balance an ethic of care approach with a disability rights approach to analysing care Hughes *et al.* assert that personalisation schemes "reverses the master/slave relation and effectively closes off the possibility of an ethic of care and responsibility in which many feminists place much hope" (Hughes *et al.* 2005, p. 263). This appears to rest upon an assumption that an ethic of care is incompatible with notions of choice and control embedded in personalisation schemes. However, I would contend that the evidence in this paper suggests that personalisation schemes offer instead a reconciliation between a feminist demand for an ethic of care on the one hand, and a disability rights demand for empowerment on the other.

If we consider the evidence from the different schemes it becomes apparent that they can be classified according to a typology which is a type of measure of empowerment, emancipation and protection for both users and carers. Those schemes which offer the most protection for *carers* (formal and informal) also tend to offer the most positive outcomes for *users* (in terms of choice and control, and quality of care offered). Those schemes which highlight the most concerns for carers (such as lack of protection) also offer poorer outcomes for users (in terms of quality, control over, and flexibility of care offered). A simplistic, but nevertheless useful way of grouping the different schemes can be depicted as shown in Figure 1.

What does this evidence tell us about the reconciliation of an ethic of care, and empowerment, choice and control? Firstly, there are legitimate concerns that personalisation schemes give the state the opportunity to step back from its moral and physical responsibilities under an ethic of care, particularly in schemes that are about (re)familiaising care. Secondly, the drive towards cost containment means that the risks of such schemes are devolved onto users and managed by them and their families. Cost-containment pressures also mean that payments are set low, which results in carers often working long hours for low pay with little employment protection. In these situations, both users and carers are vulnerable to exploitation and abuse. In the poor protection/poor outcomes box, low-paid carers run the risk of being trapped into care work with little prospect of employment protection or skills development. Although there is potentially a high 'empowerment' score in personalisation schemes which are undergoverned

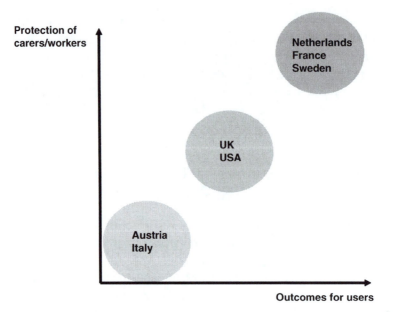

Figure 1. Personalisation schemes: balancing user and carer outcomes.

(because users can control what they spend the money on), the dangers of a lack of protection and governance of the care provided can lead to potentially poor outcomes.

Personalisation schemes introduce cash into relationships that were potentially characterised by disempowering obligations, 'burdens of gratitude' and inflexible state-provided services. This cash can provide a route to empowerment for users *and* carers by introducing an element of choice and flexibility into both sides of the caring relationship. Allowing disabled and older people to choose who provides care and support, and how and when that care and support is provided, frees them up to exercise choice and control over their lives, enabling them to participate more fully in society. At the same time, introducing payments allows carers to exercise more choice and control over the kind of care they provide (including its frequency and intensity) which can free them up to exercise choice and control over their lives (including choosing to engage in non-caring work), which in turn enables them to participate more fully in society. Freeing both carers and the cared-for from disempowering obligations enables an ethic of care to benefit both sides: the moral and emotional aspects of being caring and being cared-for can be made stronger when both parties have an element of choice and control.

The pressures of rising demands for care means that personalisation schemes will continue to form a significant part of care policies across developed welfare states. The evidence in this paper suggests that where personalisation schemes are developed the state should play a significant role in the governance of them in order to ensure that both an ethic of care *and* the empowerment of disabled and older people can be protected. It is not necessarily the commodification of care that is of concern, it is the unchecked, undergoverned commodification of care that leaves both carers and the cared-for vulnerable, disempowered and exploited. The evidence from the good protection/good outcomes box (France, the Netherlands and Sweden) indicates that a benign but powerful welfare state has a significant role to play in balancing an ethic of care with empowerment.

References

Bettio, F. & Platenga, J. (2004) 'Comparing Care Regimes in Europe', *Feminist Economics*, Vol. 10, no. 1, pp. 85–113.

Bresse, S. (2004) 'Le personnel des services d'aide à domicile en 1999', *Etude et Résultats*, no. 297.

Brisenden, S. (1996) 'Independent Living and the Medical Model of Disability', *Disability, Handicap & Society*, Vol. 1, no. 2, pp. 173–8.

Ellis, K. (2004) 'Dependency, Justice and the Ethic of Care', in *The Ethics of Welfare: Human Rights, Dependency and Responsibility*, ed. H. Dean, Policy Press, Bristol, pp. 29–49.

Ferguson, I. (2007) 'Increasing User Choice or Privatizing Risk? The Antinomies of Personalization', *British Journal of Social Work*, Vol. 37, no. 3, pp. 387–403.

Fisher, B. & Tronto, J. (1991) 'Toward a Feminist Theory of Care', in *Circles of Care: Work and Identity in Women's Lives* eds E. Able & M. Nelson, State University New York Press, Albany, pp. 35–62.

Fraser, N. (1994) 'After the Family Wage: Gender Equity and the Welfare State', *Political Theory*, Vol. 22, no. 4, pp. 591–618.

Galvin, R. (2004) 'Challenging the Need for Gratitude: Comparisons between Paid and Unpaid Care for Disabled People', *Journal of Sociology*, Vol. 40, no. 2, pp. 137–55.

Gilligan, C. (1982) *In a Different Voice: Psychological Theory and Women's Development*, Harvard University Press, Cambridge, MA.

Gori, G. & Da Roit, B. (2007) 'The Commodification of Care: The Italian Way', in *Cash for Care in Developed Welfare States* eds C. Ungerson & S. Yeandle, Palgrave Macmillan, Basingstoke, pp. 60–81.

Hughes, B., McKie, L., Hopkins, D. & Watson, N. (2005) 'Love's Labours Lost? Feminism, the Disabled People's Movement and an Ethic of Care', *Sociology*, Vol. 39, no. 2, pp. 259–75.

Keigher, S. (2007) 'Consumer Direction in an Ownership Society: An Emerging Paradigm for Home and Community Care in the United States', in *Cash for Care in Developed Welfare States*, eds C. Ungerson & S. Yeandle, Palgrave Macmillan, Basingstoke, pp. 166–87.

Kreimer, M. & Schiffbaenker, H. (2005) 'The Austrian Care Arrangement and the Role of Informal Care for Social Integration', in *Care and Social Integration in European Societies* eds B. Pfau-Effinger & B. Geissler, Policy Press, Bristol, pp. 173–94.

Kroger, T. (2009) 'Care Research and Disability Studies: Nothing in Common?', *Critical Social Policy*, Vol. 29, no. 3, pp. 398–420.

Le Bihan, B. & Martin, C. (2006) 'A Comparative Case Study of Care Systems for Frail Elderly People: Germany, Spain, France, Italy, United Kingdom and Sweden', *Social Policy and Administration*, Vol. 40, no. 1, pp. 26–46.

Lewis, J. (2002) 'Gender and Welfare State Change', *European Societies*, Vol. 4, no. 4, pp. 331–57.

Lister, R. (2002) 'The Dilemma of Pendulum Politics: Balancing Paid Work, Care and Citizenship', *Economy and Society*, Vol. 31, no. 4, pp. 520–34.

Lloyd, L. (2000) 'Caring about Carers: Only Half the Picture?', *Critical Social Policy*, Vol. 20, no. 1, pp. 136–50.

Mahoney, K. J., Simone, K. & Simon-Rusinowitz, L. (2000) 'Early Lessons for the Cash and Counselling Demonstration and Evaluation', *Generations*, Vol. 24, no. 3, pp. 41–6.

Morris, J. (ed.) (1996). *Encounters with Strangers: Feminism and Disability*, The Women's Press, London.

Morris, J. (2004) 'Independent Living and Community Care: A Disempowering Framework', *Disability and Society*, Vol. 19, no. 5, pp. 427–42.

Newman, J. (2005) *Remaking Governance: People, Politics and the Public Sphere*, Policy Press, Bristol.

Oesterle, A. (2001) *Equity Choices and Long-term Care Policies in Europe: Allocating Resources and Burdens in Austria, Italy, the Netherlands and the United Kingdom*, Ashgate, Aldershot.

Oliver, M. (2009) *Understanding Disability: From Theory to Practice*, Palgrave Macmillan, Basingstoke.

O'Reilly, D., Connolly, S., Rosato, M. & Patterson, C. (2008) 'Is Caring Associated with an Increased Risk of Mortality? A Longitudinal Study', *Social Science and Medicine*, Vol. 67, no. 8, pp. 1282–90.

Pateman, C. (1988) *The Sexual Contract*, Polity Press, Cambridge.

Pavolini, E. & Ranci, C. (2008) 'Restructuring the Welfare State: Reforms in Long-term Care in Western European Countries', *Journal of European Social Policy*, Vol. 18, no. 3, pp. 246–59.

Pierson, C. (2001) *New Politics of the Welfare State*, Oxford University Press, Oxford.

Rummery, K. (2006) 'Disabled Citizens and Social Exclusion: The Role of Direct Payments', *Policy and Politics*, Vol. 34, no. 4, pp. 633–50.

Rummery, K. (2007) 'Caring, Citizenship and New Labour: Dilemmas and Contradictions for Disabled and Older Women', in *Women and New Labour: Engendering Politics and Policy* eds C. Annesley et al., Policy Press, Bristol, pp. 175–93.

Rummery, K. (2009) 'A Comparative Discussion of the Gendered Implications of Cash-for-care Schemes: Markets, Independence and Social Citizenship in Crisis?', *Social Policy and Administration*, Vol. 43, no. 6, pp. 634–48.

Sevenhuijsen, S. (2000) 'Caring in the Third Way: The Relation between Obligation, Responsibility and Care in the Third Way Discourse', *Critical Social Policy*, Vol. 20, no. 1, pp. 5–37.

Spandler, H. (2004) 'Friend or Foe? Towards a Critical Assessment of Direct Payments', *Critical Social Policy*, Vol. 24, no. 2, pp. 187–209.

Tronto, J. (1994) *Moral Boundaries: A Political Argument for an Ethic of Care*, Routledge, New York.

Ungerson, C. (1987) *Policy is Personal: Sex, Gender and Informal Care*, Routledge, London.

Ungerson, C. (1997) 'Give them the Money: Is Cash a Route to Empowerment?', *Social Policy and Administration*, Vol. 31, no. 1, pp. 45–53.

Vogler, C. & Pahl, J. (1993) 'Social and Economic Change and the Organisation of Money within Marriage', *Work, Employment and Society*, Vol. 7, no. 1, pp. 71–95.

Walker, A. & Lowenstein, A. (2009) 'European Perspectives on Quality of Life in Old Age', *European Journal of Ageing*, Vol. 6, no. 2, pp. 61–6.

Weekers, S. & Pijl, M. (1998) *Home Care and Home Allowances in the European Union*, NIZW, Utrecht.

Abandoning Care? A Critical Perspective on Personalisation from an Ethic of Care

Marian Barnes

The adoption of personalisation as the principle on which policy and practices for social care in England should be developed has been hailed as marking a fundamental transformation in the nature of social care and the experiences of service users. This article examines both the discourse of personalisation and the practices that are being adopted to implement this from an ethic of care perspective. It adopts an approach based on Sevenhuijsen's 'Trace' analysis to trace the normative frameworks in key policy documents (in particular Putting People First), noting that critics of care have largely succeeded in relegating care to a marginal position within policy discourse and that a relational sensibility is largely absent within this. The article considers the practices associated with personalisation in relation to the moral principles of an ethic of care and conceptions of the 'individual' within these. It addresses the implications of this approach for broader political and policy issues: the universality of provision, collective responsibility for welfare and well-being, and broader issues of social justice in conditions of vulnerability.

Introduction

In this article I examine the personalisation agenda in social care in England from an ethic of care perspective. Following Gilligan's (1982) early articulation of the debate between care and justice as a basis for moral decision making, feminist political philosophers have questioned the notion that care and justice are mutually exclusive modes of thinking. In doing so they have proposed an ethic of care that can be applied to interpersonal relationships, to political decision making and to specific social policies. In this article I apply an analytical framework (Trace) developed by Selma Sevenhuijsen (2003) specifically to

Marian Barnes is Professor of Social Policy at the University of Brighton.

interrogate policy documents from this perspective and to evaluate the normative frameworks of care contained within them.

This is of particular interest in view of the devaluing of care in favour of principles of rights and choice within the contemporary social care context. An early claim by the disability movement was that 'The concept of care seems to many disabled people a tool through which others are able to dominate and manage our lives' (Wood 1991, p. 199). Strategies to recognise disabled people's capacity to make their own decisions about how to live their lives and what support they need in order to do so have often been couched as claims for rights rather than care. Whilst some disabled activists have sought to embrace an ethic of care together with a human rights-based approach (Morris 2001), others have recognised the tension between the collectivism of the disability movement and the individualism of proposed solutions to the 'problem' of care (Shakespeare 2000). Another position dismisses care as a value on which support might be based: 'The term "care" ... has exceeded its sell-by date. It is undermined by its association with inequality and discrimination' (Beresford 2008, p. 1). Such positions reinforce the moral boundaries between care and justice that Tronto (1993) sought to dismantle. This article considers the consequences of retaining such boundaries for the way in which the policy of personalisation has been conceived.

What is 'Personalisation'?

Campaigning by service users directed at ensuring greater involvement in decision making about service delivery led to 'personalisation' being adopted as the big new idea for public service reform across a number of areas of human service delivery in England, including education, children's services, health and social care. It is considered to mark a radical shift in the relationship between citizens and government, mediated through the way in which people are able not only to use but also to choose and purchase the services they wish to receive. This is hailed as marking a fundamental transformation in the nature of social care and in the experiences of service users:

> Across Government, the shared ambition is to put people first through a radical reform of public services. It will mean that people are able to live their own lives as they wish; confident that services are of high quality, are safe and promote their own individual needs for independence, well-being, and dignity. (http://www.dh.gov.uk/en/SocialCare/Socialcarereform/Personalisation/DH_079373)

Personalisation is hailed not only as the final solution to the problem of over-professionalised, bureaucratic and paternalistic welfare services, and the best way of resolving service provision challenges associated with a growing number of and increasingly assertive older people, but also as evidence of the success of campaigns waged by disabled people's movements to gain control over their lives. Decisions about the types of support services people receive, when, how and by whom they are delivered, are central to this. The organisation 'In Control'—a social enterprise committed to creating 'a new welfare system in which everyone is in control of their own lives as full citizens' (http://www.in-control.org.uk)—has become a key player in and sponsor of government action to secure the transformative change heralded by what has come to be called the personalisation agenda. The implementation of this approach has also led to formal recognition of what are now being referred to as User Led Organisations (ULOs) within official discourse as key players in the process for delivery (Prime Minister's Strategy Unit 2005, recommendation 4.3).

It is now official policy to support ULO development through financial help and capacity-building initiatives. A key role for ULOs is to support disabled people to take advantage of Direct Payments and Individual or Personal Budgets in order to 'self-direct' services: 'Professionals help an individual assess their need and once this is done, the person is given an indicative budget they can use to design the service solutions that make sense to them' (Leadbeater *et al*. 2008, p. 10). Thus workers employed by statutory social care agencies should no longer determine what services people use. Personal budgets are the key mechanism through which personalisation is to be delivered. They are the financial resource assessed as entitlement in order to meet identified need (within the context of overall criteria determining eligibility to publicly funded social care—the Fair Access to Care (FACS) criteria). The argument is that individuals decide where this money should be spent and make their own plans for how their needs should be met: individuals become their own service commissioners. ULOs can support people who may be uncertain about their ability to make these choices and decide where to seek support services and they can also keep registers of people who work as personal assistants to assist in the process of recruitment. The underlying intention of this approach is that support services are focused on and built around the individual, who is 'in control' of what help they receive, when and how.

Personalisation in social care has been the subject of critiques relating both to principles and practical implementation (Ferguson 2007; Lymbery 2010). Early research evidence also suggested that a number of policy, funding, charging and practice issues needed to be resolved, and was cautious about the extent to which significant change in outcomes was evident in the pilot projects that preceded full-scale implementation (Glendinning *et al*. 2008). My focus here is not on how the policy is being implemented and with what effect, but on what it reveals about the way in which 'care' is being addressed in 'social care' policy.

Trace

The goal of Trace analysis is to

> trace the normative framework(s) in policy reports in order to evaluate and renew these from the perspective of an ethic of care. The background motivation

to this approach is the wish to further develop care into a political concept and to position care as a social and moral practice in notions of citizenship. (Sevenhuijsen 2003, p. 1)

It is thus not a neutral endeavour. It derives from feminist scholarship that has sought to 'de-privatise' and 'de-gender' care, but also to expand our concept of citizenship through including care within this. This is evident not only in Sevenhuijsen's own work (Sevenhuijsen 1998, 2000) but also, in particular, in the work of Tronto (1993) and Kittay (1999) and I will draw primarily on these sources in developing this analysis.

The Trace framework is an articulation of the process adopted to interrogate Dutch policy documents: 'Choices in Health Care', equal opportunities policies and reports on ageing societies and family politics (Sevenhuijsen 1998). Sevenhuijsen (2000; Sevenhuijsen *et al.* 2003) has also applied it to an analysis of South African welfare policy and UK parenting policy. It calls attention to claims by policy analysts that policy is or should be based on facts rather than values; the way in which moral concepts and arguments are concealed— sometimes within empirical statements, rather than made explicit; and the way in which values and moral arguments are often taken as self-evident. Sevenhuijsen notes that policy is often the result of complex compromises and one consequence is that there are likely to be contradictions and inconsistencies in the normative frameworks of policy documents.

Policy formulation does not follow an orderly process, adopting precisely defined, uncontested and consistent ideas about positions on social problems that determine an unambiguous strategy intended to address these. Rather, policy embodies different and sometimes competing discourses that may enable co-operation or alliances in service delivery between those who adopt different ideological positions, but which may also contain the seeds of unsustainable differences. Hence an analysis based solely on official texts has limitations. Worker agency and increasingly the agency of service users and citizens can result in 'policy failure' as they resist or subvert official policy, often by taking advantages of such contradictions and inconsistencies (Barnes & Prior 2009). Thus we cannot fully understand how 'care' is being employed within personalisation without looking at how both workers and service users negotiate personalisation in practice.

However, we can establish how normative frameworks are at work within policy texts in order to construct the possibilities within which front-line negotiations take place. In order to do this the Trace analysis considers:

- How the text was produced.
- How it defines the problem to be addressed.
- What are the leading values at work within it.
- What suppositions about human nature are contained within the text.
- How care is defined and elaborated.

- Whether the role of gender in caring arrangements is acknowledged.
- How the role of the state vis-à-vis responsibilities of individuals and private institutions is defined.
- And finally, how a focus on the rhetorical characteristics of the text can support this analysis.

This is the process I applied to *Putting People First* (HM Government 2007), the policy document that sets out the 'vision' for transformation of social care through personalisation. *Putting People First* (PPF) needs to be read in conjunction with other policy and guidance, e.g. the most recent carers' strategy (HM Government 2008). I consider what these documents reveal in relation to an ethic of care under a number of headings and reflect on what this suggests about broader issues relating to the delivery of welfare and the achievement of social justice for disabled people, older people and others who need more than usual support in order to live their lives.

What Sort of People?

A focus on the way in which policy documents conceive of 'human nature' alerts us to the importance of considering how PPF understands the 'people' it seeks to address. What concept of the 'individual' is assumed by personalisation and to what extent does this reflect the lives and circumstances of social care service users and those who care for them? In many places the document is explicit about this—but it is important to make clear and evaluate the assumptions that underpin these explicit statements.

The people addressed include the increasing numbers of those living to old age whose health problems mean they need social care as well as health care; people living with dementia or chronic illness. Whilst they may 'depend on social care for their quality of life and capacity to have full and purposeful lives' (PPF, p. 1), they have high expectations not only that the services they depend on will treat them with dignity and respect but also that they will be treated as equal citizens within services and beyond. As well as needing the support of social care services there is an assumption that people are not socially isolated, and that many are in paid work: 'interdependent on family members, work colleagues, friends and social networks' (PPF, p. 3). However 'the alleviation of loneliness and isolation' is seen as a major priority (PPF, p. 3). This is one of a number of indications that the policy fails to fully engage with the diversity of circumstances in which older and disabled people live their lives. The position of isolated older people experiencing chronic mental or physical ill health is not distinguished from that of a disabled adult who is in paid employment and has a significant social network.

Whilst there is recognition of the significance of interdependence there is also an assertion that people want to live independently. Family members who identify as carers may in some cases 'deny a family member the chance to experience maximum choice and control over their own life.' (PPF, p. 4) Although the carers' strategy (HM Government 2008) recognises and seeks to promote actions to support carers in their own right, the recognition of carers as 'partners in care' is conditional on their not being seen to deny the wishes of the person they care for. Indeed, a key role for carers is to enable 'the person they support to be a full and equal citizen' (PPF, p. 16) (see Barnes 2011). In these formulations caring relationships receive little attention. The focus is on individuals whose needs and interests may be opposed to each other, rather than on the relationships through which support (often reciprocal) is given and received and in the course of which complex moral decision making is necessary to enable both care givers and care receivers to live a good quality of life (Barnes 2006).

That those who use social care services want to exercise choice and control over those services is central to personalisation. For those unable to exercise control it may be necessary to prioritise 'care and protection'. Consultations in relation to a parallel policy of 'safeguarding adults' highlights the importance of establishing an 'appropriate balance between safeguarding and personalisation' (Department of Health 2009a, p. 6). But PPF is clear that there is an expectation that people both want to and are capable of managing budgets, and planning and directing their own support. In the case of those who are already used to other ways of receiving services, there is an expectation that they can and will change their behaviour so that more people will be prepared and able to shape and commission their own services.

Elsewhere I have summarised the image of the 'people' summoned by PPF as implying: '... a high level of self knowledge and reflexivity; substantial predictability in relation to needs and the circumstances in which they may be met, and a willingness to take on responsibility of constantly reviewing whether the support and help being given is enabling the achievement of objectives' (Barnes 2008, pp. 156–57). 'People' are addressed in gender-neutral terms. The only specific reference to gender is obliquely via cited examples in which women are more often identified as care givers than men. There is no explicit recognition of the gendered nature of 'caring responsibilities', nor any discussion of the way in which gender, class and culture impact on and give meaning to the experience of both care giving and receiving. The image of the independent choice maker summoned by PPF embodies masculinised 'virtues' in contrast with the feminised, dependent welfare subject (Fraser & Gordon 2002). It reflects Tronto's observations concerning the ability of those in powerful positions not only to ignore the needs of others for care but also to ignore the importance of receiving care to enhance people's own capacity to live their lives as they wish. This position is both gendered and raced (Tronto 1993, p. 174).

What Sorts of Values?

Putting People First is suffused with explicit statements of the values that shape the policy. These relate to:

(1) The nature of the society to which it is intended to contribute: one which is socially just, which enables equality of citizenship and promotes active citizenship.

(2) The service system to be put in place. This is one that should be 'fair and sustainable'; which enables universal access to high-quality support; is accessible and responsive; is characterised by partnership and encourages innovation from outside the statutory sector; and which has citizens at its heart.

(3) The nature of available services. These should have 'dignity and respect at their heart'; emphasise 'prevention, early intervention, enablement and high quality personally tailored services' (PPF, p. 2), and be subject to maximum choice, control and power exercised by those who use them.

(4) How people should live their lives: independently, empowered, self-determining, in control, within sustained family units.

Reference to care in the section on *Values* reflects an association between care, paternalism and reaction:

> The time has now come to build on best practice and replace paternalistic, reactive care of variable quality with a mainstream system focused on prevention, early intervention, enablement and high quality personally tailored services. (PPF, p. 2)

Care, in this formulation, is not 'mainstream' but rather something to be evoked only in exceptional circumstances:

> to provide care and protection for those who through their illness or disability are genuinely unable to express needs and wants or exercise control. (PPF, p. 2)

Hence PPF constructs two distinct groups of 'people': the first, the mainstream majority, who are capable of and willing to embody the values of independence and self-determination, who have no need of 'care' and indeed would find this restrictive and possibly oppressive. The others are a marginal group, namely people who are unable to live up to the autonomous expectations on which the policy is built and thus for whom paternalism is acceptable. Care elides with protection and little attention is given to how the needs and wants of such people might be understood and responded to in a care-full manner. Beresford's (2008) assertion that care is undermined by its association with inequality and discrimination is reinforced by this discursive construction of care as incompatible with choice, and inevitably linked to protection. Tronto (1993) specifically addresses the difference between care and protection, and warns against conflating the two in precisely the way in which PPF appears to do. 'Careandprotection' is the booby prize if people can't exercise 'choiceandcontrol'.

This construction of care as something that is exceptional and only to be invoked in situations where people are unable to articulate their needs and wants is fundamentally at odds with insights offered by a feminist ethic of care. Rather than recognising care as a practice deeply embedded in everyday life, and a political idea necessary to the creation of circumstances in which we can live well together, it reflects an antipathy that Tronto claims reinforces subordination and inequality:

> In contemporary American society, where a great emphasis is placed on autonomous individual life, we perceive neediness as being a burden on those who must help us meet our needs. We often resent needing the help of others, and translate that need into a resentment towards those who are in a position to help. (Tronto 1993, p. 141)

If care is deemed relevant only to the most needy, then both they and care become devalued. If, however, we understand care as something that we all need and receive at some stages of our lives, and we recognise that 'individuals can only exist because they are members of various networks of care and responsibility, for good and bad' (Sevenhuijsen 2000, p. 9) then the challenge is not how we can *replace* care but how we can create the conditions in which good care can flourish.

This relates to the moral choices that are associated with care giving and receiving. Choice, as understood in the context of personalisation, relates to choice over what services are to be bought, from whom and how support should be given. It is undoubtedly the case that the opportunity to exercise such choices is something that many users of social care services value. However, limiting understanding of choice to decisions about what support services to buy is to offer an impoverished view of what is necessary for a good quality of life. It ignores the significance of moral and ethical choices associated with care at both the personal and collective level.

The next section of this article considers the mechanisms through which personalisation in social care is being delivered and the broader implications of this approach for welfare provision and social justice.

Planning and Buying Support

The 1990 NHS and Community Care Act introduced the practice of social care assessments that were intended to be needs led and involve the person being assessed in the process (Barnes 1997). PPF describes this as having been 'well-intentioned' but leading to a complex system that 'too often fails to respond to people's needs and expectations' (p. 1). One objective of personalisation is to shift the emphasis from professionally driven assessment to self-assessment, leading in turn to individual commissioning of services.

To support service users becoming commissioners, local councils are expected to develop markets to ensure a range of providers that users can buy services from. Specific reference is made in the circular to a 'community equipment service, consistent with the retail model' (PPF, p. 6). But it is also expected that voluntary organisations will be encouraged to provide services that demonstrate the values of personalisation and thus are likely to be attractive to and chosen by these new individual commissioners. Social care staff need to be trained and 'empowered' 'to be able to work with people to enable them to manage risks and resources and achieve high quality outcomes' (PPF, p. 6). Family members and other carers need to be trained to be 'expert care partners' (PPF, p. 5). In making these and other changes councils will also be expected not only to demonstrate effective use of resources but also to deliver 3 per cent efficiency targets.

That these changes reflect the dominance of a neo-liberal market-based approach to welfare is self-evident. Applying an ethic of care perspective suggests rather different questions need to be asked of such developments than is typically the case in analyses that focus on the political economy of care. The process of 'renewing' that the Trace analysis encompasses requires application of the moral principles of an ethic of care to this. These principles—attentiveness, responsibility, competence and responsiveness—were developed by Tronto (1993) to give ethical content to the four phases of care: caring about; taking care of; care giving and care receiving.

Whilst such principles are constructed around what are typically understood to constitute personal caring relationships, they have been developed in a way that also demonstrates their significance in addressing political questions about ways in which we determine needs and how they will be met. As Tronto (1993) notes, virtually all needs can potentially be met through the market, but does this mean that we do not need to depend on others in an ongoing relationship? More broadly—if 'support' is something that can be bought and sold, what does this mean for our moral sensibilities and our sensitivities concerning the needs of others? And if the provision of support follows a series of individual commissioning decisions, how does this affect collective understandings of responsibilities to ensure justice, well-being and citizenship for those who are vulnerable to discrimination and marginalisation?

Thus in the final section of this article I consider the implications of the personalisation approach to the personal circumstances of individual disabled people, people who live with mental health problems, long-term illness and their family, friends and lovers, and also to broader political and policy issues about the nature of welfare and social justice.

The Personal

Whilst the precise needs and circumstances of disabled people, those who live with chronic ill health or with enduring mental health problems are as varied and individual as the people themselves, qualitative research and personal accounts reveal the shared dimensions of such experience. These encompass not only practical support and financial needs but also those associated with the personal and interpersonal emotional impacts of illness or impairment, with the building or re-building of identities in response to changed or unanticipated circumstances; and needs associated with negotiating social relationships in the face of discrimination or exclusion. In this context, the strength of the personalisation agenda is its promise of ensuring person-centred responses to diverse needs. But it does so by relegating care to a marginal position, and by giving little attention to the relationships through which help and support is given.

Two examples offer a useful perspective on this issue. I have selected these because both involve a situation in which individuals (in each case a family member) has commissioned care and support. They demonstrate a form of 'personalisation' in times and places before it became official policy. My argument is that they demonstrate the significance and indeed the centrality of care within this context, rather than offering evidence that it has 'exceeded its sell-by date' (Beresford 2008, p. 1).

The first example comes from *Love's Labor* (Kittay 1999). Here, American philosopher Eva Kittay tells the story of her own disabled daughter. Sesha was born with severe brain injury and has no speech. She is very affectionate and can communicate her love and joy, but needs constant stimulation and attention. She is frequently ill, has frightening seizures and cannot communicate what hurts her or where she is in pain. Kittay realised early on that she and her partner would not be able to provide the full-time level of care that Sesha needed and thus they employed workers to assist them. She describes the model that they evolved as a system of 'distributed mothering' involving herself, her partner, various temporary care givers and Peggy, a woman who came as an agency worker, but who stayed to provide long-term care for Sesha. In contemporary English terminology Peggy and the other temporary workers could be considered personal assistants, in this instance paid for not from direct payments or an individual budget but directly from the professional salaries of Sesha's parents. But the work that they do is clearly 'care work' embodying the moral principles that Tronto (1993) has outlined: it involves attentiveness to Sesha's needs, but also awareness of her responses to the care she is given and the capacity to learn from her how best to help her. It involves preparedness to take on the responsibility for ensuring her needs are met and to do so in competent ways that reflect awareness of the impact of the care that is given. For Eva and Peggy the practice of caring for Sesha in this way involves choices and dilemmas, not only in how to care for Sesha but also how to negotiate their own relationship and how to ensure space and opportunity for their own leisure and fulfilment.

The second example is a story told in my book *Caring and Social Justice* (Barnes 2006). Alan had worked as a mental health nurse, social worker and manager within social care services. When his mother developed a form of early-onset dementia he respected her wishes not to be admitted to a nursing home, moved her into his house and used his professional contacts to put together a team of care workers, becoming the 'team manager' himself. He gave up his job in order to do this and took on occasional independent work. Once again we can understand this as a form of 'personalised support' commissioned by a family carer who also provided 'hands-on' care and offered significant emotional support. In Alan's case this focused around his mother's need in her final years to reconstruct an image of herself as a 'good mother' after an unhappy marriage, a history of heavy drinking and a conflict that had left Alan as the only one of her five children who was still prepared to have contact with her. He reflected on the importance of 'caring values' defining both professional and lay care: 'I never believed from being an 18 year old student nurse about the crap about controlled emotional involvement and professional distance . . . ' (Barnes 2006, p. 112). But he also noted that he had surprised his brother by saying that his motive to care did not come from his love for his mother: 'I didn't like her and there were times when I hated her' (Barnes 2006, p. 66). Alan's story indicates that care ethics are not inevitably linked to love.

Both these stories are told from the perspective of family carers, not from the perspective of a disabled child and a mother with dementia. We do not know whether either Sesha or Alan's mother Catherine would reject the construction of the support they were given as 'care', although there is little evidence in either story that they resented being recipients of care. But my point here is that it would be wrong to assume that the relationships created via the mechanisms of personalisation cannot or should not be characterised by 'care'. Purchasing support does not necessarily mean that the workers who provide support do not care—just as there is evidence that those employed by local authorities as home helps, providing domestic and personal support, often 'cared' for their elderly clients (Warren 1990). But stories such as these reveal the perversity of attempts to 'remove' care from the characterisation of the type of relationships necessary to support those for whom social care services are designed. The danger in such a situation is that workers are not trained or supported to care, and that the skills that are valued are those of brokerage rather than the moral, practical and relational sensibilities of care (Barnes 2006, chap. 9).

The Social

Kittay notes that the model of 'distributed mothering' she adopted to care for Sesha was a privatised model, characterised by 'discomforts and difficulties . . . attributable to lack of social services, services provided in other nations more attuned to dependency concerns' (1999, p. 160). In England one origin of personalisation lies in the perception not of a lack of service but of publicly provided services insufficiently attuned to individual needs and wishes. Those critiques were first articulated in relation to collective provision within residential care and have more recently spread to a range of services provided directly by public authorities, including day-care and personal support services. Hence one aspect of the problem that PPF seeks to address is that of poor-quality services apparently unable to demonstrate respect and dignity. The solution, as we have seen, is to create individual commissioners who will purchase only those services that they think can offer this. This, in turn, requires 'market building'—encouraging innovation in the voluntary sector as well as in private-sector services. It also involves prioritising access to 'mainstream' activities rather than promoting services such as day-care services designed specifically for older or disabled people.

Another aspect of personalisation is thus to undermine the actual and potential value of collective provision. I have noted that Shakespeare expressed some disquiet about the individualising implications of strategies adopted by the disability movement, and awareness of the potential for this was also evident in earlier research I undertook with disabled people's organisations (Barnes 1999). More recently, colleagues and I were surprised when women living with mental health problems used a consultation event to seek support for their campaign to save a day centre they attended (Barnes *et al.* 2006). Much received wisdom was that day centres were a poor substitute for 'mainstream' activities. But for these women 'their' centre was a space where they could get away from the tensions in their personal lives and receive support from others who shared similar experiences. Such experiences are also evident within mental health and other service-user groups (Barnes 2007) and the contribution of such collective, if segregated, spaces to the evolution of the disability movement has been demonstrated (Groch 2001).

From an ethic of care perspective we need to ask what might be the longer term implications of strategies that may undermine both the public provision of services and opportunities for people who live with mental health problems, older people and others to come together and share both social activity and support with each other. Will this be compensated by genuine acceptance and integration within mixed social spaces, or will it contribute to a weakening of a collective sense of responsibility for ensuring the well-being of those in need of more than usual support? And to what extent does this represent the dominance of particular white, middle-class (male?) values that prioritise the individual over more collective values and understandings of what constitutes quality of life?

The Political

The latter points hint at the necessity to assess the personalisation agenda beyond its impact on specific individuals who use social care services. The political significance of an ethic of care embraces a number of important perspectives. First is Kittay's point that we do not all start from a position of equality:

> ...the conception of society as an association of equals masks the inevitable dependencies and asymmetries that form part of the human condition—those of children, the aging and the ailing—dependencies that often mark the closest human ties. Therefore the presumption effectively obscures the needs of dependents within society and women's traditional role in tending to those needs. (1999, p. 14)

Devaluing care risks devaluing those in need of care, and what the personalisation agenda appears to offer is a re-drawing of a boundary that could reinforce the marginalisation of those who are most vulnerable. Rather than asserting the importance of linking care and social justice through challenging what Tronto (1993) refers to as a 'false dichotomy' between the perceived particularistic and compassionate characteristic of care, and the universalistic and rational qualities of justice, personalisation is in danger of prioritising service models that relegate emotionality and messy moral dilemmas to a private sphere from which public decision making is excluded. Social justice will not be achieved by starting from an assumption that we are all equal—precisely because this ignores the real inequalities experienced by those who are dependent on others' support for their very survival. Citizenship cannot be enabled by ignoring the limitations of rights-based models in complex situations where both care givers' and receivers' needs are interwoven (Brannelly 2004).

Adoption of this approach also has implications for collective responsibilities for unknown others. What will be the consequences of the widespread adoption of a model of individual service commissioning for the preparedness of those able to assert 'privileged irresponsibility' to commit to ensure public funding of high-quality welfare provision? A positive analysis suggests that one impact of personalisation will be to expand the range of people who experience the consequence of impairment, mental health difficulties or chronic poor health in old age through contacts resulting from more dispersed access to support services. This may expand and enrich understanding of the significance of care in everyday life. However, at a system level O'Brien and Duffy (2009) have argued that one consequence of self-directed support *should* be that we abandon the search for more effective partnerships between services because this may limit individuals' choices. Does this mean we should abandon the principles of universality of provision, geographical equity and public responsibility to ensure good co-ordination and effective collaboration in services? Ethic of care principles applied to public decision making imply a responsibility to ensure not only the delivery of care but also that the consequences of this are beneficial. When responsibilities for assessing impact are delegated to individuals, collective learning and accountability become more difficult to achieve.

Conclusion

Substantial claims have been made for personalisation in social care on the basis of very limited evidence and experience in practice. Whilst acceptance of personalisation as the basis on which disabled people should receive help can be seen as marking the dominance of an individualised approach to support that is the antithesis of the relational character of care, we do not know enough about how these new procedures and practices will be negotiated to conclude that the *practice* of care has been abandoned. But the discursive construction of care as marginal, inevitably associated with paternalism and protection and subordinate to choice and control, reinforces precisely those moral boundaries that Tronto (1993) sought to dismantle to argue for the necessity of care to social justice.

The devaluing of care within 'social care' policy suggests that those committed to policies and practices that embody a relational sensitivity and that recognise care as a necessary component of social justice have failed to convince. One reason for this is that care continues to be relegated to policies that focus exclusively on those considered to be vulnerable and in need of particular support. The broad definition of care offered by Tronto and Fisher (quoted in Tronto 1993, p. 103) has not been sufficiently developed, either theoretically or in policy terms, to offer a way of understanding what is necessary to live well together and with the material world. This is a task for another paper!

References

Barnes, M. (1997) *Care, Communities and Citizens*, Addison Wesley Longman, Harlow.

Barnes, M. (1999) 'Users as Citizens: Collective Action and the Local Governance of Welfare', *Social Policy and Administration*, Vol. 33, no. 1, pp. 73–90.

Barnes, M. (2006) *Caring and Social Justice*, Palgrave, Basingstoke.

Barnes, M. (2007) 'Participation, Citizenship and a Feminist Ethic of Care', in *Communities, Citizenship and Care: Research and Practice in a Changing Policy Context*, eds S. Balloch & M. Hill, Policy Press, Bristol, pp. 59–74.

Barnes, M. (2008) 'Is the Personal No Longer Political?', *Soundings*, no. 39, pp. 152–9.

Barnes, M. (2011) 'Caring Responsibilities: The Making of Citizen Carers', in *Participation, Responsibility and Choice. Summoning the Active Citizen in European Welfare States*, eds J. Newman & E. Tonkens, University of Amsterdam Press, Amsterdam.

Barnes, M., Davis, A. & Rogers, H. (2009) 'Women's Voice, Women's Choices: Experiences and Creativity in Consulting Women User of Mental Health Services', *Journal of Mental Health*, Vol. 15, no. 3, pp. 329–41.

Barnes, M. & Prior, D. (eds) (2009) *Subversive Citizens. Power, Agency and Resistance in Public Services*, Policy Press, Bristol.

Beresford, P. (2008) *What Future for Care?*, Joseph Rowntree Foundation, York, available at: <www.jrf.org.uk> (accessed 5th January 2009).

Brannelly, P. M. (2004) 'Citizenship and Care for People with Dementia', PhD thesis, University of Birmingham.

Department of Health (2009a) *Safeguarding Adults. Report on the Consultation on the Review of 'No Secrets'*, Department of Health, London.

Department of Health (2009b) *Transforming Adult Social Care*, LAC (DH) (2009) 1.

Ferguson, I. (2007) 'Increasing User Choice or Privatising Risk? The Antimonies of Personalisation', *British Journal of Social Work*, Vol. 37, no. 3, pp. 387–403.

Fraser, N. & Gordon, L. (2002) 'A Genealogy of Dependency: Tracing a Keyword of the US Welfare State', in *The Subject of Care: Feminist Perspectives on Dependency*, eds E. F. Kittay & E. K. Feder, Rowman & Littlefield, Lanham, MD, pp. 14–39.

Gilligan, C. (1982) *In a Different Voice: Psychological Theory and Women's Development*, Harvard University Press, Cambridge, MA.

Glendinning, C. *et al.* (2008) *Evaluation of the Individual Budgets Pilot Programme. Final Report*, SPRU, University of York, PSSRU, Social Care Workforce Research Unit.

Groch, S. (2001) 'Free Spaces: Creating Oppositional Consciousness in the Disability Rights Movement', in *Oppositional Consciousness: The Subjective Roots of Social Protest*, eds J. Mansbridge & A. Morris, University of Chicago Press, Chicago.

HM Government (2007) *Putting People First: A Shared Vision and Commitment to the Transformation of Adult Social Care*, Department of Health, London.

HM Government (2008) *Carers at the Heart of 21st-century Families and Communities: 'A Caring System on your Side. A Life of your Own'*, Department of Health, London.

Kittay, E. F. (1999) *Love's Labor: Essays on Women, Equality and Dependency*, Routledge, New York and London.

Leadbeater, C., Bartlett, J. & Gallagher, N. (2008) *Making it Personal*, Demos, London.

Lymbery, M. (2010) 'A New Vision for Adult Social Care? Continuities and Change in the Care of Older People', *Critical Social Policy*, Vol. 30, no. 1, pp. 5–26.

Morris, J. (2001) 'Impairment and Disability: Constructing an Ethics of Care that Promotes Human Rights', *Hypatia*, Vol. 16, no. 4, pp. 1–16.

O'Brien, J. & Duffy, S. (2009) "Self-directed Support as a Framework for Partnership Working', in *International Perspectives on Health and Social Care: Partnership Working in Action*, eds J. Glasby & H. Dickinson, Wiley-Blackwell, Chichester, pp. 136–51.

Prime Minister's Strategy Unit (2005) *Improving the Life Chances of Disabled People*, HMSO, London.

Sevenhuijsen, S. (1998) *Citizenship and the Ethics of Care: Feminist Considerations of Justice, Morality and Politics*, Routledge, New York and London.

Sevenhuijsen, S. (2000) 'Caring in the Third Way: The Relation between Obligation, Responsibility and Care in Third Way Discourse', *Critical Social Policy*, Vol. 20, no. 1, pp. 5–37.

Sevenhuijsen, S. (2003) 'Trace: A Method for Normative Policy Analysis from an Ethic of Care', paper prepared for the Care and Public Policy seminar, University of Bergen, 19–11 November.

Sevenhuijsen, S., Bozalak, V., Gouws, A. & Minnaar-McDonald, M. (2003) 'South African Social Welfare Policy: An Analysis Using the Ethic of Care', *Critical Social Policy*, Vol. 23, no. 3, pp. 299–321.

Shakespeare, T. (2000) *Help*, Venture, Birmingham.

Tronto, J. (1993) *Moral Boundaries: A Political Argument for an Ethic of Care*, Routledge, New York and London.

Warren, L. (1990) '"We're Home Helps because we Care": The Experience of Home Helps Caring for Elderly People', in *New Directions in the Sociology of Health*, eds P. Abbott & G. Payne, Falmer, London.

Wood, R. (1991) 'Care of Disabled People', in *Disability and Social Policy*, ed. G. Dalley, Policy Studies Institute, London.

Care Ethics and Carers with Learning Disabilities: A Challenge to Dependence and Paternalism

Nicki Ward

People with learning disabilities are one of the most excluded groups of people in British society and have historically been positioned as being in need of lifelong care, incapable of looking after themselves. In this context people with learning disabilities have been positioned as the recipients of care; always the cared for and never the carer. However, more recent policy initiatives have meant that they are now more able to exercise some control over their lives. In addition, changes in institutionalised care, increases in life expectancy, and the growing number of people with learning disabilities who are living with partners have all resulted in more and more people with learning disabilities becoming carers. Nevertheless, they are still a largely hidden group about whom little is known. This paper utilises a personal narrative taken from the author's own life to contextualise the issue. Drawing on this experience, and further research on carers with learning disabilities, the author moves from the personal to develop a philosophical and theoretical discussion which demonstrates the way in which a political ethic of care can serve to reposition the lives of people with learning disabilities as valued and respected citizens. Drawing on the work of key commentators, the paper considers the concepts of collective agency, caring citizenship, moral agency, interdependency and relationality, to explore the positioning of people with learning disabilities in Western society and demonstrate the way in which relationships of care may be used to forward claims for citizenship and social justice for people with learning disabilities.

Introduction

Jaggar (1995), in discussing some of the early debates around care ethics, suggests that care's emphasis on immediate need and the particularities of the

Nicki Ward is a lecturer in social work in the School of Social Policy at the University of Birmingham. Before joining academia Nicki worked for over 20 years with people with learning disabilities.

individual obscures social structural inequalities and could prevent social change. However, as feminists involved in second- and third-wave feminism demonstrated, exploration and analysis of the personal can lead to change being achieved. Tronto (1993), in developing an argument for a political ethic of care, suggests that assessing care in relation to other values can serve to illuminate public life. This paper draws on that notion to analyse the personal experience of care, from the perspective of carers with learning disabilities, to explore how an analysis based on care ethics can be used to make visible the experience of people with learning disabilities who are carers and to demonstrate how this could enable people with learning disabilities to be accorded recognition as active citizens within civic society. As such, this paper is an endeavour in moral inquiry in which theory is considered and adjusted in the light of experience (Held 1995, p. 156).

Historically, people with learning disabilities have been positioned as passive recipients of care and have had their opportunities for participation in civil society constrained. They have been the subject of a variety of negative social values (Williams 2009), including their being cast as sick, a menace and/or a burden to society, and an object of pity (Wolfensberger 1969). These perceptions informed policy towards people with learning disabilities who were protected from the rigours of society, and society from them, through institutionalisation and segregated services. Although the latter part of the twentieth century saw a shift in policy, with the learning disability rights movement calling for greater independence and control, and their voice being incorporated into more recent policy developments (DoH 2001; HM Government 2009), they continue to be marginalised within the realms of civil society.

In 2003 it was estimated that around £4.6 billion was being spent in the United Kingdom on services for children and adults with learning disabilities. For adults most of this spending is on residential and day services (Foundation for People with Learning Disabilities 2003). Adults with learning disabilities are more likely to be living with their parents or in residential accommodation and are far less likely to live independently or with a partner than the rest of the population. People with learning disabilities are more likely than the general population and the disabled population to be unemployed. In the United Kingdom, of the 800,000 adults of working age with learning disabilities, only 11 per cent of these are estimated to have a job (Morgan & Beyer 2005) and of those who are working most are working part time; one study found that 28 per cent of men and 47 per cent of women with learning disabilities who were in paid employment worked less than 16 hours a week (Emerson et al. 2005). People with learning disabilities are more likely to have experienced verbal abuse, and for those people with learning disabilities who are from black and minority ethnic groups they are also likely to face racism (DoH 2001). In this context the UK government has recognised that the learning disabled population is amongst the most socially excluded in our society (DoH 2001; HM Govt 2009).

My interest in carers with learning disabilities was stimulated by the life of a neighbour, and a chance meeting and conversation between her mother, my mother and me. My perceptions of the way in which our lives intersected, and that meeting, are presented here in order to provide the reader with a picture of this event and to foreground the discussion which follows.

Intersecting Lives: My Mother and Me, Amy and Mrs Freeman

As a young child one of my playmates was a fellow child, named 'Lisa', from our neighbourhood. Lisa had a number of siblings including a younger sister. Lisa's sister Amy had learning disabilities though this wasn't something I was aware of at the time; it was something I became aware of as my life progressed. Some of my early memories include Lisa and I playing at being teachers and Amy was often the subject of these games, being taught to do 'sums' and 'spellings'. By the time we went to senior school Lisa and I had drifted apart but my life has continued to intersect with Amy's at various intervals.

When I left school I went to work in a day centre for adults with learning disabilities; my interest in this area of work had, in part at least, been influenced by my relationship with Amy and with other people with learning disabilities who lived in our neighbourhood. Amy herself later attended the day centre where I began my career and because of this we came to have a number of acquaintances in common. Some years later when I was working elsewhere Amy would stand outside our house waiting for the bus to go to the centre and we would often chat. After I'd moved away, my mother would report that she had seen Amy in the street and that she'd always ask how I was, and on occasions when I was visiting we would sometimes have a chance meeting.

Amy's mother, Mrs Freeman, developed multiple sclerosis, a condition one of my nieces also has, and this again represented an intersection in our lives. In 2004, shortly after my father died, I was out shopping with my mother when we met Mrs Freeman, collecting for the MS Society. We stopped to talk and I asked how Amy was. Mrs Freeman explained that Amy was now her primary source of support; she did most of the shopping for her family and helped with the cooking and household chores as well as supporting Mrs Freeman with her work for the MS Society; while Mrs Freeman was in the supermarket Amy was out collecting elsewhere. During this conversation, and probably for the first time in our lives, Amy and I were suddenly, and perhaps momentarily, cast as equals. Although my life had often intersected with Amy's it had done so within a particular frame of reference where I was in many ways the one with the power; it was my position that was privileged. When we were young she was my friend's little sister, the subject of our games and our attempts to be teachers, when we got older my relationship with her was as a neighbour but it was framed within my knowledge of her as a service user, and hers of me as a social services employee, but at this point and during this discussion we were both daughters providing caring support for our mothers. This was most clearly illustrated in the conversation between our mothers, when Mrs Freeman said 'I don't know what I'd do without her' and my mother responded with 'I know what you mean, since my husband died I wouldn't have managed without her', gesturing towards me.

During and just after this interchange a number of ideas presented themselves, first and foremost the idea that this role of carer was not one that was usually seen as part of, or even potentially part of, the identity of a person with learning difficulties. As noted above, people with learning difficulties have historically been positioned as being vulnerable and in need of care and protection; within policy discourse they are the 'service users' and their parents, relatives and friends are carers. As I explored the issue it became increasingly apparent that whilst in practice people with learning difficulties were indeed 'carers' it was a role that was hidden, and largely invisible in the realms of policy and research.

To date there has been very little recognition of the existence of the growing number of carers who have a learning disability themselves (DoH 2008). This group has always existed; however, the number of carers has increased, in recent years, as an unseen consequence of successful government policies in two key areas. Firstly, independent living has enabled far more couples with learning disabilities to live together; the only major survey of people with learning disabilities to be carried out in the United Kingdom found that 6 per cent of people were married or living with a partner (Emerson *et al.* 2005). For some couples they are living together in a situation of mutual caring where each person does tasks for the other as a result of their disability, whilst for others there is a significant caring role for one partner, owing to differing abilities. Secondly, owing to better health care, people with learning disabilities are living longer despite the continued, significant failings of health services in this area (Mencap 2007). Therefore, many older people with a learning disability are still living at home with older and increasingly frail family members. As a result of this the needs of older people with learning disabilities and their families have become the subject of increasing interest in policy circles (see, for example, DoH 2001, 2003; Foundation for People with Learning Disabilities 2003). However, these discussions have tended to focus either on the changing needs of the person who has a learning disability or the need of the older carer in terms of their ability to cope and the importance of planning for the future. In addition, as Bowey and McGlaughlin (2005) note, although research has been conducted in the area of people with learning disabilities living with older family carers, the focus has been on family carers' needs and opinions rather than those of people with learning disabilities. However, according to Emerson *et al.*, 10 per cent of those people with learning disabilities living in private households are involved in caring for someone they live with. There has been increasing recognition that these family relationships are complex; as families get older caring relationships become increasingly reciprocal and consequently the roles of 'carer' and 'cared for' are less easy to differentiate (DoH 2001b; Mencap 2002). Whilst there has begun to be some acknowledgement that people with learning disabilities may themselves be family carers (Learning Disabilities Taskforce 2005), policy initiatives rarely recognise the needs of people with learning disabilities as 'carers' or acknowledge the implications of this for the older family members who have traditionally been perceived as the providers rather than the recipients of care. Where people with learning disabilities are identified as carers this is usually done informally and the information is not recorded or collated systematically (Foundation for People with Learning Difficulties 2003). Recent research conducted on behalf of two of the largest national carers organisations, namely the Princess Royal Trust for Carers (PRTC) and Crossroads—Caring for Carers, found that people with learning disabilities who are carers are indeed a significant group. Fifty-three per cent ($n = 48$) of the groups that responded to the survey stated that they did provide support for carers with learning disabilities. Almost half of those who were providing services ($n = 23$) indicated that they did not know how many carers with learning disability were being supported. Where figures were included they were usually estimations, as records were not kept; however, these estimates suggest that approximately 230 carers with learning disabilities were known to be receiving a service. As many were unable to provide figures and many people with learning disabilities are hidden from services, this is likely to be a low estimate (Holman *et al.* 2009).

The narrative presented above also demonstrates, as Williams (2001) suggests, that care is an activity which binds us all, and here the role of carer has the power to equalise, to undermine the binaries of disabled and non-disabled, carer and cared for, dependent and independent. In the context of disability studies the concept of care has been critiqued for the positioning of the 'cared for' as passive. Language is important (Parton 2003), and it has been suggested that there is a danger that the language of care creates a discourse of dependency (Shakespeare 2000) and oppression (Orme 2001). There are negative connotations to care which have traditionally been associated with charity and as potentially patronising, paternalistic and marginalising (Meagher & Parton 2004), and for many people with disabilities the concept encapsulates a history of oppression that has maintained the dependency and powerlessness of the cared for (Williams 2001). In this context, vulnerability and dependence have been part of the process of othering (Sevenhuijsen 1998a) and the service user has been cast as the dependent recipient of care. As indicated above, this has been the case for people with learning disabilities who are always perceived as the cared for. However, using an ethic of care analysis to critique this perspective, and to highlight aspects of interdependence (rather than autonomy) and reciprocity, disrupts the discourse that creates such binaries and the drivers that compartmentalise and essentialise people either as care givers or care receivers; it provides a space in which to demonstrate interdependence and to unmask the artificial boundaries of care. It is in this sense that Williams suggests that the ethic of care 'challenges the false dichotomy of carer and cared for' (2001, p. 487).

Caring and Learning Disability: An Ethic of Care Analysis

A political ethic of care moves the interrelated factions of care, dependency, vulnerability and power from the background to the foreground (Sevenhuijsen

1998b), and therefore offers a framework to explore and question both the role of people with learning disabilities as carers and how this understanding might be used to promote advocacy and self-determination for people with learning disabilities and undermine the dominant discourse of vulnerability and dependence.

Notions of dependence are part of a discourse which creates vulnerability through a false belief in the independence of those who have not been labelled learning disabled. The critiques of care that are developed by those who question the value of this notion focus on the fact that care focuses on the needs and dependence of the cared for. In this discourse independence and self-sufficiency are seen as ideals to which we should all aspire; therefore, those who are in some way dependent are seen as lesser beings, and those who need care become paternalised and are seen as being in need of protection. It is in this sense that Sevenhuijsen notes that 'too often vulnerability is turned into a deficit or a weakness that should either be denied or suppressed, or be countered by protecting those who can be constructed as vulnerable and dependent' (1998b, p. 13). An ethic of care offers an alternative analysis which acknowledges dependency and vulnerability as part of every person's human experience through which we can challenge the notions of power and powerlessness. In its infancy an ethic of care was counterposed to an ethic of justice within which moral agency is dependent upon moral principles that are chosen rationally and impartially. Such objective individualised decision making requires the individual to undertake particular cognitive applications of theoretical instruments (Walker 1995). These normative assumptions of the skills and abilities required for unilateral individualism serve to position people with learning disabilities as inadequate, incapable of moral agency, citizenship and political activity. Rather, in the framework of an ethic of justice they are positioned as passive recipients of social care. In discussing social work with older people Lloyd (2006) suggests that feminist ethics of care present a challenge to the way in which justice, autonomy and rights are conceptualised. It can do the same in the context of our views of and relationships with people with learning disabilities. Stereotypical views of people with learning disabilities and their capacity, or lack of, to care for themselves and exercise individual responsibility has positioned them as dependent and in need of protection. This in turn obscures their roles as carers and supporters of others in reciprocal and responsive care relationships.

In contrast to justice ethics, care ethics is contextual; 'moral theory and moral principles are defined not in terms of rational decisions about rights and responsibilities but in terms of relationships of care' (Tronto 1993, p. 249). In this sense an ethic of care offers an alternative moral epistemology which provides different ways of understanding and analysing 'the forms of intelligence which define responsible moral action' (Walker 1995, p. 140). It is an epistemology which recognises expressions of moral action through the practice of care and through interdependence, rather than individualised cognitive applications of abstract theories, and it therefore opens up these spaces for people with learning disabilities.

Here I will explore two particular aspects of this, namely relationality and interdependence, and caring citizenship and moral agency.

Relationality and Interdependence

Western approaches to ethics have at their centre an individual moral agent who is able rationally to consider and balance individual duties and rights (Banks 2006, p. 1243). Such assumptions of universality deny diversity, not only in relation to gender but also 'race, culture and class and the multiplicity of experiences of those who are recipients of community care. It is in this way that the ethics of justice denies reflection on connectedness and dependency represented by the ethics of care' (Orme 2002, p. 808).

Relationality and interdependence may be seen as the core concepts in the ethic of care (Sevenhuijsen 2003). A political ethic of care has at its core the notion that all people are interdependent, and this is divergent from unilateral individualism and normative assumptions embedded in moral theory and political theory. In relation to people with learning disabilities it is this emphasis, on relationships and interrelationality, which offers a challenge to notions of dependence and incapacity. Rather than the boundedness and individualism found in more traditional ethical frameworks, these concepts expose the tensions and inaccuracies of the binary opposites associated with care such as independent versus dependent and autonomy versus dependence. This is particularly important for people with learning disabilities who have been located firmly on the dependence side of this binary. Recognising and acknowl-edging their role as mutual carers has the power to relocate them as capable individuals engaged in relational autonomy. Relational autonomy enables people to develop a 'sense of self' because there are others in the world who both 'recognise and value' them as individuals and 'value their presence in the world' (Sevenhuijsen 2003, p. 184). It recognises that our sense of self develops in relation to the others who populate our worlds. For people with learning disabilities who are carers their caring activities help to reaffirm their value and make them feel autonomous. During a recent focus group interview with six people with learning disabilities who are carers, each of them noted how caring gave them a sense of being able to give something back to their family members who had always cared for them. They talked with pride, not only of providing this loving support but also of developing their own skills as they learned to take responsibility for the tasks that their family members could no longer do. For some there was also a sense that doing these things enabled them to challenge the attitudes of others who believed them incapable. Tronto (1995) notes that those who are 'cared for' are not seen by society as rational or autonomous whereas the care giver is; this gives rise to relationships of authority, dependence and inequity. Exploring the roles of people with learning disabilities as care givers disrupts these boundaries. One woman, Jenny, talked of the fact that her brother had always bullied her and told her she was useless and how, through her role as carer for her mother, she had proved to him that she was not. Through her caring role Jenny was able to challenge her brother's authority and his understanding of her as dependent. In this sense Jenny's experience echoes Williams' argument that

> A care ethic recognises that good quality care and support brings dividends for the present in terms of improved relationships, creativity, sociability, emotional wellbeing and greater self determination for both the carer and the cared for. (2004, p. 10)

The arguments presented by many commentators on the way in which care positions people with disabilities as dependent and passive have been as true for people with learning disabilities as they have for others, and this is, I would argue, one of the main reasons why people with learning disabilities who are carers are such a hidden group. However, the experience of people with learning disabilities who are carers demonstrates the value of focusing on an ethic of care analysis in order to demonstrate the interconnectedness of lives and the shifting boundaries of care and dependence apparent within all relationships. Their experience provides a sharp contrast to the historic contextualisation of care and care relationships. Noddings (1995) suggests that the obligation to care is relational, and that it requires the person either to have a relationship or see the potential for a relationship, which is embedded with the notion of reciprocity and mutuality. This, then, recognises the relationship of care not as a 'one-way' paternalising concept but as a relational dynamic. If care is conceptualised as relational, and in the context of care ethics an 'other'-regarding activity, then for people with learning disabilities who are carers the value of seeing them in this way is that it undermines historical constructions of them as passive recipients of care who are in need of protection, rather than as friends, lovers, daughters or fathers. An ethic of care analysis makes visible carers who have a learning disability.

In recent years, policy for people with learning disabilities has focused on rights, independence, choice and well-being (DoH 2001; HM Government 2009), and has promoted advocacy and person-centred service development. However, this is counterposed against an increase in individualisation and a fragmentation of services that has contributed to a loss of focus on the interpersonal and emotional aspects of people's lives, and thus the obscuring of 'care' (Lloyd 2006). In addition, the increasing focus on procedural and resource issues in assessments can prevent the views and perceptions of service users being heard (Lloyd 2006, p. 1179). Gilligan (1995) suggests that justice stands back from a situation and uses rules or principles to make decisions, whereas care enters into the situation to attend to and create a way of responding to all need. In this sense these two models, of justice and care, can be seen to correspond to procedural, as opposed to value-based, responses to need and might link to professionally defined rather than user-defined models of intervention. An example of this was given at a seminar in 2005 which focused on the needs of older families of people with learning disabilities. During this seminar one participant told the story of how one older family carer and her daughter who had learning disabilities had been subject to two separate assessments. The independent assessments had found that both mother and daughter required support with meals and, consequently, at lunch time two different home care workers, funded by two separate budgets, would visit the home to help with the preparation of lunch. Whilst it is right that assessment should give adequate attention to individual needs and desires, and choices and decisions involving others should be negotiated, the procedural division of services and budgets is likely to continue to obstruct rather than aid this process. In a situation in which the needs and roles of carers with learning disabilities are already hidden, a justice model based on rules and principles is likely to further obscure the relational aspects of need.

Walker suggests that some forms of universalist thinking lead to 'moral colonisation' in which the subjects of procedural decision making 'disappear behind uniform policies' (1995, p. 147). Such policies make it difficult to deal with the nuances of interrelationality and the vagaries of capability in the context of interdependence. For people with learning disabilities this links to their invisibility as carers, in procedures which demand that one person is the cared for and the other the carer, and that the carer should be competent. In practice this has meant that for some carers with learning disabilities, even when they are acknowledged as carers, there have been implications for their own support services. Eve Rank, one of the co-founders of the campaign group 'Who Cares For Us' found her own need for services and support as a person with a learning disability being questioned because she was so capable in her caring role for her partner (Rank 2006).

Caring Citizenship and Moral Agency

The ethic of care framework is characterised by a 'relational ontology' which notes that 'individuals can only exist because they are members of various networks of care and responsibility' (Sevenhuijsen 2000, p. 9). Responsibility and obligation in this framework are considered from the perspective of the self in the relationship (Sevenhuijsen 2000), rather than as an individual moral agent where decision making arises through rational self-government. Therefore care, as a practice demonstrated by people with learning disabilities, can be seen as representative of their role in civil society and their position as democratic citizens. In this context active citizenship is based on notions of relationality and interdependence within which care is a central practice (Sevenhuijsen 2003).

In a discussion of the relevance of the ethic of care for social policy, Sevenhuijsen suggests that new spaces will be created for practices of caring citizenship: 'practices in which people can manifest themselves as givers and receivers of care' (Sevenhuijsen 2003, p. 182). As noted above, for people with learning disabilities, changes in attitudes towards their relationships and living arrangements, and developments in health services have both contributed to the creation of new spaces in which, increasingly, they are being cast as carers as well as cared for. In these contexts, caring relationships are increasingly reciprocal and mutual. As such, these relationships are representative of caring citizenship and moral agency. Acknowledgement of citizenship through an ethic of care does indeed open up alternative spaces within which the contribution of people with learning disabilities can be recognised and acknowledged. Throughout the past decade there has been much political emphasis on the work ethic (Williams 2004), and on work as a route out of social exclusion (Ward 2009). This emphasis ignores the exclusion which people face within the field of employment and narrows the boundaries of citizenship. An ethic of care response which recognises 'the significance of people's care commitments, and the contribution these make to citizenship' broadens these boundaries, making citizenship and the practice of citizenship more inclusive (Williams 2004, p. 9).

Caring citizenship is part of a practice of collective agency (Sevenhuijsen 2003), where people can realise their connections with, and commitments to, each other, and within which people can manifest themselves as givers and receivers of care. As demonstrated above, for people with learning disabilities who are carers this can transform their self-belief and offer a challenge to the negative perceptions of others, thereby undermining the othering process. Through these practices of caring citizenship people with learning disabilities who are carers are able to participate in society as active moral agents. Within an ethic of care framework, attentiveness, as one of the core values of an ethic of care (along with responsibility, competence and responsiveness) (Sevenhuijsen 1998a; Tronto 1993) is, it has been suggested, the mark of an 'active moral agent' (Murdoch 1970 cited in Walker 1995, p. 141). People with learning disabilities, through their caring roles and relationships, are demonstrating their attentiveness and their capacity for attentiveness. This challenges the view of people with learning disabilities as vulnerable, incompetent, passive recipients of care. In the context of citizenship, people with learning disabilities are rarely seen as active and are often deemed to lack the capacity for agency. Through their roles as carers they may become visible as moral agents, with their moral agency being demonstrated not through logic and objectivity but through action. As Williams suggests, an 'energetic moral agent' is one who 'spend[s] time weighing up the pros and cons of the consequences of their actions, considering others' perspectives and needs and reflecting on the decisions they make' (2004, p. 42).

Conclusion

Recent changes in policy and practice for people with learning disabilities and their families have contributed to an increase in the number of people with learning disabilities who are themselves carers. However, traditional notions of care, within which the boundaries of care are demarcated by essentialising notions of the carer and cared for, have led to these roles being hidden. This discourse is reinforced by an ethics of justice approach that is dependent on concepts of cognition and objectivity, which further demeans the skills of people with learning disabilities who are defined as lacking such cognitive ability (DoH 2001; Williams 2009), and are therefore cast as incapable and passive.

In the context of a political ethic of care, care is a democratising process (Tronto 1996 cited in Sevenhuijsen 2003). The core concepts of interdependence and relationality expose and undermine the binaries which position people as dependent or independent, carer and cared for and which in turn construct the power relationships that render people with learning disabilities as in need of protection. By using the ethic of care to analyse the mutuality and reciprocity apparent within the care relationships of people with learning disabilities, and acknowledging their role as carers, opens up new spaces for participation and can accord carers with learning disabilities the valued role of active citizen. Through the practices of caring citizenship and attentiveness people with learning disabilities have their skills and abilities to care, and be cared for, acknowledged.

References

Banks, S. (2006) 'Critical Commentary: Social Work Ethics', *British Journal of Social Work*, Vol. 38, pp. 1238–49.

Bowey, L. & McGlaughlin, A. (2005) 'Adults with a Learning Disability Living with Elderly Carers Talk about Planning for the Future: Aspirations and Concerns', *British Journal of Social Work*, Vol. 35, pp. 1377–92.

Department of Health (DoH) (2001) *Valuing People: A New Strategy for Learning Disability for the 21st Century*, Department of Health, London.

Department of Health (DoH) (2003) *Valuing Families*, The Stationary Office, London.

Department of Health (DoH) (2008) *Carers at the Heart of 21st Century Families and Communities: A Caring System on your Side, a Life of your Own*, Department of Health, London.

Emerson, E., Mallam, S., Davies, I. & Spencer, K. (2005) *Adults with Learning Disabilities in England 2003/2004*, Office for National Statistics and NHS Health and Social Care Information Centre, London.

Foundation for People with Learning Disabilities (2003) *Planning for Tomorrow: Report on the Findings of a Survey of Learning Disability Partnership Boards about Meeting the Needs of Older Family Carers*, Mental Health Foundation, London.

Gilligan, C. (1995) 'Moral Orientation and Moral Development', in *Justice and Care: Essential Readings in Feminist Ethics*, ed. V. Held, Westview Press, Boulder. Originally published in Kittay, E. F. & Meyers, D. (eds) (1987) *Women and Moral Development*, Rowman & Littlefield, Lanham, MD, pp. 31–46.

Held, V. (1995) 'Feminist Moral Inquiry and the Feminist Future', in *Justice and Care: Essential Readings in Feminist Ethics*, ed. V. Held, Westview Press, Boulder. Originally published in Held, V., *Feminist Morality: Transforming Culture, Society and Politics*, University of Chicago Press, Chicago, pp. 153–78.

HM Government (2009) *Valuing People Now: A New Three Year Strategy for People with Learning Disabilities*, Department of Health, London.

Holman, A., Rank, E., Ward, N. & West, R. (2009) *Sharing the Caring: Finding out about Support for Carers for People with Learning Disabilities*, PRTC and Crossroads, London.

Jaggar, A. (1995) 'Caring as a Feminist Practice of Moral Reason', in *Justice and Care: Essential Readings in Feminist Ethics*, ed. V. Held, Westview Press, Boulder.

Learning Disabilities Taskforce (2005) *Annual Report 2004 'Challenging, Listening, Helping to Improve Lives'*, Learning Disabilities Taskforce, London.

Lloyd, L. (2006) 'A Caring Profession? The Ethics of Care and Social Work with Older People', *British Journal of Social Work*, Vol. 36, pp. 1171–85.

Meagher, G. & Parton, N. (2004) 'Modernising Social Work and the Ethics of Care', *Social Work and Society*, Vol. 2, no. 1, pp. 10–27.

Mencap (2002) *The Housing Timebomb: The Housing Crisis Facing People with Learning Disabilities and their Older Parents*, Mencap, London.

Mencap (2007) *Death by Indifference*, Mencap, London.

Morgan, H. & Beyer, S. (2005) *Employment and People with Learning Disabilities: A Policy Briefing*, Foundation for People with Learning Disabilities, London.

Noddings, N. (1995) 'Caring', in *Justice and Care: Essential Readings in Feminist Ethics*, ed. V. Held, Westview Press, Boulder. Originally published in *Caring: A Feminine Approach to Ethics and Moral Education*, Regents of the University of California, pp. 7–30.

Orme, J. (2001) *Gender and Community Care*, Basingstoke, Palgrave.

Orme, J. (2002) 'Social Work: Gender, Care and Justice', *British Journal of Social Work*, Vol. 32, pp. 799–814.

Parton, N. (2003) 'Rethinking Professional Practice: The Contributions of Social Constructionism and the Feminist Ethics of Care', *British Journal of Social Work*, Vol. 33, pp. 1–16.

Rank, E. (2006) 'Eve Rank's Blog', hosted at Inspired Services, available at: <http://www.inspiredservices.org.uk/blogseve.html> (accessed 3 June 2009).

Sevenhuijsen, S. (1998a) *Citizenship and the Ethics of Care: Feminist Considerations of Justice, Morality and Politics*, Routledge, London.

Sevenhuijsen, S. (1998b) *Too Good to be True? Feminist Considerations about Trust and Social Cohesion*, IWM Working Paper no. 3, Institute for Human Sciences, Vienna.

Sevenhuijsen, S. (2000) 'Caring in the Third Way: The Relation between Obligation, Responsibility and Care in Third Way Discourse', *Critical Social Policy*, Vol. 20, pp. 5–37.

Sevenhuijsen, S. (2003) 'The Place of Care: The Relevance of the Feminist Ethics of Care for Social Policy', *Feminist Theory*, Vol. 4, no. 2, pp. 179–97.

Shakespeare, T. (2000) *Help*, Venture Press, Birmingham.

Tronto, J. (1993) *Moral Boundaries: A Political Argument for an Ethic of Care*, London, Routledge.

Tronto, J. (1995) 'Women and Caring: What can Feminists Learn about Morality from Caring?', in *Justice and Care: Essential Readings in Feminist Ethics*, ed. V. Held, Westview Press, Boulder. Originally published in Jaggar, A. & Bordo, S. (1989) *Gender/Body/Knowledge*, Rutgers University Press, New Brunswick, NJ, pp. 101–16.

Walker, M. U. (1995) 'Moral Understandings: Alternative "Epistemology" for a Feminist Ethics', in *Justice and Care: Essential Readings in Feminist Ethics*, ed. V. Held, Westview Press, Oxford, pp. 139–52. Originally published in *Hypatia: A Journal of Feminist Philosophy* (1989).

Ward, N. J. (2009) 'Social Exclusion, Social Identity and Social Work: Defining Social Exclusion from a Material Discursive Perspective', *Journal of Social Work Education*, Vol. 28, no. 3, pp. 237–52.

Williams, F. (2001) 'In and Beyond New Labour: Towards a New Political Ethics of Care', *Critical Social Policy*, Vol. 21, pp. 467–93.

Williams, F. (2004) *Rethinking Families*, London, Calouste Gulbenkian Foundation.

Williams, P. (2009) *Social Work and People with Learning Difficulties*, 2nd edn, Exeter, Learning Matters.

Wolfensberger, W. (1969) 'The Origin and Nature of our Institutional Models', in *Changing Patterns in Residential Services for the Mentally Retarded*, eds R. Kugel & W. Wolfensberger, President's Committee on Mental Retardation, Washington, DC.

Care Ethics in Residential Child Care: A Different Voice

Laura Steckley and Mark Smith

Despite the centrality of the term within the title, the meaning of 'care' in residential child care remains largely unexplored. Shifting discourses of residential child care have taken it from the private into the public domain. Using a care ethics perspective, we argue that public care needs to move beyond its current instrumental focus to articulate a broader ontological purpose, informed by what is required to promote children's growth and flourishing. This depends upon the establishment of caring relationships enacted within the lifespaces shared by children and those caring for them. We explore some of the central features of caring in the lifespace and conclude that residential child care is best considered to be a practical/moral endeavour rather than the technical/rational one it has become. It requires morally active, reflexive practitioners and containing environments.

Introduction

Residential child care in the United Kingdom includes a range of provision from respite units for disabled children, children's homes and residential schools through to secure accommodation. In recent years it has faced professional antipathy towards institutional care, revelations of historical abuse and concern over poor outcomes for children and youth leaving care. It continues to be used as a last-resort service (McPheat *et al.* 2007), with those children and young people experiencing the most serious difficulties placed in care (Forrester 2008). These developments have brought residential care firmly into the complex and contentious borderland between public and private life.

Laura Steckley is a lecturer at Glasgow School of Social Work and course directs the MSc in Advance Residential Child Care. Prior to working in academia, she worked in residential treatment with adolescents in the United States and residential child care with young people in the United Kingdom. Mark Smith is senior lecturer in social work in the School of Social and Political Science at The University of Edinburgh. Before that he was a practitioner and manager in residential child care settings for almost 20 years.

Government engagement with residential child care has assumed an ever-greater managerial and regulatory focus. Despite, or perhaps because of, the surveillant gaze cast upon the sector, policy initiatives have been characterised by technical rationality. There has been a singular failure to consider what might be meant by 'care' within residential child care (Smith 2009). This failure is, we suggest, implicated in the poor state of state care.

Residential child care needs some ontological grounding. Fundamentally, it should foster growth. Noddings draws on Dewey's (cited in Noddings 2002) idea of growth to attempt to capture a holistic concept of care. For Dewey, growth incorporates intellectual, emotional, moral, social and cultural dimensions. It is a dynamic process that comes about through engaging with situations of life and with those people encountered along the way. An additional purpose of residential child care is to provide reparative environments, often for children and youth who have experienced abuse, neglect or other trauma. Without providing healing spaces for such trauma, growth (in its richer conceptualisation) is far less possible.

Across the social professions, care ethics are increasingly identified as offering an alternative to technical/rational paradigms. Orme noted in 2002 that they had rarely been addressed in the social work literature. Since then they have attracted growing interest across social work, including services for looked-after children (Barnes 2007; Holland 2009). Their application to residential child care, however, remains largely unexplored. We consider that care ethics provide a useful heuristic both to critique the state of contemporary residential child care and to (re)conceptualise it by stressing the centrality of reciprocal and interdependent relationships in the creation of environments that foster children's growth and flourishing.

Context: Shifting Discourses of Care

Over the past few decades residential child care in the United Kingdom has been subject to shifting professional and policy discourses, through domestic, professional, and managerial to regulatory. The effect of these shifts has been to alter the balance between the private and public dimensions of care. These different phases are, briefly, addressed in turn.

In England and Scotland, the Curtis (1946) and Clyde Committees (1946) recommended a shift away from large, institutionally based provision for children to smaller homes modelled on family living. In that sense, public care was considered to be an extension of or a direct alternative to the family and, like the family, was located primarily within the private domain. The task was thought of as primarily domestic.

The professionalisation of UK social work in the late 1960s saw residential child care incorporated within the new profession. Social work pursued professional status through appeal to 'logical positivist rationality' (Sewpaul 2005, p. 211). 'Professionalism', located within a casework relationship (Biestek 1961), sought to ensure an emotional distance between the cared for and the one caring. While the Central Council for Education and Training in Social Work (CCETSW), social work's governing body, declared that residential care was social work, there remained ambiguity about the professional status of those responsible for direct caring.

The emergence of neoliberal political and economic ideologies over the course of the 1980s and 1990s took care into the marketplace (Scourfield 2007). Managerial ways of working, predicated upon concerns for economy, efficiency and effectiveness, imposed more rigorous external control over residential child care, often exercised by managers with little or no experience of the sector. At another level, neoliberal ideology, which valorises independence, autonomy and competition, constructed care (with its connotations of dependency) as something to be avoided. Indeed, the term 'care' was removed from the professional lexicon. Following the 1989 Children Act (HMSO 1989) and 1995 Children (Scotland) Act (Norrie 1995), children were no longer considered to be 'in care' but were 'looked after and accommodated'.

With the election of a New Labour government in 1997, modernisation was to be achieved through a concept of governance. The governance paradigm spawned a massive increase in regulatory regimes, which entrenched managerial and bureaucratic ways of working (Humphrey 2003). This trend was reified in 2001 through Regulation of Care legislation which established regulatory bodies and inspection regimes to assess the quality of care, measured against defined care standards. The idea of the state as the corporate parent of children in care became a central idea. But while legislation set out where care was to be offered and whose duty it was to provide it, it singularly failed to define care.

Critique

The above professional and policy trends have been postulated to bring about modernisation and improvement. The reality, however, is that residential child care in the United Kingdom is not working. Its failure is, according to Cameron, because any concept of care is rarely seen as visible. She notes: '... the marked contrast between the potential for care within families as centring on control and love, and the optimum expected from state care which is around safekeeping' (2003, p. 91). Such an indictment cannot be sustained merely on a managerial prospectus of underperforming systems or staff, but, rather, is indicative of broader flaws in the conceptualisation of residential child care over recent decades.

Orme (2002) notes that regulation institutionalised the shift of care from the private to the public domain. One consequence of residential child care entering into an increasingly 'public' domain is that its perceived task has shifted away from responding to the needs of the 'concrete other' to echo broader, universalising discursive and social policy agendas. Specifically, it is subject to the dominant concerns that have come to frame approaches to children in neoliberal, anglophone societies, specifically those of risk, rights, and protection. While these may be considered 'taken for granted' ideas, they impose a particular imprint upon the nature of care offered and the ability of residential care workers to deliver it.

Risks

Webb (2006) identifies the idea of risk as the defining narrative of late modern societies. An elusive concept, risk has, nevertheless, come to dominate the thinking of policy makers, managers and practitioners (Houston & Griffiths 2000). Children in residential care are increasingly constructed as being 'a risk' or 'at risk'. Being deemed 'a risk' brings more and more children into the criminal justice system (Goldson 2002), while being 'at risk' triggers inclusion within a child protection discourse. Discourses of protection are not necessarily benign but involve 'a very different conception of the relationship between an individual or group, and others than does care. Caring seems to involve taking the concerns and needs of the other as the basis for action. Protection presumes bad intentions and harm' (Tronto 1994, pp. 104–05).

In residential child care, ideas deriving from risk and protection discourses permeate care. They inhibit what ought to be everyday recreational and educational activities, requiring that staff undertake disproportionate and prohibitive risk assessment schedules before they can take children for a picnic or to go paddling on the beach (Milligan & Stevens 2006). At another level they cast a veil of suspicion over adult/child relationships. This suspicion is evident in prescriptions and injunctions applied to staff boundaries (particularly related to physical touch) and will be discussed more fully in the next section. The upshot of this is that staff and organisations have come to take their own safety as the starting point for 'professional' interactions with children (McWilliam & Jones 2005), employing various 'technologies' such as ensuring that office or bedroom doors are kept open or that children are asked for permission before any physical contact is initiated.

Rights

The other central principle applied to residential child care is that of children's rights. The rights discourse, as it has developed in the anglophone world, is consistent with wider neoliberal positioning of the individual (Harvey 2005), reflecting an 'increasing recourse to law as a means of mediating relationships . . . premised on particular values and a particular understanding of the subject as a rational, autonomous individual' (Dahlberg & Moss 2005, p. 30). As such it can be inimical to conceptions of care that stress interdependence, reciprocity and affective relations. Care, moreover, involves relationships that are generally non-contractual. A consequence of attempts to render them contractual 'undermine[s] or at least obscure[s] the trust on which their worth depends' (Held 2006, p. 13). Trust is a quality often missing from simplistic conceptions of rights, which can distort thinking into adversarial terms (e.g. staff rights versus young people's rights or rights versus responsibilities), stripping out the context and complexity of relationships.

Bubeck (1995, p. 231) claims that public care is 'shaped by the requirement of impartiality', and as such carers are expected not to allow relatedness to influence their actions. There has been a subsequent privileging of methods and techniques, based upon increasingly abstract managerial principles, over practical and relational encounters between carers and those cared for. Whan (1986, p. 244), however, argues that there is a need 'to define the daily encounter with clients not as a matter of technique or method, but as a practical-moral involvement'. Vesting (or arguably, abrogating) responsibility for children's care to abstract principles or technologies may in fact dissipate any wider moral impulse towards relationally based care, for as Bauman contends: 'When concepts, standards and rules enter the stage moral impulse makes an exit' (1993, p. 61). The plethora of rules and regulations that increasingly surround residential child care are not just minor but necessary irritants. They fundamentally reshape the nature of that care towards the instrumental and away from the relational.

Professionalised Care

From a care ethics perspective, 'professionalised' care privileges what Noddings calls 'caring about' over 'caring for' (1984, 2002). 'Caring about' reflects a general predisposition to see that children are well treated but does not require the provision of direct care. 'Caring for' requires carers to become involved in the actual practices of care. At policy and professional levels, the way in which residential child care has developed in the United Kingdom privileges 'caring about' over 'caring for'. External managers, professionals who see a child for 15 minutes to prescribe medication, or visiting social workers are unlikely to be involved in direct acts of 'caring for'.

Yet merely 'caring about' can, according to Noddings (2002, p. 22), 'become self-righteous and politically correct. It can encourage dependence on abstraction and schemes that are consistent at the theoretical level but unworkable in practice'. An over-reliance on abstract concepts such as risk, protection and rights essentially reduces nitty gritty, particularist and relational acts to universal principles. This faith in abstraction is arguably inimical to moral thinking, which 'requires a process of concretization rather than abstraction' (Ricks 1992).

Unlike other areas of social work where workers may get by with 'caring about' children, residential child care requires that workers are called, primarily, to 'care for' children. They work at the level of the face-to-face encounter, engaging in embodied practices of caring such as getting children up in the mornings, encouraging their personal hygiene, participating in a range of social and recreational activities with them and ensuring appropriate behaviours and relationships within the group. They are also confronted with the intensity of children's emotions and get involved in the messy and ambiguous spaces around intimacy and boundaries.

Fisher and Tronto (1990) and Tronto (1994) extend Noddings' definition of care to include the category of care receiving. This important development makes visible the person being cared for and her particular responses to that care. Rather than being seen as a one-way dynamic where care is 'done to' the cared for by the carer, care receiving conceives of care as a reciprocal relationship. It can be assumed within an instrumental policy discourse that residential care workers are dispensers of care. Such an assumption reinforces a view of young people as passively at risk (or simply a risk), denying their active involvement in caring relationships and their agency in shaping their own lifepaths. An appreciation of care as reciprocal brings an awareness of the complex psychodynamic processes that emerge within particular relationships, which will rarely be amenable to managerial claims to 'evidence' or 'best practice'.

Within the legalistic and instrumental discourses that dominate public policy, children have become more 'cared about' than 'cared for'—subject to a benign neglect and denied the more intimate relational care that they need. The corporate parenting role that is perhaps the centrepiece of policy initiatives in respect of children in care is conceived of in primarily administrative terms through the application of 'universalised systems of assessment, monitoring and review' (Holland 2010, p. 1677). Such a focus 'can serve to de-emphasise the relational aspects of the corporate parent's involvement with the child in care' (2010, p. 1677). Holland concludes that an ethic of justice rather than one of care has come to predominate policy and practice in relation to children in care.

Attempts to date to apply care ethics perspectives to work with looked-after children, however, foreground 'caring about'. This identifies care as largely dispositional. Care ethics literature, by contrast, emphasises that care is both an activity and a disposition (Tronto 1994), a practice and a value (Held 2006). According to Held 'a caring person not only has the appropriate motivations in responding to others or in providing care but also participates adeptly in effective practices of care' (2006, p. 4).

Workers in residential child care are required to become involved in effective practices of care. These, if they are to be effective, depend upon the development of caring relationships between the cared for and the one caring, centring on 'an expressive rather than instrumental relationship to others' (Brannan & Moss 2003, p. 202). Maier (1987) argues that, in order to become a medium for children's growth, physical care needs to be transformed to caring care. A conceptualisation of the central features of such care, one that is more grounded in the complex realities of the residential child care context, is discussed in the next section.

CARE ETHICS

Central Features of Residential Child Care

The Lifespace

Residential workers' central task can be seen as promoting children and youth's growth and healing. This requires establishing loving and appropriately containing environments. The arena for promoting growth is the lifespace: the physical, social and psychological space shared by children and those who work and live within them (Smith 2005). The volume and intensity of time spent with young people enables, and often demands, a highly intimate level of care. As a fellow former residential worker reflected, there are not many other contexts in which one might reasonably practice in one's pyjamas.

Key to good practice in the lifespace is the caring utilisation of everyday events as opportunities for therapeutic benefit (Ward 2000). Maier (1975, pp. 408–09) describes the 'critical strategic moments when child and worker are engaged with each other in everyday tasks' and how these 'joint experiences constitute the essence of development ...' These daily events of wake-up and bedtime routines, of shared meals, chores and recreation, and the inevitable crises they often bring, all provide rich opportunities for bonding, strengthening attachments, working through fears or resentments, and developing a sense of competence and basic worth.

Within these events, attention to the minutiae is required (Garfat 1998). This can be illustrated by the sometimes profound significance of a cup of tea. Knowing how someone likes her tea is a powerful symbol of knowing and caring about her; sharing a cup, a medium for being in relationship together; correctly preparing it for another, a gesture to express the far-too-difficult words 'I'm sorry' or 'I care'. It is reciprocal, the exchanges going both ways between workers and young people. While seemingly anecdotal or idiosyncratic, this well-known dynamic has been highlighted in recent research (Dorrer et al. 2008). Yet the power of good care as it manifests in the minutiae has become increasingly overshadowed by more instrumental approaches (e.g. anger management programmes or elaborate systems of rewards and undesirable consequences).

Within lifespace contexts, issues of dependency are highly relevant. Dependence is necessary for attachment and healthy development; secure dependence enables independent functioning (Maier 1979). Yet for many young people in residential child care, their dependencies have all too often been neglected or exploited, making it difficult for them to depend on adults in developmentally appropriate ways. This struggle is compounded by adult reactions that exaggerate or suppress dependencies based on fear, convenience or personal or organisational interests (Ward 2007). All this plays out within an overarching discourse that valorises independence, distorting conceptions of how healthy relationships are achieved and often positioning children's independence, rather than their growth and flourishing, as the primary purpose of care.

Another key element of the lifespace is the group. Ward (2006) connects simplistic conceptualisations of the needs of children in residential care with the trend towards increasingly smaller residential units, highlighting the associated risk of losing the peer group. Emond (2002) points to the predominantly negative depiction of residential peer groups, the current emphasis in the United Kingdom on individual work in research and practice, and the lack of evidence for this position. She found, however, that young people placed significant value on the peer group for information, security and care. Whether formal, informal, fleeting or more fixed, the various groups within the larger group context have a profound effect on the lifespace and the quality of care within it. They take the complexity of the relationship between worker and child, and multiply it exponentially. Related skills, knowledge and adept use of self are all required to tap into its powerful benefits and minimise its destructive potential, yet within current discourses the group is almost invisible.

Love and Right Relationship

The intimacy of the lifespace makes close relationships between adults and children inevitable. Relationship has long been seen as the heart of residential child care practice (Ward 2007). Staff often challenge models of relationship that, while functional in helping young people survive, no longer serve them in their daily functioning or longer term happiness. This challenge is set primarily in the way in which the worker is in relationship with the young person. It is a gradual, non-linear process, rarely amenable to prescription. In this context Noddings draws on Uri Bronfenbrenner's oft-quoted assertion that a child needs 'the enduring, irrational involvement of one or more adults in care and joint activity... Somebody has to be crazy about that kid' (cited in Noddings 2002, p. 25). When an adult is crazy about a kid and that kid knows it, he can, in Noddings' terms, 'glow and grow'. Such relationships could be reasonably described and understood as loving, yet love in a professional context is generally seen as inappropriate or even taboo. White (2008), however, has recently resurrected the word in relation to residential child care. His conception of love is that of 'right relation', legitimising the centrality of love in ethical relationships.

Achieving and being *in relationship*, however, is ambiguous and not easily measured, thus making it difficult to regulate and evaluate (indicators of value in the current lexicon). It is also challenging and complex. Workers must contend with young people's tendencies to replicate previous, often damaging relationships. These tendencies can manifest in seductive or rejecting behaviour, and maintaining related boundaries while preserving the relationship can be difficult. For this to be possible, workers must manage their own natural feelings of aversion, attraction or counter-aggression, as well as any issues of their own that can often be triggered. This requires high levels of self-awareness and reflection, and appropriately supportive organisational cultures.

Highlighting the risk averse and bureaucratic nature of steadily emerging technical-rational approaches to practice, Ruch (2005) argues that child care social workers require containing contexts in order to manage the anxieties triggered by the contentious, complex and uncertain nature of care. If inadequately contained, these anxieties interfere with clear thinking and, thus, the ability to effectively reflect on practice. Her model of containment includes emotional support, forums for making sense of the complexities of practice, and clarity of policies and procedures; rather than replacing caring and discursive processes, the procedural facet is positioned alongside them in a supportive function.

Much of the work of reflective practice centres on relationship boundaries. Notions of professionalism predicated upon distance and detachment further complicate efforts to make sense of, establish and maintain these boundaries. A recent discussion thread on CYC Net, an international online forum for workers in child and youth care, offers an illuminating example that reflects the contentious, complex and uncertain (yet vitally important) nature of relationship boundaries. It focused on the question of whether it is okay to say 'I love you' to a child in one's care and stimulated an extremely active and long-running discussion. Answers covered the spectrum from unacceptable to highly desirable.

Those who advocated for the possibility of 'I love you' being acceptable in practice included context, attunement and discursive approaches in their contributions to the thread. The possibility of love emerging from connections formed in care settings suggests that public care needs to move beyond its assumption of impartiality to acknowledge the irredeemably emotional nature of caring relationships. European traditions of social pedagogy offer a simple, tripartite model for understanding use of self called the Three P's: the private, the personal and the professional (Bengtsson *et al.* 2008). This is a useful shift away from more dichotomous constructions of a personal/professional divide that can inhibit authenticity and spontaneity within relationships.

Working with Challenging Behaviour

Responding to problematic behaviour—part and parcel of daily practice— reflects many of the complexities of lifespace and relationship. Anglin (2002) identifies psycho-emotional pain as being at the core of difficult behaviour and argues that the central challenge for residential workers is to respond to this pain without unnecessarily inflicting further pain through controlling or punitive reactions. Managing reactions that may be triggered by challenging behaviour requires a tolerance for uncertainty. This can be extremely difficult in practice, where there is pressure for quick and decisive action.

When working with challenging behaviour, residential workers enter the most common interface between their responsibilities of care and control. Justice orientations have supported the tendency to view care and control as competing values, with one 'trumping' another in certain circumstances (Yianni 2009). Codes and recommendations, based on justice orientations, offer little help with difficult moral choices involving elements of control (Beckett 2009). Yet, as in good parenting, good residential child care requires an integrated, rather than dichotomous, approach to care and control. Evidence indicates the need for moderate levels of control, embedded in warm, emotionally available relationships for young people to develop self-control, efficacy and self-esteem (Mann 2003). At times, this can be straightforward. At other times, when young people's behaviour poses a serious threat of imminent harm, extreme measures of control are required and often take the form of physical restraint. While there is evidence that physical restraint is experienced by some young people as helpful, it is more often experienced negatively. Impacts can be severe and long lasting, particularly on young people but also on staff (Steckley & Kendrick 2008). Conversely, simplistic efforts to avoid restraint can abandon young people to their own destructive patterns (Steckley 2010) or abdicate intervention to local police, with whom the young person has no relationship. Ultimately, it is the 'relationships between young people and staff ... [that are] significant in how young people experienced and made sense of their experiences of restraint' (2010, p. 124).

Such an ethically complex area of practice clearly requires discursive forums in which staff and young people can make sense of dilemmas, meanings and impacts on relationships. When debriefing is simply another box to tick, or complaints procedures are a consistent immediate consideration and early choice for managing difficulties, important processes of relationship repair (and related necessary supports) can be completely bypassed.

Touch

Possibly the best example of a culmination of the complexities of relationship, lifespace and working with challenging behaviour is the issue of touch. Touch can be a primary medium for the expression of affection. Lifespace work can (and sometimes should) involve touching interactions, and some children in residential care have more pronounced touch-related needs due to previous experiences of neglect. When working with challenging behaviour, touch can reassure and defuse aggression in some young people.

Yet organisations that serve children are increasingly developing proscriptive policies and practices due to a current moral panic about touching children (Piper & Stronach 2008). Cuddles and physical play (e.g. horseplay), once seemingly natural forms of interaction between adults and children, are often banned or narrowly prescribed in residential child care (e.g. side-hugs only). At the same time, children may also have experienced abusive or otherwise transgressive forms of touch, making it more difficult for them to initiate and accept being touched. Skilful attunement, reflexivity and confidence are required to manage such a delicate area of practice. In current climates, however, staff can lack the confidence to connect with children using touch at the time they may need it most.

Residential Child Care in a Different Voice

Gilligan (1982, 1993, p. xvi) identifies voices that are 'resonant with or resounded by others, and ... voices that fall into a space where there is no resonance, or where the reverberations are frightening, where they begin to sound dead or flat'. The voice of residential child care has been flattened by a lexicon that has not resonated with the realities of caring for children.

Attending to the personal, developmental needs in children and young people's lifespaces, normally considered the domestic, private domain of the family, within wider professional, bureaucratic and political contexts is fraught with difficulties. Care, according to Bauman (1993), is incurably aporetic—it has a dark side that can lead to the domination and, in extreme cases, the overt abuse of those to be cared for. The managerial and regulatory impulse evident over recent decades has sought to eradicate the darker side of care. An unintended consequence of this, however, has been to dissipate the moral impulse that draws people to want to care in the first place. A justice voice that speaks a language of risk, rights, protection, best practice, evidence, standards and inspection crowds out a care voice that struggles to murmur of love, connection and control.

Approaches dominated by a justice orientation, however, have not delivered enhanced experiences of care or improved life chance for children. This is due, in large part, to their dissonance with the complexities of caring for traumatised children. Those complexities, as we have discussed, require an understanding of what is involved when those cared for and those caring enter into relationship within the particular and intense environment of the lifespace. The lexicon of care ethics far better serves a conceptualisation of residential child care as a practical/moral endeavour.

Care ethics emphasise the importance of listening (Koehn 1998), interpretation, communication and dialogue (Parton 2003). Not only are these vital for effective (i.e., ethical) relationships, but the aforementioned processes of attunement, maintaining boundaries and containing contexts are impossible without them. The power and moral relevance of the minutiae, invisible in current constructions, are brought centre stage by care ethics' primary focus on attending to and meeting needs (Held 2006). The agency of children is better acknowledged by notions of reciprocity and care receiving. The messy, complex, ambiguous nature of relationships and use of self are far better served by notions of interpersonal responsibilities and concrete circumstances (Gilligan 1982, 1993). Residential workers should not be conceived as autonomous, self-interested and independent but as relational, embedded, encumbered and interdependent (Held 2006).

Fallibility, flexibility (Hamington 2006) and humility, other qualities of care, require more prominence in constituting ethical practice. *Fallibility* refers to the space made for mistakes and *flexibility* the ability to learn from them and adapt accordingly. Humility underlies both characteristics; it is also required for the aforementioned suspension of knowing and tolerance of ambiguity. In lifespace work, children's mistakes are often seen as opportunities for growth and learning. This approach is only effective, however, when the residential cultures can hold and promote a congruent perspective about the errors of staff. Practice can often be distorted by cultures of blame, making it unsafe to acknowledge mistakes. Yet there is something very human about fallibility. Mistakes made in an earnest attempt at caring are not only forgivable but can foster an even stronger bond if they are admitted to and dealt with in their proper context (ibid, p. 116). Notions of fallibility, flexibility and the underpinning humility, with their solid grounding in relationship, offer a potential remedy.

Relinquishing the future of residential child care to woolly notions of 'care' and 'relationship' is likely to be a bridge too far for the modernist mind with its need for checks and balances. This is why Held suggests that 'we need an *ethics* of care, not just care itself. The various aspects and expressions of care and caring relationships need to be subjected to moral scrutiny and *evaluated*, not just observed and described' (Held 2006, p. 11). In this sense care ethics may offer a more ethical and effective means to address issues of poor practice and abuse than managerial and regulatory ones. It does so by placing good care (rather than merely following the rules) at the heart of the moral endeavour. Moral development emerges from reforming practices rather than simply reasoning from abstract rules (ibid). Ethics need to be re-personalised within morally active practitioners (Husband 1995).

Residential child care adds yet another layer to the idea of the morally active practitioner, that of the morally active community. Residential care workers 'live a personal and collective inquiry into each others beliefs and values that in turn models or lives an ethic of caring for and learning about each other' (Ricks & Bellefeuille 2003, p. 125). This enables co-creation not only of meanings but also of cultures within which members of the home can live differently together.

The promotion of sharing, understanding and living values alongside children and families marks a significant shift away from focusing on changing behaviour to enabling collective creation of new ways of being together. It moves away from a paradigm of 'individual moral endeavour to community moral endeavour' (2003, p. 122), one that can hold the complex network of relationships (and groups) within its moral boundaries.

We began this section on the theme of voice and end it by suggesting that residential child care needs to find a different voice. Moss and Petrie (2002, p. 79) offer some possibilities that might find a place in its vocabulary:

> Joy, spontaneity, complexity, desires, richness, wonder, curiosity, care, vibrant,
> play, fulfilling, thinking for yourself, love, hospitality, welcome, alterity,

emotion, ethics, relationships, responsibility— ... are part of a vocabulary which speaks about a different idea of public provision for children ...

Conclusion

By critiquing current conceptual frameworks around residential child care, we are not arguing for the elimination of rights, protection or accountability but for their realignment. We contend that their current pre-eminent positioning obscures the centrality and complexity of caring for children with serious difficulties. Notions of safety and outcomes have come to eclipse growth and flourishing, yet growth and flourishing are the higher imperatives of residential child care. Care ethics offer a more resonant, confident voice for reconceptualising residential child care and more meaningfully informing policy and practice.

References

Anglin, J. P. (2002) *Pain, Normality, and the Struggle for Congruence: Reinterpreting Residential Child Care for Children and Youth*, Haworth Press, New York.

Barnes, V. (2007) 'Young People's Views of Children's Rights and Advocacy Services: A Case for Caring Advocacy?', *Child Abuse Review*, Vol. 16, no. 3, pp. 140–52.

Bauman, Z. (1993) *Postmodern Ethics*, Blackwell, Oxford.

Beckett, C. (2009) 'The Ethics of Control', *Ethics and Social Welfare*, Vol. 3, no. 3, pp. 229–33.

Bengtsson, E., Chamberlain, C., Crimmens, D. & Stanley, J. (2008) *Introducing Social Pedagogy into Residential Child Care in England*, NCERCC/SET, London.

Biestek, F. (1961) *The Casework Relationship*, Allen & Unwin, London.

Brannan, J. & Moss, P. (2003) 'Conclusion: Some Thoughts on Rethinking Children's Care', in *Rethinking Children's Care*, eds J. Brannan & P. Moss, Open University Press, Buckingham, pp. 198–209.

Bubeck, D. (1995) *Care, Gender and Justice*, Oxford University Press, Oxford.

Cameron, C. (2003) 'An Historical Perspective on Changing Child Care Policy', in *Rethinking Children's Care*, eds J. Brannan & P. Moss, Open University Press, Buckingham, pp. 80–95.

Clyde Committee (1946) *Report of the Committee on Homeless Children*, Cmd 6911, HMSO, Edinburgh.

Curtis Committee (1946) *Report of Care of Children Committee*, Cmnd 6922, HMSO, London.

Dahlberg, G. & Moss, P. (2005) *Ethics and Politics in Early Childhood Education*, RoutledgeFalmer, London.

Dorrer, N., Emond, R., McIntosh, I. & Punch, S. (2008) Food and the Creation of Relationship Opportunities, paper presented at the Scottish Institute for Residential Child Care national conference, Crieff, 12–13 June.

Emond, R. (2002) 'Understanding the Resident Group', *Scottish Journal of Residential Child Care*, Vol. 1, no. 1, pp. 30–40.

Fisher, B. & Tronto, J. (1990) 'Towards a Feminist Theory of Caring', in *Circles of Care: Work and Identity in Women's Lives*, eds E. K. Abel & M. Nelson, State University of New York Press, Albany, pp. 35–62.

Forrester, D. (2008) 'Is the Care System Failing Children?', *Political Quarterly*, Vol. 79, no. 2, pp. 206–11.

Garfat, T. (1998) 'The Effective Child and Youth Care Intervention', *Journal of Child and Youth Care*, Vol. 12, no. 1–2, pp. 1–168.

Gilligan, C. (1982, 1993) *In a Different Voice: Psychological Theory and Womens Development*, Harvard University Press, Cambridge, MA.

Goldson, B. (2002) 'New Labour, Social Justice and Children: Political Calculation and the Deserving–Undeserving Schism', *British Journal of Social Work*, Vol. 32, no. 6, pp. 683–95.

Hamington, M. (2006) 'An Inverted Home: Socializing Care at Hull-House', in *Socializing Care: Feminist Ethics and Public Issues*, eds M. Hamington & D. C. Miller, Rowman & Littlefield, Oxford, pp. 105–210.

Harvey, D. (2005) *A Brief History of Neoliberalism*, Oxford University Press, Oxford.

Held, V. (2006) *The Ethics of Care: Personal, Political, Global*, Oxford University Press, New York.

HMSO (1989) *The Children Act*, HMSO, London.

Holland, S. (2010) 'Looked after Children and the Ethic of Care', *British Journal of Social Work*, Vol. 40, no. 6, pp. 1664–80.

Houston, S. & Griffiths, H. (2000) 'Reflections on Risk: Is it Time for a Shift in Paradigms?', *Child and Family Social Work*, Vol. 5, no. 1, pp. 1–10.

Humphrey, J. C. (2003) 'New Labour and the Regulatory Reform of Social Care', *Critical Social Policy*, Vol. 23, no. 1, pp. 5–24.

Husband, C. (1995) 'The Morally Active Practitioner and the Ethics of Anti-racist Social Work', in *Ethical Issues in Social Work*, eds R. Hugman & D. Smith, Routledge, London, pp. 84–103.

Koehn, D. (1998) *Rethinking Feminist Ethics: Care Trust and Empathy*, Routledge, London.

Maier, H. W. (1975) 'Learning to Learn and Living to Live in Residential Treatment', *Child Welfare*, Vol. 54, no. 6, pp. 406–20.

Maier, H. W. (1979) 'The Core of Care: Essential Ingredients for the Development of Children Home and Away from Home', *Child Care Quarterly*, Vol. 8, no. 3, pp. 161–73.

Maier, H. W. (1987) *Developmental Group Care of Children and Youth: Concepts and Practice*, Haworth Press, New York.

Mann, V. (2003) 'Attachment and Discipline', *Relational Child and Youth Care Practice*, Vol. 16, no. 3, pp. 10–4.

McPheat, G., Milligan, I. & Hunter, L. (2007) 'What's the Use of Residential Childcare? Findings of Two Studies Detailing Current Trends in the Use of Residential Childcare in Scotland', *Journal of Children's Services*, Vol. 2, no. 2, pp. 15–25.

McWilliam, E. & Jones, A. (2005) 'An Unprotected Species? On Teachers as Risky Subjects', *British Educational Research Journal*, Vol. 31, no. 1, pp. 109–21.

Milligan, I. & Stevens, I. (2006) 'Balancing Rights and Risks: The Impact of Health and Safety Regulations on the Lives of Children in Residential Care', *Journal of Social Work*, Vol. 6, no. 3, pp. 239–54.

Moss, P. & Petrie, P. (2002) *From Children's Services to Children's Spaces: Public Policy, Children and Childhood*, RoutledgeFalmer, London.

Noddings, N. (1984) *Caring: A Feminine Approach to Ethics and Moral Education*, University of California Press, Berkeley.

Noddings, N. (2002) *Starting at Home: Caring and Social Policy*, University of California Press, Berkeley.

Norrie, K. M. (1995) *Children (Scotland) Act 1995 (Greens Annotated Acts)*, Green/Sweet & Maxwell, Edinburgh.

Orme, J. (2002) 'Social Work: Gender, Care and Justice', *British Journal of Social Work*, Vol. 32, no. 6, pp. 799–814.

Parton, N. (2003) 'Rethinking Professional Practice: The Contributions of Social Con-structionism and the Feminist "Ethics of Care"', *British Journal of Social Work*, Vol. 33, no. 1, pp. 1–16.

Piper, H. & Stronach, I. (2008) *Don't Touch! The Educational Story of a Panic*, Routledge, London.

Ricks, F. (1992) 'A Feminist's View of Caring', *Journal of Child and Youth Care*, Vol. 7, no. 2, pp. 49–57, available at: <www.cyc-net.org/features/ft-ricks-fem.html> (accessed 2 May 2010).

Ricks, F. & Bellefeuille, G. (2003) 'Knowing: The Critical Error of Ethics in Family Work', in *A Child and Youth Care Approach to Working with Families*, ed. T. Garfat, Haworth Press, New York, pp. 117–30.

Ruch, G. (2005) 'Reflective Practice in Contemporary Child-care Social Work: The Role of Containment', *British Journal of Social Work*, Vol. 37, no. 4, pp. 659–80.

Scourfield, P. (2007) 'Are there Reasons to be Worried about the "Cartelisation" of Residential Care?', *Critical Social Policy*, Vol. 27, no. 2, pp. 155–81.

Sewpaul, V. (2005) 'Global Standards: Promise and Pitfalls for Re-inscribing Social Work into Civil Society', *International Journal of Social Welfare*, Vol. 14, no. 3, pp. 210–7.

Smith, M. (2005) *In Residence No 2: Working in the Lifespace*, Scottish Institute for Residential Child Care, Glasgow.

Smith, M. (2009) *Rethinking Residential Child Care*, Policy Press, Bristol.

Steckley, L. (2010) 'Containment and Holding Environments: Understanding and Reducing Physical Restraint in Residential Child Care', *Children and Youth Services Review*, Vol. 32, no. 1, pp. 120–8.

Steckley, L. & Kendrick, A. (2008) 'Hold On: Physical Restraint in Residential Child Care', in *Residential Child Care: Prospects and Challenges*, ed. A. Kendrick, Jessica Kingsley, London, pp. 152–65.

Tronto, J. (1994) *Moral Boundaries: A Political Argument for an Ethic of Care*, Routledge, London.

Ward, A. (2000) *Opportunity Led Work*, University of East Anglia, Norwich.

Ward, A. (2006) 'Models of "Ordinary" and "Special" Daily Living: Matching Residential Care to the Mental-health Needs of Looked after Children', *Child and Family Social Work*, Vol. 11, no. 4, pp. 336–46.

Ward, A. (2007) *Working in Group Care: Social Work and Social Care in Residential and Day Care Settings*, 2nd edn, Policy Press, Bristol.

Webb, S. (2006) *Social Work in a Risk Society: Social and Policy Perspectives*, Palgrave, Basingstoke.

Whan, M. (1986) 'On the Nature of Practice', *British Journal of Social Work*, Vol. 16, no. 2, pp. 243–50.

White, K. (2008) *The Growth of Love*, Bible Reading Fellowship, Abingdon.

Yianni, C. (2009) 'Aces High: My Control Trumps your Care', *Ethics and Social Welfare*, Vol. 3, no. 3, pp. 337–43.

Care as Regulated and Care in the Obdurate World of Intimate Relations: Foster Care Divided?

Andrew Pithouse and Alyson Rees

This paper outlines briefly care as a formal construct of a highly regulatory approach to being looked after in the setting of foster care. It then moves on to consider care and its expression within the interdependencies and everyday moral 'workings out' between people in caring relationships. These relationships are informed partly by exterior regulation, but also emerge predominantly from care as a social process and daily human activity in which the self exists through and with others. Drawing from an in-depth qualitative study of 10 foster families supported by local authorities or independent agencies in Wales, the paper examines the meaning of care in what is often a nebulous mix of paid and unpaid fostering. The moral texture of the foster family is revealed in regard to three areas of everyday domestic life that are often taken for granted and rarely researched: the symbolism of food, issues of the body, and aspects of touch. The paper concludes with a brief reprise of foster care as relational, constitutive and contextual in contrast with care as a professional and regulatory discipline.

Introduction

While we have seen an increasingly interventionist approach to the family in the United Kingdom over recent decades, policy still tends to view the family as a private arrangement in which the state should only intervene directly in order to offer essential support. By contrast, the safeguarding of vulnerable children has been built on a much more standards-based, regulatory and controlling

Andrew Pithouse is Director of Research at the School of Social Sciences, Cardiff University and has researched and published extensively in children's social work services. Alyson Rees is a lecturer in social work at the School of Social Sciences, Cardiff University, teaching on the MA in Social Work. She was a practising social worker and probation officer for many years. She has undertaken research in the areas of domestic violence, foster care, neglect and working with complex families.

framework with regard to parenting and child development (Smith *et al.* 2004). In this context, foster families must straddle the assumptions and sentiments of the private family as well as serve the statutory requirements and public scrutiny that accompanies their role as carers. As Erera notes: 'More than any other family type, it [the foster family] is shaped by laws, policies and practice approaches that are often in contention from differing ideological perspectives' (2002, p. 21).

The rise of both professionalisation and governance in the United Kingdom regarding the fostering task has been noted for some time (Wilson & Evetts 2006). Fostering has come to be viewed as a skilled and effective intervention and we have seen a trend towards fee paying in both the statutory and (particularly) the independent sector and a more professionalised approach taken towards the role and identity of carers (Sellick 2002). A UK-wide decline in residential care together with welfare pressures towards family reunification (which have often failed) have meant that foster care must cope with increasing numbers of children with complex needs (Farmer *et al.* 2005). Accompanying these trends has been greater regulation and scrutiny of foster carers and their activities in order to satisfy the ever-present backdrop of risk with regard to child, family and community. This gradual shift from care as some unquantifiable private sentiment of altruism to care as a contractual and regulated activity has not occurred unnoticed nor without regret (Orme 2002, p. 802).

Care as Codes and Prescriptions

Wilson and Evetts note how fostering has shifted 'from an ordinary activity to one which requires regulation and by extension training' (2006, p. 40). Over recent decades, this gradual encoding of foster care as a formal set of laws, purposes, types, standards and practices calls forth particular personal qualities and characteristics in those who seek to foster and must be matched against these criteria. These laminations of policy and guidance have now assumed a form of complex governance that prescribes, in general terms, how children may come to be fostered and for how long, as well as the nature of the fostering task and who may foster. This regulatory matrix, by no means coherent or straightforwardly applicable, nonetheless has laid down with increasing precision the requirements for foster care services. Its most prominent expression in legislation in England and Wales can be seen in the Children Act (1989) S22; Fostering Services Regulations (Department of Health 2002), the Care Standards Act (2000) and National Minimum Fostering Standards (Department of Health 2003).

The embodied and lived world of care cannot, of course, be grasped or restrained via such protocols and pre-defined categories, which serve other purposes around accountability and control. For example, many of the fostering regulations focus on the protection of children (Department of Health 2002, p. 12), yet there is little detail about how one *actually* protects within the fostering environment. The formal encoding of the fostering task cannot conceivably map the extraordinary diversity of activities, actors and relationships that make up this field of public care nor provide performative requirements for all contingencies. Instead, the regulations focus on 'the procedure to be followed in the event of any allegation of abuse or neglect' (Department of Health 2002, 12.1). In summary, the regulatory apparatus serves broad purposes around bureaucratic control, risk management and service quality and operates at the boundary of the foster family.

The distinction we wish to draw, as in Tronto's (1994) depiction of care, is the fundamental point that regulation and the professionalisation of fostering describes a duty *of* care rather than a duty *to* care. Policy and guidelines address how we should care *for* the generalised vulnerable child. By contrast, foster carers care *about* a particular child. This raises important questions about how well care is understood by those who define and oversee the fostering task. In short, the formal governance of fostering tends to underplay, if not ignore, many of the interdependences and everyday moral 'workings out' between people in caring relationships in family settings.

Yet it is precisely in this interior, typically unobserved, world of intimacy, affect and subjectivity that care is created by the participants in fostering. Complex ties and interplays of affection are for most of us a daily taken-for-granted aspect of our lives (Sevenhuijsen 2000, p. 9). Children and young people can be seen as active agents who can consider the implications of their actions in relation to others. We would argue, therefore, that care, as intuitively understood within family settings, is based typically upon informality, mutuality and reciprocity and that this also obtains in many fostering settings. Indeed, we argue that it is an ethic of care linked to relationality within a private family setting that provides the single distinctive characteristic of fostering. In understanding better this interior world of care we may also learn more about those aspects of day-to-day life that make for a sense of valued membership and attachment for the fostered child.

Care in Fostering: Complicated, Contrary and Contingent

Foster families have typically been cast as variants of a nuclear family, hosting an additional member and operating in the context of child welfare. Such families, or more typically the adult carers, have been conceptualised as engaged in a 'gift-relationship' (Titmuss 1970, p. 60), giving to the stranger irrespective of their social worth and motivated by a strong value disposition towards childhood and caring (Rees & Pithouse 2008). Carers' actual motives to foster are, of course, more complicated than a basic desire to give. Schofield and Beek's research (2005) reveals three broad influences: wanting a second family, wanting to be a family builder or wanting an occupational role in the caring professions. More populist stereotypes view foster parents as saints and martyrs, dedicated altruistic and idealised parent figures who are able to handle burdens that ordinary parents are not capable of bearing. Erera (2002) claims that such stereotypes can be an isolating factor for foster parents; if they are so gifted, then they do not need support and nurturing. It is expected that they will somehow resolve the child's problems, expending unusual effort in tutoring, mentoring and helping the child function in school and in interpersonal relations. They are not expected to voice their own needs or complain about children as other parents do. Contrariwise, there can be negative conceptions of carers as motivated only by financial gain (Chapman 2004), or who become carers in order to adopt by the 'backdoor' (Rees 2009).

Foster carers are not substitute parents, but if they fail to act 'as a parent would' they are unlikely to provide the sorts of affect and boundaries that are deemed essential to a child's social and emotional development (Erera 2002). Moreover, the foster family must maintain its own identity and cohesion while also maintaining open family boundaries that can facilitate some degree of reciprocal attachment to the fostered child as well as managing the eventual departure of this child. Indeed, it is evident that not all families or all foster children simply withdraw their affect once the child leaves the home (Happer et al. 2006). Such polarised stereotypes reveal the way in which popular (mis)conceptions (as with the formulations of broad policy) become a distorting gloss on the empirical world of fostering.

Thus foster care is not necessarily time limited and contractually bestowed, but more open ended and contingent upon human interdependencies which call forth an emotional disposition that assumes some form of ongoing connection. This can be seen in Tronto's formulation of care which describes a process from caring about someone with needs, to taking responsibility for the need, then meeting the need by caring for the person, who in turn will respond to the care received (1994, pp. 108–09). As Tronto and others point out, care has long been closely connected to women and thereby presumed to be socially constituted within the household, so that it generally becomes the work of the least well off (Finch & Groves 1983; Orme 2002). Those who are wealthy are likely to pass on the work of caring to others. Gender, race and class are related to caring in terms of those who are often found in the caring roles. Care work, then, has often been overlooked or devalued because it is associated with the private and the emotional. By contrast, technical rationality, autonomy and material accomplishment have been cast by an individualising Western culture as ideal human attributes (Tronto 1994, p. 117). Yet as Parton observes, 'care is central to everyone; it is not a parochial concern of women alone' (2003, p. 11). Hence, part of the professionalisation of the fostering agenda has been about promoting the intrinsic worth of the caring role, yet this, as noted above, has also been accompanied by a less welcome regulatory approach to fostering that is deemed inimical to the caring impulse (Parton 2003, p. 2). We must look to the empirical character of care in specific settings if we are to understand its multiple, varied and often practical manifestation. We find these particularly in the mundane events and rhythms of family living, which we now present selectively from the following study.

A Study of Everyday Care

Our study (see Rees 2009) comprises a small-scale, in-depth, multi-method qualitative analysis of a purposive sample of stable foster care placements. We defined 'stable' as families having provided placements that had not been disrupted for at least one child and where they had been carers for over a year. Our assumption was that stable placements provided by experienced carers might make for easier access and participation, which in turn could facilitate a more revealing encounter in which the mundane processes of day-to-day care-based relationships could be jointly explored and illuminated. We do not assume, however, that placements that lack stability somehow also lack the care elements and qualities that we describe below. The carers were chosen from three types of providers of mainstream foster care in the United Kingdom: an independent agency; a local authority with an extra support service provided by the voluntary sector; and a local authority with no specialist support service. While agency context was a relevant variable in the study, we do not address this aspect here in any detail, but instead focus on a delimited field of everyday family activities in which care relations are constituted.

Ten foster families took part in the study, eight of whom were heterosexual couple-carers and two single female carers. Their ages ranged from 39 to 61 (mean 50.2) and all were white British. They had been carers for an average of 9.5 years. Eight of the families had birth children as well as foster children. Although many birth children were over 18 years of age, all families with birth children had at least one still living at home. There were 16 foster children aged 9–16 who we refer to interchangeably as children or young people living with the families. Six of the young people were from ethnic minorities and ten were white British.

Over a period of 18 months the research aimed to gain the shifting perspectives of all members of the foster families via a variety of sequential data-generation techniques. Initially, carers completed questionnaires exploring motivation and capturing demographic details. In-depth semi-structured inter-views were then carried out with 15 carers, some lasting up to three and a half hours. Seventeen children were then interviewed: eight foster children, eight birth children and one adopted child. All children and carers were invited to complete audio diaries over a one-week period and seven carers, two birth children, one adopted child and four foster children participated. Another foster child completed a written diary. In all, nearly 60 hours of audio-recorded interviews and audio diaries were transcribed and subjected to qualitative methods of coding and thematic analysis. Pseudonyms were used throughout the study and other potential identifiers were omitted to preserve anonymity. From these sources we offer a small number of insights into aspects of mundane daily living that both constitute and mediate care: food and meal times and issues of the body such as appearance and touch. Our findings depict care as temporal, jointly constructed, commonsensical, but profound in its consequences for the child's sense of identity and well-being.

Food and Meal Times

The meaning of food and everyday activity surrounding meal times has rarely been examined for children 'looked after' in foster or residential care, with the exception of practical training (Hamil 2007). Guidelines for foster carers tend to emphasise nutrition, with the social aspects of meals and eating mentioned relatively briefly (see, for example, The Caroline Walker Trust 2001). With the exception of diet being mentioned as a possible health need, there is little explicit mention of food in the National Minimum Fostering Standards (Department of Health 2003). Gillen *et al*. note that food is of considerable symbolic and cultural significance in that 'eating in families is immersed in social contexts that provide meaning' (2008, p. 12). In essence, meal times allow families to enact and display family life and are fundamental to the way people recognise themselves as not only being in a family but in a particular class of family (Finch 2007; Ashley *et al*. 2004, p. 128).

Meal times thus help to structure and demarcate family life. Children who have suffered neglect and chaotic parenting may display some ambivalence towards food and shared meal times, which they have come to experience as sites of anxiety and potential distress. Hence, the way that food and meal times are managed by foster families can be vital in helping the young person feel secure in their new setting. Brannen *et al*. (1994) note that eating together is a particularly important way of incorporating new household members and a means of helping to develop a sense of cohesion between reconstituted families. Thus food and meal times are an important medium through which children can become known and accepted by a family, or, in some instances perceived as different and unwelcome. Foster carers in our study used a number of strategies around food and meals in order to enable children to feel part of their family. Giving children choice about food was seen as important by carers and children. Carers were deliberate in their deployment of choice to signal interest and affect when children first arrived:

> When Lilly first came, I said 'What do you like? I know what Jayne (other foster child) likes, I like pizza, but what do you like?' So it softens the blow a bit. Food is important to give them what they like. You got to take it, these kids have been uprooted into foster care, just dropping on somebody's doorstep. Imagine if it was kids of mine ... (Female foster carer, family ten)

Responding to preferences became an indicator of recognition and affirmation, which oiled the wheels of family relations and helped legitimate the foster child's position in the family. Such adaptation might not be appropriate in all family circumstances, but seemed to be functional in the foster family. Families seemed to be able to strike a balance between indulgence and providing a tailored response to the needs and desires of the child, who in turn adapted to the social mores of the family. As Mennell *et al.* observe succinctly: 'Feeding children gets caught up in loving and pleasing them, expressed by, among other things, acquiescence to their demands for one food rather than another' (1992, p. 107).

Knowledge of the child's 'food persona' (Brannen *et al.* 1994, p. 162) was part of getting to know a child and catering for their needs. Food was one of the most commonly raised themes emerging, often unprompted, in the interviews with adults and children. Children especially talked about food, particularly in the audio diaries in which they recounted their day. The type and amount of food consumed appeared to help them understand the structure of daily family life and seemed to have greatly enhanced their enjoyment of the day. One young person contrasted a much more stressful history of meal times with his new life:

> I used to have to eat very quickly because if I didn't there would be hands in, nicking bits of food because there was so many of us ... we used to fight for food and stuff ... Now I don't have to fight for the food but I still eat very, very quickly ... (Male foster child, family eight)

In a later interview, his foster carer describes her approach to this child and how she uses meal times to engage with the children in her family more generally:

> [He] attaches a lot of importance to his food. He has a good appetite but I don't think he has beaten me yet! The evening meal is the one time we are all together. The family meal on a Sunday is a good time to talk to the whole family. They are sitting targets then once the food is on the plates, they are not going to leave ... (Female foster carer, family eight)

Food has the potential on many levels to create a warm, physical and satisfying experience and carers across the study provided numerous insights into the way food and meal times operated subtly as a mechanism for communication, affirmation, membership, joy and laughter as well as opportunities for conflict and tension. The child becomes part of the enactment of family by their very doing of a communal activity such as a shared meal. Food is a neglected topic and merits more analytic focus with regard to the foster home and the child's incorporation into the family network (Hamil 2007).

Issues of the Body

The body, while central in social science literature (Douglas 1984; Morgan 1996), has rarely been examined within fostering and other social work. Nor does the body per se feature in fostering standards and procedures other than by implication in more general statements about developmental needs, health, safeguarding and self-care. In recent years there has been an increased *sociological* focus on body matters relating to children (James *et al.* 1998). Intellectually, notions of the body and childhood have moved from measuring to meaning; to what the body represents culturally rather than measuring its size and changes to it.

Usually in foster care the child as 'stranger' becomes a family intimate in a relatively short period of time. Indeed, it is somehow assumed that the child stranger can enter a family with relative ease (doubtless with some discomfort) without first understanding the nuanced and subtly negotiated arena of the new family. The family, in this sense, comprises both physical and emotional practices that have to be learned by the foster child. At the same time, the family has to learn to respond to the child and their needs and demands. It is the recognition and careful consideration of the ways of dealing with corporeal issues that contribute to successful fostering and foster care relationships. These aspects of both physical intimacy and emotional work rarely surface within empirical sources about fostering, nor within much of the procedural and administrative discourse of fostering. This absence is curious. Family practices are, to a very large extent, bodily practices (birth, death, sexuality, hygiene) (Morgan 1996, p. 113). Indeed, the theme of bodily comfort arose often in data from the children. For example, the importance and symbolic nature of bodily care and the harmful impact of its absence (see Cameron & Maginn 2008, p. 1156) was noted by the foster children, particularly the girls who found the ordered routine of personal, physical care comforting and reassuring and valued its nurturing aspects.

Foster children need to learn that they can be nurtured and enjoy it. They can then, in turn, develop self-nurturing capacities as well as learn to nurture others. This much was evident from the data that revealed the critical importance of bodily care as a basic indicator of warmth and inclusion in the family. For example, from the audio diary data the following extract from a young girl typified the sorts of ordinary events around bodily care that helped reinforce a sense of order, warmth and security:

> Now I'm in bed and after dinner we had some chocolate chip ice cream. Then I went up for a nice warm bath and washed my hair. Then I done my teeth and went downstairs to say goodnight ... and then I jumped in bed ... I am going to have a very nice sleep. Night, night. (Female foster child, family three)

Carers felt that boys also appreciated physical comforts and the affect this expressed:

> He returned [after running away] and he hadn't washed or anything ... I said have a hot shower, look after yourself and go to bed because it looks as if you haven't slept for days ... (Female foster carer, family eight)

Here the foster carer demonstrates her care for the young person, regardless of his behaviour, by putting his physical needs first. There were similar accounts from other carers about physical care as a prime display of caring, despite a child's problematic behaviour in or outside the home.

In her study of families, Backett-Milburn (2000) suggests that children's bodies often need fewer resources and care to maintain them, as children are naturally active and healthy. However, an emphasis on bodily care within fostering serves far more than to maintain the body and acts as a clear display of caring. Our data revealed predictable differences with regard to the way in which gender informed carer approaches to bodily caring. Girls seemed to benefit from physical care that was gender sensitive, involving the female carer and female child in more encounters than was the case between boys and carers:

> This morning was spent with the girls, washing hair, having baths and talking.
> (Audio diary extract, female foster carer, family one)

Not only bodily care but children's clothing is gender linked (Barnes & Eichler 1992). One carer in particular made reference to gender and the need for the female body to reflect the femininity of the child in question. While this could of course be cast as some unreflective promotion of a gender stereotype, it has to be understood in the context of carer assumptions about their role. For example, the carer described a girl who came to her wearing 'scruffy, boyish'-looking clothes and with her head having been shaved; the girl came to the placement with 'pitifully few belongings in a plastic bin bag'. The carer perceived a need for the girl to re-define herself and her gender, so that she could begin to find a secure positive identity and to value herself. This also helped the child to feel that she could fit in with others. Finding her sense of femininity and a feminine identity appeared to be part of this:

> We grew her hair, we went out, we bought her new clothes, pinks and lilacs and, we got rid of everything from before and we went out and fitted her out in all the girl colours. I mean, we couldn't do anything with her hair, so we bought some slides and one thing and another and slowly she came to be this little girl.
> (Female foster carer, family three)

This example of long-term gender-specific nurturing was by no means unique and is cited here to point to the way attention to the exterior of the body can express affect. The child's visible appearance is acted upon by others, as it provides an acceptable surface; it exhibits the status of its carers and is also a moral statement of adult achievements and failures (Christensen 2000, p. 48; Morgan 1996, p. 128). Given the pressure on the acquisition of commodities in late modern society, there is a tendency for individuals to place ever more importance on the appearance and presentation of the body as constitutive of self-identity (Williams & Bendelow 1998, p. 73). Yet the provision of clothing was typically understood by carers much more as representative of thoughtful nurturing and care rather than a display of 'status'. For example, one respondent prided herself on the foster children being indistinguishable from her own children with respect to their external appearances:

> They never ever get it right. People who don't know us very well but know we foster, never ever once have got it right [i.e. can distinguish fostered child from carer's own children]. (Female foster carer, family three)

Privacy and Touch

Rules around uncovering the body were explicit in all of the families in this study. The revealing of the body was often restricted to private space. Bedroom space was clearly delineated and all families had a clear rule that everyone knocks on a bedroom door before entering; in some of the families the rule was that nobody enters anyone else's bedroom. While the gender of the foster children coming to the home was central to the functioning of the family, all carers spoke of a shared norm of being dressed, irrespective of the child's gender:

> For a start you can't walk around in pyjamas like you would with your own child; making sure everyone has their bedroom door shut when they go to bed. It just comes natural; it is just part and parcel of life now ... (Female foster carer, family seven)

These explicit and implicit rules impacted upon birth children too and inevitably influenced their behaviour. It is difficult to imagine being as mindful of the body at all times within one's home as is the young respondent below:

> You can't just lay around in your pyjamas watching telly and eating chocolate. (Male birth child, family six)

A sense of potential risk lay behind much of these explicit and tacit rulings that made the body a self-conscious object in day-to-day domestic arrangements. Several carers spoke of caring for children who had been abused and who had been abusers. All families had developed over time a set of house rules and practices that constituted a 'curriculum' for the body (Simpson 2000) and covered aspects of dress, privacy, personal hygiene, access to rooms and movement at night. The covering of the body and the heightened sense of privacy in relation to the body in foster homes raises questions of how touch occurs. Touch is vital for all people as reassurance and a means of communication. Yet because of the risk of allegations about carers by foster children (Sinclair *et al.* 2004) and because of the bureaucratisation of the caring role, it may be that some children in foster care are rarely touched.

Foster children and birth children noted the importance of touch as signifying care and concern over and above that which had been anticipated. Those carers who were willing to engage in this way were deemed by some young people to be demonstrating exceptional care. This was the case for boys and girls alike:

> He [foster carer] is a real people person. He is a very funny person and a very serious person as well. I found living with him he'd mess about 'do you want a fight' just messing around we just got on so well from the moment I came here. He was very hands on, he'd put his arms round me and stuff. Hazel [female carer] would be a motherly hug. (Male foster child, family eight)
>
> ... during the first 6–8 months, I wouldn't say that Susie [foster child] and I had had a conversation. I tried very hard but nothing at all. Now she has started to talk to me ... Some children want this want that, she is not like that. I don't know what makes it work. She just loves being cuddled [now]. Susie was never like that but now I often give her a cwtch [Welsh for cuddle]. I tug her hair a little bit, playful you know and she loves it ... (Female adult birth child, family seven)

In the latter extract we have an adult birth child reflecting on the needs of the child in foster care and on how, as the child's confidence had grown, she benefited increasingly from physical touch. By contrast, the social work profession has become much less likely to use touch as a means of reassurance to children within the care relationship. Piper *et al*. see this lack of touch as part of a culture of concern about the body and risk, and some distance from a traditional culture of care in social work (2006, p. 151). However, this fear of allegation and its negative impact on a more spontaneous caring interplay has been noted in focus groups undertaken with male foster carers (Gilligan 2000, p. 67).

While there is official recognition within policy that touch can be therapeutic (Department of Health 2002), many child-related settings are becoming no touch zones for fear that touch is misinterpreted. Touching is still nevertheless regarded as vital to children's emotional and physical development. Many children in the care system have come not to expect physical contact with their carers and this makes it difficult for them to express emotion. Regulations on touch avoidance and safe working in care settings stem from and reinforce a risk-averse and fear culture in social work that not only polices professional touch but the possibility of touch (see Piper *et al*. 2006, p. 154). While we have seen an increase in regulations around safe care, the number of false allegations against professionals in social care has remained more or less static (Piper *et al*. 2006). Nonetheless, such allegations are a major cause of stress for carers and play a part in their giving up fostering (Wilson *et al*. 2000).

Carers, aware of risks around allegations of improper touch, acknowledged the need to be selective with whom and when they would cuddle, offering a tailored and individualised approach. It is thought that girls generally touch or are touched more than boys (Coffey & Delamont 2000). By contrast, there is an implicit assumption that men are more of a risk to children than are women or older girls (Piper *et al*. 2006). This risk and safe care discourse stands in some opposition to that which invites and encourages men to develop 'caring masculinities' (Jones 2001) and arguably undermines men's work with children, thus resisting change to occupation and family sex roles (Piper *et al*. 2006, p. 159). While positive touch in fostering can be beneficial, it remains a challenging everyday aspect of care to be constantly navigated against a backdrop of uncertainty and potential risk.

Conclusion

This difficult duality—the body as a site of both care and risk—cannot easily be resolved by some blanketing regulatory requirement that hermetically insulates the child from the foster family. Carers and their birth children in this study drew upon an amalgam of experience, formal training and lay theorising about what might be appropriate physical comfort and contact with a specific child at a particular moment or stage. This largely tacit reasoning or 'interactional expertise' (Collins & Evans 2007) stemmed from immersion within the discursive social life of the foster home and its immediate network of kin, friends and key professionals. From this community of interest, the carers and their children developed their own assumptions and pragmatic rules of thumb about fostering, which for them was caring as an applied art of everyday living. Thus care was not understood as some abstract disinterested ethic of altruism, or as some distanced professional intervention devoid of intimacy. Instead, care was understood as a practical and emotional application of concern and affect, expressed in mundane everyday ways as instanced here; through food and food choices and the togetherness of meal times, through personal clothing and, where trust and risk allowed, through touch. These sorts of nuanced and subtle aspects of day-to-day care cannot, of course, be legislated and somehow encoded in procedures and guidance. Yet, as Horlick-Jones (2005) observes more generally of public services, the more externally driven systems of procedural control fail to recognise and integrate tacit sources of understanding that underlie everyday practice, the less effective these will be. Quite how this growing divide between care defined in the regulatory universe of law, procedures and guidance can mesh more usefully with care as produced in the sensuous and complex world of fostering is something of a conundrum, and likely to remain so.

References

Ashley, B., Hollows, J., Jones, S. & Taylor, B. (2004) *Food and Cultural Studies*, Routledge, London.

Backett-Milburn, K. (2000) 'Children, Parents and the Construction of the Healthy Body in Middle Class Families', in *The Body, Childhood and Society*, ed. A. Prout, Macmillan, Basingstoke, pp. 79–100.

Barnes, R. & Eichler, J. (1992) *Dress and Gender: Making and Meaning in Cultural Contexts*, Berg, Oxford.

Brannen, J., Dodd, K., Oakley, A. & Storey, P. (1994) *Young People, Health and Family Life*, Open University Press, Buckingham.

Cameron, R. J. & Maginn, C. (2008) 'The Authentic Warmth Dimension of Professional Childcare', *British Journal of Social Work*, Vol. 38, no. 6, pp. 1151–72.

Care Standards Act (2000) Available at: <http://www.opsi.gov.uk/acts/acts2000/ukpga_20 000014_en_1> (accessed 20 July 2010).

Caroline Walker Trust, The (2001) *Eating Well for Looked After Children and Young People: Nutritional and Practical Guidelines. Report of an Expert Working Group*, The Caroline Walker Trust, St Austell.

Chapman, T. (2004) *Gender and Domestic Life: Changing Practices in Families and Households*, Palgrave, Basingstoke.

Christensen, P. (2000) 'Childhood and the Cultural Constitution of Vulnerable Bodies', in *The Body, Childhood and Society*, ed. A. Prout, Macmillan, Basingstoke, pp. 38–67.

Coffey, A. & Delamont, S. (2000) *Feminism and the Classroom Teacher: Research, Praxis and Pedagogy*, RoutledgeFalmer, London.

Collins, H. & Evans, R. (2007) *Rethinking Expertise*, University of Chicago Press, Chicago.

Department of Health (2002) Fostering Services Regulations, available at: <http://www.opsi.gov.uk/si/si2002/20020057.htm> (accessed 20 July 2010).

Department of Health (2003) National Minimum Fostering Standards, England, available at: <http://www.dh.gov.uk/assetRoot/04/03/43/84/04034384.pdf> (accessed 20 July 2010).

Douglas, M. (1984) *Food and Social Order*, Russell Sage Foundation, New York.

Erera, I. P. (2002) *Family Diversity. Continuity and Change in the Contemporary Family*, Sage, London.

Farmer, E., Lipscombe, J. & Moyers, S. (2005) 'Foster Carer Strain and its Impact on Parenting and Placement Outcomes for Adolescents', *British Journal of Social Work*, Vol. 35, no. 2, pp. 237–53.

Finch, J. (2007) 'Displaying Families', *Sociology*, Vol. 41, pp. 65–8.

Finch, J. & Groves, D. (eds) (1983) 'Introduction', in *A Labour of Love; Women, Work and Caring*, Routledge & Kegan Paul, London, pp. 1–10.

Gillen, J., Accorti Gamannossi, B. & Hancock, R. (2008) '"A Day in the Life": Relating Understandings of "Eating Events" to the Concept of "Literacy Events" as Cultural Activities in the Lives of Two-year Old Girls in Diverse Global Communities', paper presented at the International Society for Cultural Activity Research conference, 8–13 September.

Gilligan, R. (2000) 'Men as Foster Carers: A Neglected Resource?', *Adoption and Fostering*, Vol. 24, no. 2, pp. 63–9.

Hamil, J. (2007) 'The Symbolic Significance of Food in the Treatment, Care and Recovery of Emotionally Damaged Children', presentation to Fostering Network, London.

Happer, H., McCreadie, J. & Aldgate, J. (2006) *Celebrating Success: What Helps Looked After Children Succeed*, Social Work Inspection Agency, Edinburgh, available at: <www.scotland.gov.uk/Resource/Doc/129024/0030718.pdf> (accessed 20 July 2010).

Horlick-Jones, T. (2005) 'Informal Logics of Risk: Contingency and Modes of Practical Reasoning', *Journal of Risk Research*, Vol. 8, no. 3, pp. 253–72.

James, A., Jenks, C. & Prout, A. (1998) *Theorising Childhood*, Polity Press, Cambridge.

Jones, A. (ed) (2001) *Touchy Subject: Teachers Touching Children*, Otago University Press, Dunedin.

Mennell, S., Murcott, A. & Otterloo, A. H. (1992) *The Sociology of Food: Eating, Diet and Culture*, Sage, London.

Morgan, D. (1996) *Family Connections: An Introduction to Family Studies*, Polity Press, Cambridge.

Orme, J. (2002) 'Social Work: Gender, Care and Justice', *British Journal of Social Work*, Vol. 32, no. 6, pp. 799–814.

Parton, N. (2003) 'Rethinking Professional Practice: The Contributions of Social Constructionism and the Feminist Ethics of Care', *British Journal of Social Work*, Vol. 33, no. 1, pp. 1–16.

Piper, H., Powell, J. & Smith, H. (2006) 'Parents, Professionals and Paranoia: The Touching of Children in a Culture of Fear', *Journal of Social Work*, Vol. 6, no. 2, pp. 151–67.

Rees, A. (2009) 'The Inner World of Foster Care: An In-depth Exploration', unpublished PhD thesis, Cardiff University.

Rees, A. & Pithouse, A. (2008) 'The Intimate World of Strangers—Embodying the Child in Foster Care', *Child and Family Social Work*, Vol. 13, pp. 338–47.

Schofield, G. & Beek, M. (2005) 'Risk and Resilience in Long-term Foster Care.', *British Journal of Social Work*, Vol. 35, no. 8, pp. 1283–301.

Sellick, C. (2002) *Foster Care Services in the Independent Sector*, Nuffield Foundation, London.

Sevenhuijsen, S. (2000) 'Caring in the Third Way: The Relation between Obligation, Responsibility and Care in the Third Way Discourse', *Critical Social Policy*, Vol. 20, no. 1, pp. 5–37.

Simpson, B. (2000) 'The Body as a Site of Contestation in School', in *The Body, Childhood and Society*, ed. A. Prout, Macmillan, Basingstoke, pp. 60–78.

Sinclair, I., Gibbs, I. & Wilson, K. (2004) *Foster Carers: Why they Stay and Why they Leave*, Jessica Kingsley, London.

Smith, F., Brann, C., Cullen, D. & Lane, M. (2004) *Fostering Now: Current Law Including Regulations, Guidance and Standards*, BAAF, London.

Titmuss, R. (1970) *The Gift Relationship: From Human Blood to Social Policy*, reprinted by the New Press (reissued with new chapters in 1997, John Ashton & Ann Oakley, LSE Books).

Tronto, J. K. (1994) *Moral Boundaries: A Political Argument for an Ethic of Care*, Routledge, London.

Williams, S. J. & Bendelow, G. (1998) *The Lived Body: Sociological Themes, Embodied Issues*, Routledge, London.

Wilson, K. & Evetts, J. (2006) 'The Professionalisation of Foster Care', *Adoption and Fostering*, Vol. 30, no. 1, pp. 39–47.

Wilson, K., Sinclair, I. & Gibbs, I. (2000) 'The Trouble with Foster Care: The Impact of Stressful Events on Foster Carers', *British Journal of Social Work*, Vol. 30, no. 2, pp. 193–209.

An Ethic of Care in Nursing: Past, Present and Future Considerations

Martin Woods

The purpose of this article is to re-examine an ethic of care as the main ethical approach to nursing practice in light of past and present developments in nursing ethics, and to briefly speculate whether or not it will survive within nursing in the future. Overall, it is maintained throughout that the terms 'caring', 'nursing' and an 'ethic of care' are inextricably linked. This is because, it is argued, professionally focused nursing practices are based predominantly on a well-recognised moral commitment to deliver expert care, and that a care-based ethic is the major factor in the construction and maintenance of these practices. Subsequently, the influences and developments of a caring ethic in nursing are firstly re-examined, and the discussion is supported by evidence from more recent nursing research and theoretical developments. Consideration is given to the philosophical underpinnings of both care theory and caring ethics, and the fundamental importance of caring in nursing, as an interpersonal relationship and as an appropriate ethical response, is made transparent. Finally, an outline of the future possibilities that may affect an ethic of care in nursing is offered.

Introduction

There are few better examples of the potential value of an ethic of care than in the profession of nursing. Nursing has been theorised as the caring profession par excellence throughout the twentieth century, if not from Nightingale's time (Mortimer & McGann 2004). Indeed, several nurse philosophers and theorists have always maintained that caring is the philosophical, theoretical, practical *and* ethical foundation of nursing, and furthermore that a care ethic was an integral, if not an intrinsic, part of nursing practices (Benner & Wrubel 1989; Leininger

Martin Woods has been involved in nursing education for more than thirty years and in particular with the teaching of nursing ethics, law and related subjects to students at all levels. He is also the New Zealand representative for Ethics & Human Rights for the international Council of Nurses.

1990; Bishop & Scudder 1991; Boykin & Schoenhofer 1993; Watson 2008; Benner *et al.* 2009). Hence, nursing has its own carefully evolved theories, discernible practices and ethical concerns that are different from those of medicine (Tan-Alora 2004; Davis *et al.* 2006). It follows, then, that if nursing is *the* caring profession, that some sort of care-based ethic may be associated with the modus operandi of its practitioners. Yet, as many skilful and highly professional nurses will testify, the value of their caring practices, and most certainly their ethical capabilities, is frequently downplayed by socio-political forces within the healthcare system, and in society in general (Liaschenko 1995; Kelly 1998; Woods 1999; Gordon 2005; Miller 2006; Makaroff *et al.* 2010). It is also evident that even within nursing itself there are those who regard the entire debate about nursing as a mainly caring practice with its own variation on caring ethics as potentially a futile blind alley (Paley 2002). Nevertheless, several nurses realise that regardless of these polarising viewpoints, the healthcare context itself is becoming an ever more complex and difficult arena in which to deliver safe, efficient and ethical care. This has forced them to continue to take stock of not only their caring practices within the healthcare system but also of their moral capacity to respond via care-based ethics as well. In turn, nurses at all levels, and particularly in nursing education, have re-examined the universally recognised main elements of nursing, namely the nurse–patient relationship (Benner 1997; Bergum 2004) and the moral ideal of nursing as caring (Gastmans *et al.* 1998; Tuck *et al.* 1998; Tschudin 2003), from within the context of modern nursing practices. Perhaps unsurprisingly, numerous nurses continue to support the concepts of care and caring in nursing, but a complementary care-based ethic remains as much a controversial and very much unfinished debate now as it was 20 years ago. To understand why this should be so, and to rebuild the case for a nursing ethic of care from all of its diverse beginnings, it is necessary to briefly re-visit the foundations of this ethic in nursing.

The Foundations of a Nursing Ethic of Care

An ethic of care reflects contributions from a variety of care-related philoso-phical sources such as Buber (1970), Mayerhoff (1971) and Blustein (1991), and sometimes diverse ones such as Spinoza (O'Brien 2005), Hume (Slote 2007) and even Aristotle (Curzer 2007). Nevertheless, it has been more closely related to feminist moral philosophy (Noddings 1984, 2002; Tronto 1994; Walker 1998; Alcoff & Kittay 2007), relational ethics (Gadow 1999; Kendrick & Robinson 2002; Bergum 2004; Sevenhuijsen 2003; MacDonald 2007) and also to virtue ethics (Oakley & Cocking 2001), where the virtuous characteristics of nursing—such as courage, trustworthiness and practical wisdom—merge relatively seamlessly with the main attributes of an ethic of care (Benner 1997; Sellman 2007). However, the main philosophical catalyst was Carol Gilligan's significant challenge to mainstream moral theorising that followed her influential research into the moral development of women (Gilligan 1982). Gilligan's recognition of the factors that could affect moral decision making *and guide* the nature of the moral response, such as the difficulty of abstract thought in concrete moral situations, the value of meeting the needs of others through relationships within particular contexts, and the centrality of caring and the prevention of harm, was in stark contrast to Kohlberg's popular view that ethical decision making was based on abstracted, rational, and reason-based thought (Kohlberg 1981). Subsequently, the 'ethic of care' that she identified as associated primarily with feminine ways of reasoning has been subject to considerable scrutiny because such an ethic is perceived to be a radical departure from the principle-based ethics approach that continues to be promoted for use in healthcare ethics, bioethics, medical ethics and most nursing ethics texts (Beauchamp & Childress 2001; Volbrecht 2001; Thompson *et al.* 2006).

It is perhaps unsurprising that nursing, a profession that is still comprised predominantly of females, and is firmly established on notions of care and commitment towards the (healthcare) needs of others, adopted an ethic of care with considerable enthusiasm. It was, after all, an ethic that showed consider-able promise as it appeared to offer confirmation of the main arguments that were emerging from care-based research and theoretical conceptualisation into nursing practice, as well as an explanation of the ethical difficulties that nurses were experiencing in the medically dominated healthcare context. Subsequent research projects and conceptual commentaries showed that nurses greatly valued the crucial importance of caring as a moral impetus to act (Watson 1990) but did not particularly attach similar value to abstract thought or moral principles as a guide to ethical responsiveness in concrete or particular moral dilemmas (Woods 1999). Nurses also argued that they well understood the centrality of the caring emphasis on meeting the needs of others through particular relationships (Euswas 1991; Gastmans et al. 1998; Tschudin 2003), but also that they were experiencing moral quandaries in practice. These related to the ever-present realities of contextual influences such as socio-cultural, hegemonic, or socio-political factors that affected the nature of their moral responses (Liaschenko 1995). Several other nursing researchers have since argued along similar lines by claiming that various aspects of an ethic of care represent a common thread within nursing practices and moral decision making in particular, but that this ethic is unappreciated or unrecognised (von Essen & Sjödén 1991; Schreiber & Lützen 2000; Rodney *et al.* 2002; Barnes & Brannelly 2008). Thus, the well-established arguments of several influential nursing scholars and research-ers, i.e. that to be a professional nurse required participation in the care of others in ways that were heavily relational, particular or situational and personally involving, confirmed that nursing practice had a greater voice through an ethic of care than perhaps any other approach.

Yet for all of the initial enthusiasm that admittedly arose from predominantly nursing sources, attempts to promote a nursing ethic of care based on a combination of Gilligan's and other theorists' ideas, and from the ideological position of nursing as caring, have met with mixed success. This is because whilst there has been a significant amount of material supporting such an ethic since its inception, there has also been an almost equal number of voices of doubt or dissent. Critics from both within nursing and in related fields such as medicine and bioethics remain largely unconvinced by such arguments, arguing that the term 'care' and its subsequent use in contemporary nursing theory is not a strong enough foundation upon which to construct a nursing ethic of care (Tarlier 2004). One commonly seen major criticism focuses on the need for healthcare professions to adhere to the continuing use of the 'four main principles', with or without the inclusion of normative moral theories such as deontology, utilitarianism or libertarianism (Gillon 2003). Others argue that the interpreted meaning of the philosophical sources of an ethic of care is a rather limited set of primary sources; that research on nursing's moral reasoning is not rigorous enough; and that nursing's attempts to promote an ethic of care as an alternative approach to moral reasoning is either too obscure, ill-founded, or hopelessly vague for use in practice (Allmark 1995; Crigger 1997; Kuhse 1997; Paley 2006). The most protracted argument stubbornly remains that an ethic of care within nursing is a highly suitable general attitude, but not an appropriate approach to ethical decision making for nurses *in practice*.

It is the argument of this paper that it is entirely possible to claim that the use of an ethic of care is not only desirable within nursing practice but also that, overall, it continues to guide both the moral ideals and ethically focused practices of competent and committed nurses. This claim is pared down to the two most fundamental elements of nursing as a caring ethic, namely that good nursing practice is itself an observable result of the recognised (or even unrecognised) use by nurses of an ethic of care, and that the interpersonal caring activities that are apparent in nursing supply the profession with ample explanations of its caring ethic.

Nursing Practice as an Ethic of Care

In 1990, a detailed analysis of 35 nursing authors provided at least five major conceptual categories/s of caring *as used in nursing practice* (Morse *et al.* 1990), namely caring as a human trait; caring as an affect; caring as an interpersonal relationship; caring as a therapeutic intervention, and *caring as a moral imperative or ideal*. In the mid-1990s, a selected review of caring research and theoretical works of major nurse theorists revealed that there was a vast amount of reliable research and theorising about caring in nursing (Lea & Watson 1996). In later years, research was conducted that measured caring in many different nursing environments including surgery, oncology, psychiatric care and critical care (Larson & Dodd 1991; Macey & Bouman 1991; Lützen & Nordin 1994; Andrews *et al.* 1996; Wu *et al.* 2006; O'Brien *et al.* 2007; Watson 2008). Research has also been applied to an assessment of conceptually specific nurse-centred caring practices such as the use of touch, listening, and appreciating the patient's self-knowledge (von Essen & Sjödén 1991, 1995).

Yet, whilst care and caring practices have been well philosophised and theorised in nursing, it must be understood that research based evidence supporting a parallel care-based ethics within nursing was still regarded by some as unconvincing. Nonetheless, in recent times the ethical values and practices of student nurses, new practitioner nurses and experienced nurses have been researched in greater depth. For instance, Woods (1999) argues that his research amongst experienced nurses revealed that there was evidence that 'morally committed nurses' exhibited a distinct *nursing ethic* in their approach to practice rather than one that mirrored standard medical or bioethical sources. In this regard, nurses brought a number of moral refinements to bear on their practices that included elements such as exhibiting appropriate nursing values and moral character; establishing purposeful relationships; being personally involved; maintaining trust; advocating for others; and, most importantly, being committed to delivering expert care. Such qualities are clearly closely related to a care-based ethic, because to care in a professionally focused practice-based sense requires caring in a moral sense. Other nursing researchers with similar findings have argued that such an ethic has both validity and reliability as an adequate explanation of nurses' moral motives and practices in a variety of settings (Vallence 2003; Rodney *et al.* 2002; MacDonald 2007; Barnes & Brannelly 2008). One all-embracing and unifying element in all of the research noted previously is that nursing cannot function beyond a very basic and ultimately ineffective level without the maintenance of a high level of interpersonal care.

Nursing as Interpersonal Caring within a Care Ethic

Nursing may be described as a professional response to the requirements of a basic but vital human phenomenon, i.e. the universal need for care (Reich 2001). Nurses do indeed 'have a care of' and 'care for' their patients, and this is evident in the amount of attention that they are expected to pay to the needs of others who are in receipt of their services. In this regard, human need, particularly when nursing care is required, is a universal and self-evident social requirement that is met through commitments to care for others (Blustein 1991; Walker 1998; Kittay *et al.* 2005). However, nurses exhibit a distinct moral *commitment* to caring for others in the form of a social 'investment' in the welfare of their patients, i.e. they care for and have a care of others because they care *about* others.

Caring about another person involves an attitude, feeling, or state of mind that is directed towards another's *situation* through a relationship with them (Blustein 1991; Walker 1998). This commitment to care, this investment in a caring relationship, manifests itself in nursing in various ways: for instance, caring nurses aim to offer skilful care to their patients; they seek to do this in rational but compassionate ways; they have concerns for the well-being of their patients; and, most of all, they strive to conduct their practice virtuously for the good of those with whom they come into contact in the caring setting (Woods 1999). Here is evidence of not only an ethic of care but also a clear connection to virtue ethics, and therefore to the longstanding moral ideals of professional nursing that began with Nightingale and continues into present-day nursing practices. In brief, nurses *care about* their patients because they accept the inherent moral commitment to caring that is nursing as practised. It may be argued that a nurse may have overplayed the interpersonal and relational importance of their practices and are merely delivering an objective or 'evidence-based' service, but this is to miss the point. The type of care that humans require from nurses is multifaceted, e.g. it ranges constantly between basic *and* complicated levels, subjective *and* objective, rational *and* emotional, and certainly between the mundane *and* the profound. Hence, amongst other terms, it has been described as 'embodied' (MacDonald & McIntyre 2000), 'engrossed' (Noddings 1984), 'intimate' (as in that type of care needed during 'the most intimate life and death events' (Zalumas 1995, p. 5), and more commonly as an 'interpersonal' and appropriate moral attitude (Gastmans 1999). In the latter case, it may be seen that nursing care is not just an observable entity, it is also an applied morality: it is a willingness to care, and a commitment to care regardless (or *regardful*) of all circumstances. An ethic of care is, in short, an ethic where moral situations are defined not in terms of rights and responsibilities but in terms of relationships of care often within challenging contextual circumstances (Tronto 1994; Bergum 2004; Goethals *et al.* 2010).

The Future of a Care-based Ethic in Nursing

In this article, it has been suggested that the most appropriate response from the nursing profession will always include an endorsement of a care-based approach that is both a valid depiction of ethical nursing practices and an accurate representation of the vital interpersonal aspects of the profession that separates nursing practices from others. Yet if nursing is to survive future ethical challenges in health care with its moral foundations and preferred ethical practices intact, then nurses will no doubt have to find ways not only to maintain such an ethic but to promote it within the brave new world of post-modern uncertainties. In this age, health-related ethics will no doubt continue to be beset by major discursive contradictions that will continue to plague biomedicine and health care in general. Topics such as genetics, information technology, stem cell research and oncology care advances will continue to emerge as major developments within health care. For example, genetic engineering within medical practices has now reached the stage where a myriad of potential diseases may be predicted in any given individual at any life stage. Undoubtedly, nurses will be increasingly involved in genetic counselling, and thus, by implication, with ongoing debates about human rights and social justice, the use of scarce resources, the boundaries of medical interventions, and much more. In each case, nurses will be challenged to re-examine their practices from their own ethical perspectives but ever mindful of the contextual barriers that may prevent them from responding according to their ethical ideal.

Subsequently, even biomedicine, which is likely to remain widely regarded as an applied science, will be increasingly challenged by a far greater range of socio-cultural discourses that are increasingly resistive towards techno-rational explanations (Lupton 2003). Perversely, this development may finally allow nurses to maintain that their viewpoint on a nursing ethic of care actually allows for such apparent challenges, and incorporates them into an ethic that may be of considerable value to all healthcare professionals. Admittedly, in such an age, care-based ethics approaches may struggle to survive unchanged and unrefined, but with its emphasis on human relationships, meeting human need within and ever mindful of particular social contexts, an ethic of care approach should always have a place in such debates. Indeed, it may prove invaluable in counterbalancing some of the potential excesses and threats to human dignity that future healthcare services may experience as the need for humane and ethically driven care is counterbalanced against overall cost effectiveness and service delivery expediencies.

Conclusion

It may be seen that a 'nursing ethic of care' is an entirely adequate explanation of moral responsiveness based on the long-established caring role of nurses in society. However, the most important characteristic of an ethic of care in nursing is *not* the nurse's ability to utilise moral reasoning or moral theory; nor is to be regarded as a perfunctory guide for practice, or even just a desirable moral attitude. In nursing, an ethic of care is a complete moral response based on professional caring that is as much an integral part of nursing practice as any other aspect. The use of an ethic of care in nursing enhances nurses' abilities to respond to the needs of their patients in ways that are grounded in the particular welfare and situation of each individual patient. Furthermore, because con-textual factors are fully recognised within a caring ethic, the nurse's responses to the needs of each patient will always be sensitive to the other person's situation. In doing so nurses will continue to take into account the hegemonic, economic and cultural realities that face each of their patients, and act accordingly.

It may be argued that in the clinical setting, which has often been regarded as ethically problematic for nurses because of a long history of various restraints to their practices within 'the system', it is not easy for nurses to practise using a care-based ethics. Yet however problematic the healthcare context may be, the social, cultural and moral contexts that nurses are required to operate within *require* that nurses focus their care on each of their patients' *particular* situations and *particular* needs if the nursing care is to be successful. Good practice in an increasingly uncertain and bureaucratic healthcare climate therefore requires considerable courage and commitment from present-day nurses. As healthcare settings and practices continue to change at a rapid pace, the need for adequate nursing responses to the ethical issues that confront members of the profession on a daily basis will become even greater.

References

Alcoff, L. M. & Kittay, E. F. (2007) *The Blackwell Guide to Feminist Philosophy*, Blackwell, Oxford.

Allmark, P. (1995) 'Can there be an Ethics of Care?', *Journal of Medical Ethics*, Vol. 21, pp. 19–24.

Andrews, L. W., Daniels, P. & Hall, A. (1996) 'Nurse Caring Behaviors: Comparing Five Tools to Define Perceptions', *Ostomy/Wound Management*, Vol. 42, no. 5, pp. 28–30.

Barnes, M. & Brannelly, T. (2008) 'Achieving Care and Social Justice for People with Dementia', *Nursing Ethics*, Vol. 15, no. 3, pp. 384–95.

Beauchamp, T. L. & Childress, J. F. (2001) *Principles of Biomedical Ethics*, 5th edn, Oxford University Press, Oxford.

Benner, P. (1997) 'A Dialogue between Virtue Ethics and Care Ethics', *Theoretical Medicine*, Vol. 18, pp. 47–61.

Benner, P., Tanner, C. A. & Chesla, C. A. (2009) *Expertise in Nursing Practice: Caring, Clinical Judgement and Ethics*, 2nd edn, Springer, New York.

Benner, P. & Wrubel, J. (1989) *The Primacy of Caring*, National League for Nursing Press, New York.

Bergum, V. (2004) 'Relational Ethics in Nursing', in *Toward a Moral Horizon: Nursing Ethics for Leadership and Practice* eds J. L. Storch, P. Rodney & R. Starzomski, Pearson Education Canada, Toronto, pp. 485–503.

Bishop, A. H. & Scudder, J. R. (1991) *Nursing: The Practice of Caring*, National League for Nursing Press, New York.

Blustein, J. (1991) *Care and Commitment*, Oxford University Press, London.

Boykin, A. & Schoenhofer, S. (1993) *Nursing as Caring: A Model for Transforming Practice*, National League for Nursing Press, New York.

Buber, M. (1937/1970) "*I. & Thou*". Trans. (1970) W. Kaufman, T. & T. Clark, Edinburgh.

Crigger, N. J. (1997) 'The Trouble with Caring: A Review of Eight Arguments against an Ethics of Care', *Journal of Professional Nursing*, Vol. 13, no. 4, pp. 217–21.

Curzer, H. J. (2007) 'Aristotle: Founder of the Ethics of Care', *Journal of Value Enquiry*, Vol. 41, pp. 221–43.

Davis, A., Tschudin, V. & de Reave, L. (eds) (2006) *Essentials of Teaching and Learning in Nursing Ethics: Perspectives and Methods*, Churchill Livingstone/Elsevier, London.

Euswas, P. (1991) 'The Actualized Caring Moment: A Grounded Theory of Caring in Nursing Practice', unpublished PhD thesis, Massey University, New Zealand.

Gadow, S. (1999) 'Relational Narrative: The Postmodern Turn in Nursing Ethics', *Scholarly Inquiry for Nursing Practice: An International Journal*, Vol. 13, no. 1, pp. 57–70.

Gastmans, C. (1999) 'Care as a Moral Attitude in Nursing', *Nursing Ethics*, Vol. 6, no. 3, pp. 214–23.

Gastmans, C., Schotsmans, P. & Dierckx de Casterle, B. (1998) 'Nursing Considered as Moral Practice: A Philosophical-Ethical Interpretation of Nursing', *Kennedy Institute of Ethics Journal*, Vol. 8, no. 11, pp. 43–69.

Gilligan, C. (1982) *In a Different Voice: Psychological Theory and Women's Development*, Harvard University Press, Cambridge, MA.

Gillon, R. (2003) 'Ethics Needs Principles—Four can Encompass the Rest—and Respect for Autonomy Should be "First among Equals"', *Journal of Medical Ethics*, Vol. 29, pp. 307–12.

Goethals, S., Gastmans, C. & Dierckx de Casterlé, B. (2010) 'Nurses' Ethical Reasoning and Behaviour: A Literature Review', *International Journal of Nursing Studies*, Vol. 47, pp. 635–50.

Gordon, S. (2005) *Nursing against the Odds: How Health Care Cost-cutting, Media Stereotypes, and Medical Hubris Undermine Nursing and Patient Care*, Cornell University Press, Ithaca, NY.

Kelly, B. (1998) 'Preserving Moral Integrity: A Follow up Study with New Graduate Nurses', *Journal of Advanced Nursing*, Vol. 28, pp. 1134–45.

Kendrick, K. D. & Robinson, S. (2002) 'Tender Loving Care" as a Relational Ethic in Nursing Practice', *Nursing Ethics*, Vol. 9, no. 3, pp. 291–300.

Kittay, E. F., Jennings, B. & Wasunna, A. A. (2005) 'Dependency, Difference and the Global Ethic of Long Term Care', *Journal of Political Philosophy*, Vol. 13, no. 4, pp. 443–69.

Kohlberg, L. (1981) *The Philosophy of Moral Development: Moral Stages and the Idea of Justice*, Harper & Row, San Francisco.

Kuhse, H. (1997) Caring: Nurses, Women and Ethics, Blackwell, Maldon, MA.

Larson, P. J. & Dodd, M. J. (1991) "The Cancer Treatment Experience: Family Patterns of Caring", in *Caring, the Compassionate Healer* eds D. A. Gaut & M. M. Leininger, National League for Nursing, New York, pp. 61–78.

Lea, A. & Watson, R. (1996) 'Caring Research and Concepts: A Selected Review of the Literature', *Journal of Clinical Nursing*, Vol. 5, no. 22, pp. 71–7.

Leininger, M. M. (ed.) (1990) *Ethical and Moral Dimensions of Care*, Wayne State University Press, Detroit.

Liaschenko, J. (1995) 'Artificial Personhood: Nursing Ethics in a Medical World', *Nursing Ethics*, Vol. 2, no. 3, pp. 185–96.

Lupton, D. (2003) *Medicine as Culture: Illness, Disease and the Body in Western Societies*, 2nd edn, Sage, London.

Lützen, K. & Nordin, C. (1994) 'Modifying Autonomy—a Concept Grounded in Nurses' Experiences of Moral Decision Making in Psychiatric Practice', *Journal of Medical Ethics*, Vol. 20, pp. 101–7.

MacDonald, H. (2007) 'Relational Ethics and Advocacy in Nursing: Literature Review', *Journal of Advanced Nursing*, Vol. 57, no. 2, pp. 119–26.

Macey, B. A. & Bouman, C. C. (1991) 'An Evaluation of Validity, Reliability, and Readability of the Critical Care Family Needs Inventory', *Heart and Lung-The Journal of Critical and Acute Care*, Vol. 20, no. 4, pp. 398–403.

Makaroff, K. S., Storch, J., Newton, L., Fulton, T. & Stevenson, L. (2010) 'Dare We Speak of Ethics? Attending the Unsayable amongst Nursing Leaders', *Nursing Ethics*, Vol. 15, no. 5, pp. 566–76.

Mayerhoff, M. (1971) *On Caring*, Harper & Row, New York.

McDonald, C. & McIntyre, M. (2000) 'Reinstating the Marginalized Body in Nursing Science: Epistemological Privilege and the Lived Life', *Nursing Philosophy*, Vol. 2, no. 3, pp. 234–9.

Miller, J. F. (2006) 'Opportunities and Obstacles for Good Work in Nursing', *Nursing Ethics*, Vol. 13, no. 5, pp. 471–87.

Morse, J. M., Solberg, S. M., Neander, W. L., Bottorf, J. L. & Johnson, J. L. (1990) 'Concepts of Caring and Caring as a Concept', *Advances in Nursing Science*, Vol. 13, no. 1, pp. 1–19.

Mortimer, B. & McGann, S. (eds) (2004) *New Directions in Nursing History: International Perspectives*, Routledge, New York.

Nightingale, F. (1964) *Notes on Nursing: What it is and What it is No*, Lippincott, Philadelphia.

Noddings, N. (1984) *Caring, a Feminine Approach to Ethics and Moral Education*, University of California Press, Berkeley.

Noddings, N. (2002) *Starting at Home: Caring and Social Policy*, University of California Press, Berkeley.

O'Brien, A. P., Woods, M., Watson, P. & Alpass, F. (2007) 'The Development of a Trans-cultural Instrument Designed to Measure Registered Nurse Attitudes to Caring, Technology and Professional Self: New Zealand in a Multicenter Study', *Asian Journal of Nursing*, Vol. 10, no. 4, pp. 219–27.

O'Brien, R. (2005) *Bodies in Revolt: Gender, Disability and Workplace Ethics of Care*, Routledge, New York.

Oakley, J. & Cocking, D. (2001) *Virtue Ethics and Professional Roles*, Cambridge University Press, Cambridge.

Paley, J. (2002) 'Caring as Slave Morality: Nietzschean Themes in Nursing Ethics', *Journal of Advanced Nursing*, Vol. 40, pp. 25–35.

Paley, J. (2006) "Past Caring. The Limitations of One-to-one Ethics", in *Essentials of Teaching and Learning in Nursing Ethics* eds A. J. Davis, V. Tschudin & L. De Raeve, Churchill Livingstone/Elsevier, London, pp. 149–64.

Reich, W. T. (2001) 'The Care-based Ethic of Nazi Medicine and the Moral Importance of What We Care About', *American Journal of Bioethics*, Vol. 1, no. 1, pp. 64–74.

Rodney, P., Varcoe, C., Storch, J. L., McPherson, G., Mahoney, K., Brown, H., Pauly, B. & Starzomski, R. (2002) 'Navigating Towards a Moral Horizon: A Multisite Qualitative Study of Ethical Practice in Nursing', *Canadian Journal of Nursing Research*, Vol. 34, no. 3, pp. 75–102.

Schreiber, R. & Lützen, K. (2000) 'Revisiting Nursing in a Non-therapeutic Environment', *Issues in Mental Health Nursing*, Vol. 21, pp. 257–67.

Sellman, D. (2007) 'On Being of Good Character: Nurse Education and the Assessment of Good Character', *Nurse Education Today*, Vol. 27, pp. 762–7.

Sevenhuijsen, S. (2003) 'The Place of Care: The Relevance of the Feminist Ethics of Care for Social Policy', *Feminist Theory*, Vol. 4, no. 2, pp. 179–97.

Slote, M. (2007) *The Ethics of Care and Empathy*, Routledge, New York.

Tan-Alora, A. (2004) 'Humane Medicine', *Philippine Journal of Microbiology and Infectious Diseases*, Vol. 33, no. 3, pp. 89–93.

Tarlier, D. S. (2004) 'Beyond Caring: The Moral and Ethical Bases of Responsive Nurse–Patient Relationships', *Nursing Philosophy*, Vol. 5, pp. 230–41.

Thompson, I. E., Melia, K. M., Boyd, K. M. & Horsburgh, D. (eds) (2006) *Nursing Ethics*, 5th edn, Elsevier/Churchill Livingstone, Edinburgh.

Tronto, J. C. (1994) *Moral Boundaries: A Political Argument for an Ethics of Care*, Routledge, New York.

Tschudin, V. (2003) *Ethics in Nursing: The Caring Relationship*, 3rd edn, Butterworth Heinemann, Oxford.

Tuck, I., Harris, L., Renfro, T. & Lexvolds, L. (1998) 'Care: A Value Expressed in Philosophies of Nursing Services', *Journal of Professional Nursing*, Vol. 14, no. 2, pp. 92–6.

Vallence, E. (2003) 'Navigating Through: A Grounded Theory of the Ethical Context of Undergraduate Nursing Education', unpublished master's thesis, Massey University, New Zealand.

Volbrecht, R. M. (2001) *Nursing Ethics: Communities in Dialogues*, Prentice Hall, Upper Saddle River, NJ.

von Essen, L. & Sjödén, P. O. (1991) 'The Importance of Nurse Caring Behaviors as Perceived by Swedish Hospital Patients and Nursing Staff', *International Journal of Nursing Studies*, Vol. 28, no. 3, pp. 267–81.

von Essen, L. & Sjödén, P. O. (1995) 'Perceived Occurrences and Importance of Caring Behaviours among Patients and Staff in Psychiatric, Medical and Surgical Care', *Journal of Advanced Nursing*, Vol. 21, pp. 266–79.

Walker, U. M. (1998) *Moral Understandings: A Feminist Study in Ethics*, Routledge, New York.

Walker, U. M. (2003) *Moral Contexts*, Rowman & Littlefield,, Oxford.

Watson, J. (1990) 'Caring Knowledge and Informed Moral Passion', *Advances in Nursing Science*, Vol. 13, no. 1, pp. 15–24.

Watson, J. (2008) *Assessing and Measuring Caring in Nursing and Health Sciences*, 2nd rev. edn, Springer, New York.

Woods, M. (1999) 'A Nursing Ethic: The Moral Voice of Experienced Nurses', *Nursing Ethics*, Vol. 6, no. 5, pp. 423–33.

Wu, Y., Larrabee, J. H. & Putman, H. P. (2006) 'Caring Behaviors Inventory: A Reduction of the 42-Item Instrument', *Nursing Research*, Vol. 55, no. 1, pp. 18–25.

Zalumas, J. (1995) *Caring in Crisis: An Oral History of Critical Care Nursing*, University of Pennsylvania Press, Philadelphia.

Ethics and the Street-level Bureaucrat: Implementing Policy to Protect Elders from Abuse

Angie Ash

As an independent researcher, registered social worker and erstwhile long-term, long-distance carer, the care of older people and protection of elders from abuse had been constant professional and personal foci for me for many years. Commissioned to review a case involving the serious abuse of an elder where official safeguarding procedures had not been used, I puzzled why this had been managed 'informally' by social services and partner agencies (i.e. outside adult safeguarding procedures), with vague unspecified 'monitoring' (AEA 2006). Why was there this apparent gap between policy intention and implementation? That question led to research on which this essay is based.

Introduction

This essay describes a research journey that discovered ethics at its core. The abuse of older people, and other groups of vulnerable adults, crept over the UK professional and policy radar in the 1990s (Homer & Gilleard 1990; Slater & Eastman 1999; SSI 1993). In 2000, governments in England and Wales issued guidance on the protection of vulnerable adults (DH 2000; NAfW 2000); local policies deriving from that guidance required staff to implement adult safeguarding (or protection) procedures when abuse was disclosed, suspected or witnessed. This 'implementation' may not result in intervention, but it required agencies to communicate under the procedures, pool information and reach a decision about action to be taken. However, this did not always happen (Preston-Shoot & Wigley 2002).

For example, commissioned to review a case involving the serious abuse of an elder where safeguarding procedures had not been used, I puzzled why this had

Angie Ash is a principal of the research consultancy Angela Ash Associates. She completed her doctorate at the School for Policy Studies, University of Bristol in 2009.

been managed 'informally' by social services and partner agencies (i.e. outside adult safeguarding procedures), with vague unspecified 'monitoring' (AEA 2006). Why was there this apparent gap between policy intention and implementation? What factors influenced whether or not social workers used adult safeguarding procedures?

In trying to figure out why what happened had happened, Lipsky's (1980) thesis of street-level bureaucracy seemed worth a re-visit. This 'street-level approach' to examining policy implementation has been held to be useful in situations involving the use of discretion by front-line workers, and complex decision making in a context of ambiguity and uncertainty (Brodkin 2000). Lipsky argued that the routines and devices that street-level bureaucrats (who include social workers) adopt to manage the ambiguities and dissonance arising from their implementation of public policy in human services effectively, become the policy implemented at local level. This seemed to offer some analytical potential in understanding the case I was reviewing. However, had Lipsky's thesis of street-level bureaucracy contemporary relevance more widely?

The research this question prompted was carried out in a statutory social services department in Wales. The accounts of social workers and their managers in this authority were riddled with the dilemmas and accommodations they made in planning, managing and delivering services to older people generally, and when dealing with potential elder abuse in particular. Rare, however, was reference to these dilemmas being matters of ethics and morality: rather, they were framed, variously, as problems of inadequate or inappropriate service provision, poor service standards, or difficulties of multi-agency joint working.

This paper considers this missing ethical dimension in implementation of policy to protect elders from abuse. Firstly, Lipsky's thesis of street-level bureaucracy is outlined, to situate what follows within its originating context. Secondly, some research findings are described leading, thirdly, to consideration of Tronto's (1993) four elements of an ethic of care, and the location of the missing ethical voice within those findings. Finally, some ways are proposed by which a stronger ethical presence can be imprinted into policy making, regulation, planning and delivery of services to older people, as well as safeguarding more specifically. The terms 'adult protection' and 'adult safeguarding' are used interchangeably; the former is more commonly used in Wales.

Street-level Bureaucracy and a Corrupted World of Service

Although published in 1980, Lipsky's *Street-level Bureaucracy* (subtitled *Dilemmas of the Individual in Public Services*) has a contemporary ring to it. Lipsky said policy making was insufficiently understood by looking at the actions of policy makers, as what he called street-level bureaucrats have to exercise discretion to undertake their work. Instead, he claimed policy is actually made in the crowded offices and daily encounters of street-level workers and that insights are gained into how and why organisations often perform contrary to their own rules and goals by discerning how the rules are experienced by workers in the organisation (Lipsky 1980, pp. xi–xii). Lipsky's thesis was, essentially, that:

> the decisions of street level bureaucrats, the routines they establish, and the devices they invent to cope with uncertainties and work pressures, effectively *become* the public policies they carry out. (Lipsky 1980, p. xii; emphasis in original)

He suggested that street-level bureaucrats experience dissonance as they struggle with dilemmas inherent in the structure of their work and 'a corrupted world of service' (Lipsky 1980, p. xiii). People enter public-sector work with some commitment to service, but become disillusioned. Aspirations are defeated by large workloads, inadequate resources, and ambiguous, conflicting or vague agency policy. Agencies devote energy 'to concealing lack of service and generating appearances of responsiveness' (Lipsky 1980, p. 76) perpetrating a 'myth of altruism' that remains unexamined within the street-level bureaucracy (Lipsky 1980, p. 71).

This provided the conceptual framework for the research which set out to understand the dilemmas that social workers faced when concerns about potential abuse of an older person were raised. It aimed to understand factors influencing social workers in their implementation of safeguarding procedures to protect older people, and the extent to which they and their managers shared similar understandings of the intention and implementation of the procedures. Using a mixed-methods design, national and local statistical data and relevant internal documentation were analysed, and all staff and managers working with older people and in adult protection were interviewed, either individually or in focus groups.

The following section describes some of the research findings, and the discovery of the missing ethical voice within them.

Missing Ethics

'Ethics' and 'ethical' were not an initial focus of the research design. References to an ethic of care in social work (e.g. Houston 2003; Parton 2003; McBeath & Webb 2002) made only fleeting appearance in the research proposal and early literature review. Nor did the findings suggest that the words 'ethics' and 'ethical' were much used by the social workers and managers in this study.

As data analysis got underway, the silent 'ethical voice' in the stories and accounts of street-level bureaucrats and their managers became audible. Elder abuse referral rates were low in this authority; domestic abuse in old age was rarely mentioned, despite Wales having the highest UK rate of reported elder abuse, and of physical, sexual and emotional abuse perpetrated by partners and those known to the elder (O'Keefe *et al.* 2007). Respondents in the study spoke of 'barely acceptable' care homes—'the whole place is an abuse' was a social worker's chilling description of one; of home situations where care arrangements were fragile and prone to collapse; of a lack of appropriate continence pads for older people (who had to make do with unsuitable alternatives), or of domestic abuse in old age that was neither recognised nor supported by age-appropriate services. The culture of the authority was, intriguingly, described as 'encouraging challenge' and 'questioning', and as one where the exercise of professional discretion was valued. Yet none of the dilemmas recounted by social workers were framed as *ethical* dilemmas, still less ones requiring an assertive professional voice to challenge.

Instead, such situations were construed as ones that, day in, day out, social workers had to deal with and manage in a 'make do and mend' mode of practice. Social workers tolerated lengthy police investigations into alleged abuse, health colleagues not showing up to adult-protection meetings, and poor-quality care homes. This was, *pace* Lipsky, their 'real world'. A manager summed it up: 'you've got somebody broken down at home, the carer can't possibly cope anymore, you're going to make a placement, it meets regulatory standards, it's acceptable, but well ... that's a very real world for people'.

As Banks (2008) has observed, how practitioners frame 'the ethical' influences their perceptions of their ability to act. In social work, 'ethical issues' are usually raised in relation to difficult cases or decisions, or as something found in the profession's code of practice. The context framing ethics and decision making is often viewed as 'policy' or 'politics' (the world of hard choices, tough decisions and the like) happening 'out there', rather than here and now (Lloyd 2004; Sevenhuijsen 1998). However, 'ethics' cannot be demarcated out of decision making around elder abuse and elder care, or when securing justice for and rights of the older person. Tronto's (1993) work on moral boundaries differentiated care and protection, and its relevance to these findings is considered next.

Tronto's Four Elements of an Ethic of Care

Care, Tronto suggested, involved taking the needs of the other as a basis for action; 'protection' presumed bad intentions from another and was a response to potential harm. Defining care very widely as a 'species activity that includes everything that we do to maintain, continue and repair our "world" so we can live in it as well as possible' (Tronto 1993, p. 103) delineated four elements of an ethic of care that resonated with many of the themes of this research.

Firstly, that of *attentiveness*—noticing needs is a primary human task. *Not* seeing, *not* attending, *not* noticing are, within an ethical framework, moral failings.

Secondly, *responsibility* is central to a care ethic. Tronto suggested that this is embedded in cultural practices, not in rules, obligations and duties.

The third element—*competence*—is necessary to counterbalance notions of 'taking care of' with those of 'care-giving'. Tronto suggested that 'intending to provide care ... but then failing to provide good care, means that in the end the need for care is not met' (Tronto 1993, p. 133).

The fourth moral element is *responsiveness*; that of the care giver to the care receiver. Needing care places a person in some vulnerability: the response made to that vulnerability has moral consequences. The moral element of responsiveness requires we stay alert to 'the possibilities for abuse that arise with vulnerability' (Tronto 1993, p. 133).

Finally, for Tronto, good care required that the four phases of care (caring about, taking care of, care giving, and care receiving), and the four elements of an ethic of care (attentiveness, responsibility, competence and responsiveness) should form a whole: that is, they should *have integrity*. The means by which this happens must be more than beseeching others to do this or that, or codifying rules into policies, procedures and professional codes. This is where an ethic of care gets *personal*: 'personal' in that caring practice requires, in Tronto's words, 'a deep and thoughtful knowledge of the situation, of all the actors' situations, needs and competencies' (1993, p. 136). 'Personal' caring practice derives from social, cultural and political contexts bearing on the care giver, the care receiver, and the exchange of care. Caring involves complex judgements about needs and how to meet them; such judgements derive from personal awareness of the construction and manifestation of needs within wider social, cultural and political contexts.

Whilst open to reasonable criticism for defining care very broadly (Sybylla 2001) or for locating it too closely in the perspective of the carer, not those cared-for (Lloyd 2006), Tronto's four elements of care opens up some ethical space to see the social and political context of care and justice as matters of morality. Street-level implementation of policy to protect vulnerable elders takes place within this context: implementation has a moral dimension.

Ethical Dilemmas—Everyday Practice

Firstly, this was not a failing agency; its organisational culture was described by those working in it as supportive and collaborative; it had been open to learning from this research exercise; and the outputs of regulatory and inspection activity had not found it wanting. However, the social and political context of the work of social workers and their managers mitigated their alertness, or attentiveness, to barely acceptable situations for older people—'you calibrate what's acceptable to what you know ... you operate in that real world', as one manager put it, became the operant conditions of their 'real world'. Constructive critical challenge was not embedded into discussions, whether of elder abuse, or of service planning, management, delivery and regulation. As one manager observed 'all this activity that goes on often doesn't seem to get to the heart of how people are living and being cared for'.

Secondly, professional ways of 'seeing' and 'not seeing' elder abuse or how life was for very vulnerable older people masked what we might call the 'real world' of elders. A team manager described an 85-year-old woman with unexplained bruising, who was cared for by her 93-year-old husband—'you go from "this is abuse and is being done deliberately" to hang on a moment, to care for someone who's elderly is quite hard work'. Here, the either/or of abuse (and no doubt in other situations assessed daily by social workers) masked the 'real world' within which two very old people were living. Attentiveness and responsiveness to the lived reality of these two older people (that care of another dependent being *is* 'hard work') were constructed in the policy paradigm that social workers as street-level bureaucrats operated, and the rules—the procedural processes they followed.

Thirdly, vacant safeguarding posts and shortfalls in services for older people were a day-to-day reality in this authority and familiar to most people working in human services. They also say something more about attentiveness to elder care and elder abuse. As a senior manager recognised: 'you can add all the usual money and things like that but I think … strategically it's about giving it attention'. The moral responsibility to challenge poor practice, delays, not accepting the 'barely acceptable', requires opening up 'space as a moral agent' (Øvrelid 2008). This was not identified as practice that social workers as street-level bureaucrats or their managers routinely engaged in. Questioning *why* referral rates for elder abuse were low relative to other authorities and to the national prevalence rate, or *why* people living in some care homes would be destined to die in a place where staff swore in front of them, were not a feature of everyday discourse.

Tronto's four elements of an ethic of care therefore provided some ethical purchase in grasping how constraints and realities were experienced by social workers and their managers. For Lipsky (1980) 'dilemmas of the individual in public services' are also dilemmas of ethics—although in this research they were rarely construed as such.

Street-level Bureaucracy, Policy Making and Morality—What Do We Do?

Towards the end of *Street-level Bureaucracy*, Lipsky deliberated about the potential for reform of street-level bureaucracies but returned in the end to considering strategies to make them 'work better'. The ethical dimensions of human transactions within these strategies were not directly mentioned. To be fair, Lipsky was under no illusion that organisational 'solutions' such as more training would be more than palliative in effect, because street-level bureau-cracies were part of 'organizational relations in the society as a whole' (Lipsky 1980, p. 192).

However, if ethics are not placed in the centre of policy design and implementation to protect elders we are likely to witness a search for ever more rules, protocols and procedures, designed to make service and regulatory systems function 'better', and for responsibilities to become ever more rule based, rather than ethically driven. Tronto (1993) was perceptive in her location of 'responsibility' in cultural practices, not rules. Lipsky, too, concluded that developing more rules was likely to be futile; rather, he saw the need to 'secure or restore the importance of human interactions in services that require discretionary intervention or involvement' (Lipsky 1980, p. xv).

Mainstreaming ethics at the heart of policy formation, implementation and service delivery holds out the possibility that inadequate resourcing, poor care and 'people-processing' practices (Prottas 1979) of social workers as street-level bureaucrats, can be exposed to ethical, as well as rule-based, scrutiny. Rational, rule-based policy making may be necessary, but it is not sufficient to safeguard vulnerable elders if resourcing (cash, people, bricks and mortar) do not emanate, as it were, from a 'morality-based duty of care' to the vulnerable elder at risk of abuse. If, as Lipsky suggested, the problems of the street-level bureaucrat lie in the systems and structure of their work, then in social work those need a clear, unblinking gaze. Social workers have an ethical and moral duty to safeguard older people; the organisational and policy context within which they operate must similarly manifest this ethical and moral obligation.

Locating an ethic of care at the centre of everyday practice demands organisational cultures that not only encourage challenge to everyday (not just poor) practice, *but expect it*. Such cultures would invite *and require* critical thinking and questioning: where managers ask, routinely, why there are few, if any, whistle-blowers; and where staff would feel professionally confident in constructively challenging each other, their agency, and other professionals.

Finally, this research journey started with speculation about what influenced social workers' implementation of policy to protect elders from abuse. It found Lipsky's street-level bureaucracy has continued salience in understanding how the problems of social workers as street-level bureaucrats lie in the structure, system and organisation of their work. Along the way, the author woke up to the ethical dimension of what she was learning: Tronto's four elements of an ethic of care illuminated the need for attentiveness, responsibility, competence and responsiveness in adult protection, and older people's services more generally.

The journey ended when I had a feedback meeting with a senior manager in the authority after the research was completed. We talked about low elder abuse referral rates, 'domestic violence grown old' (Straka & Montminy 2006), about ethics and morality which include 'big' questions, hard to peg down in the action-planned, task-listed world of a street-level bureaucracy. Then the manager mentioned the old, caked vomit found on the slippers of a person living in the 'whole-place-is-an-abuse' care home investigated for abusive practices that came to light when this research was being done.

We fell silent, considering this. Lipsky's 'corrupted world of service' and the missing ethical dimension of this research journey suddenly collapsed into one image: that of old, caked vomit on an elder's slippers.

References

AEA (Action on Elder Abuse) (2006) *Adult Protection Data Collection and Reporting Requirements: Conclusions and Recommendations from a Two Year Study into Adult Protection Recording Systems in England*, Funded by the Department of Health, AEA, London.

Banks, S. (2008) 'Critical Commentary: Social Work Ethics', *British Journal of Social Work*, Vol. 38, pp. 1238–49, doi: 1210.1093/bjsw/bcn1099, Advance Access publication, July 2008.

Brodkin, E. Z. (2000) Investigating Policy's 'Practical' Meaning: Street-level Research on Welfare Policy, available at: <http://www.jcpr.org/wpFiles/brodkin3.PDF> (accessed 22 April 2006).

DH (Department of Health) (2000) *No Secrets: Guidance on Developing and Implementing Multi-agency Policies and Procedures to Protect Vulnerable Adults from Abuse*, Department of Health, London.

Homer, A. & Gilleard, C. (1990) 'Abuse of Elderly People by their Carers', *British Medical Journal*, Vol. 301, pp. 1359–62.

Houston, S. (2003) 'Establishing Virtue in Social Work: A Response to McBeath and Webb', *British Journal of Social Work*, Vol. 33, no. 6, pp. 819–24.

Lipsky, M. (1980) *Street-level Bureaucracy: Dilemmas of the Individual in Public Services*, Russell Sage Foundation, New York.

Lloyd, L. (2004) 'Mortality and Morality: Ageing and the Ethics of Care', *Ageing & Society*, Vol. 24, no. 2, pp. 235–56.

Lloyd, L. (2006) 'A Caring Profession? The Ethics of Care and Social Work with Older People', *British Journal of Social Work*, Vol. 36, no. 7, pp. 1171–85.

McBeath, G. B. & Webb, S. A. (2002) 'Virtue Ethics and Social Work: Being Lucky, Realistic and Not Doing One's Duty', *British Journal of Social Work*, Vol. 32, no. 8, pp. 1015–36.

NAfW (National Assembly for Wales) (2000) *In Safe Hands: Implementing Adult Protection Procedures in Wales*, National Assembly for Wales, Cardiff.

O'Keeffe, M., Hills, A., Doyle, M., McCreadie, C., Scholes, S., Constantine, R., Tinker, A., Manthorpe, J., Biggs, S. & Erens, B. (2007) *UK Study of Abuse and Neglect of Older People: Prevalence Survey Report*, Comic Relief, London. Prepared for Comic Relief and the Department of Health, June, available at: <http://www.comicrelief.com/docs/elderabuse/ComicRelief-ElderAbuse-Full.pdf> (accessed 15 June 2007).

Øvrelid, B. (2008) 'The Cultivation of Moral Character: A Buddhist Challenge to Social Workers', *Ethics & Social Welfare*, Vol. 2, no. 3, pp. 243–61.

Parton, N. (2003) 'Rethinking *Professional* Practice: The Contributions of Social Constructionism and the Feminist "Ethics of Care"', *British Journal of Social Work*, Vol. 33, no. 1, pp. 1–16.

Preston-Shoot, M. & Wigley, V. (2002) 'Closing the Circle: Social Workers' Responses to Multi-agency Procedures on Older Age Abuse', *British Journal of Social Work*, Vol. 32, no. 3, pp. 299–320.

Prottas, J. M. (1979) *People-processing: The Street-level Bureaucrat in Public Service Bureaucracies*, Lexington Books, Lexington, MA.

Sevenhuijsen, S. (1998) *Citizenship and the Ethics of Care*, Routledge, London.

Slater, P. & Eastman, M. (1999) 'Introduction', in *Elder Abuse: Critical Issues in Policy and Practice*, eds P. Slater & M. Eastman, Age Concern England, London, pp. ix–xvii.

SSI (Social Services Inspectorate) (1993) *No Longer Afraid: The Safeguard of Older People in Domestic Settings*, HMSO, London.

Straka, S. M. & Montminy, L. (2006) 'Responding to the Needs of Older Women Experiencing Domestic Violence', *Violence Against Women*, Vol. 12, no. 3, pp. 251–67.

Sybylla, R. (2001) 'Hearing Whose Voice? The Ethics of Care and the Practices of Liberty: A Critique', *Economy and Society*, Vol. 30, no. 1, pp. 66–84.

Tronto, J. C. (1993) *Moral Boundaries: A Political Argument for an Ethic of Care*, Routledge, New York.

Crossing the Divide between Theory and Practice: Research and an Ethic of Care

Lizzie Ward and Beatrice Gahagan

This paper explores the application of ethic of care principles to research practice. It reflects on a research partnership between a voluntary-sector organisation (VSO) for older people and a university research centre (URC). The focus is a participatory research project on older people and well-being in which older volunteers were involved as co-researchers. The shared values of the VSO's culture of practice and the participatory approach of the university researchers have enabled joint research projects to be developed within an ethic of care framework. The model sought to break down the barriers between expert and lay knowledge and encouraged the mutual recognition, sharing and validating of different areas of expertise. An ethic of care framework offers context-specific ways of understanding and responding to the ethical challenges of undertaking participatory research, and to the relational aspects of well-being identified by older people during the course of the work.

Introduction

The feminist ethic of care originated as a theoretical framework to highlight the moral dimensions of care and caring relationships by conceptualising 'care' as a political value (Tronto 1993). It has been elaborated to critique the normative notions of independence, autonomy and responsibility in social and welfare policy discourses (Sevenhuijsen 1998, 2000, 2003) and applied to question the framework of citizenship, participation and social justice predicated on individual rights and responsibilities embedded in current government policies (Barnes 2007). Providing an alternative framework to understand the ways in which people make decisions about care, family, work and relationships, an ethic of care framework has also been used to analyse policies and practice relating to welfare reform (Haylett 2003; McDowell 2004),

Lizzie Ward is a research fellow in the Social Science Policy and Research Centre, University of Brighton. Beatrice Gahagan is the Senior Manager at Age Concern, Brighton, Hove and Portslade.

family (Williams 2001, 2004), and social care (Barnes 2006). In this article we reflect on how an ethic of care framework, based on the interconnected principles of *attentiveness, responsibility, competence, responsiveness* and *trust* can be applied to develop research practice, taking as our focus a research project which considers concepts and experiences of well-being amongst older people. We explore the significance of an ethic of care both to the way in which we conduct the research and the way in which we understand the rather nebulous concept of well-being. We describe how the research relationship has evolved before going on to discuss how we have applied ethic of care principles to the research practice.

Developing the Relationship

VSO Roots and Culture of Practice

From the VSO (voluntary-sector organisation) perspective, a number of factors have been key in developing the relationship with the URC (university research centre). The VSO's mission is to improve the quality of life of older people in its locality. It does this by ensuring that older people are treated with dignity and respect; that they are offered an adequate choice of high-quality preventative and rehabilitative services; and that they are given every opportunity to exert their rights and responsibilities as local citizens. The VSO also aims to enable older people to influence policy makers at a local, regional and national level. It is committed to identifying areas of unmet need and exploring innovative ways of meeting that need, or encouraging other agencies to do so.

As an organisation focused on its client group, the VSO has developed a specific culture of practice which is based on a person-centred philosophy, originally developed by psychologist Carl Rogers in the 1930s (Thorne 1992). Rogers developed client-centred therapy, based on a non-judgemental approach and treating clients as experts on themselves. The traditionally hierarchical relationship between therapist and client is rejected in favour of a supportive, non-directive environment where the therapist is open and genuine, offering the client warmth, acceptance and understanding, trusting in the client's strengths and ability to reach their fullest potential.

The VSO encompasses a person-centred approach by:

- respecting each older person as a unique individual;
- providing a warm and caring atmosphere;
- giving each person time to explain what they want/need;
- listening non-judgementally;
- helping to improve the quality of life through the positive nature of interaction, even if it is not possible to resolve the person's problem;
- allowing and encouraging people to express their views and feelings;

- supporting people to make their own choices without imposing views or decisions on them;
- recognising the importance of autonomy and continuity for people.

Research about older people's needs and issues plays an important role in achieving the VSO's mission. Although the VSO gains large amounts of information about issues affecting older people through its work, it has increasingly sought the skills and expertise of the university as a research institution, in gaining credible research evidence to take the use of information to a more robust level. Prior to the current research relationship the VSO tended to commission professional researchers to deliver research about specific issues affecting different groups of older people. The research processes and methods were largely designed and shaped by the researcher.

URC—Participatory Approaches and Collaborative Working

From the perspective of the URC, collaborative working has always featured strongly in its work. Since its inception in 1991, the URC has been committed to developing applied research with an emphasis on participatory approaches and working in partnership with policy makers, practitioners and service users to build connections between theory, policy and practice. A major focus of the URC's recent work has been developing research on age and ageing. The commitment to participatory approaches has led URC researchers to explore theoretically informed methods which seek to address the issues and challenges of involving older people as active participants in the research process. The current collaboration with the VSO developed out of a previous project exploring older people's alcohol use. The project used a participative approach and involved older people in designing and carrying out the research as co-researchers. Working as a team we were able to draw on our different knowledge, experience and expertise to create contexts in which older people could talk about their experiences of drinking in ways that made sense to them (Ward *et al.* 2008). The positive experience of working together on the alcohol project led to the development of the current project on well-being. As the relationship has developed into an ongoing collaborative partnership the implicit link between the URC participatory research approach and the VSO's values and philosophy has become more explicit, and more overtly part of the relationship which enables ethic of care principles to be expressed in a real practice setting.

Developing an Ethic of Care Framework to Research Older People's Well-being

The model we wanted to continue to develop aims to break down the barriers between expert and lay knowledge and encourage the mutual recognition, sharing and validating of different areas of expertise. To achieve this we recruited older volunteers as members of the research team to be involved from the very beginning of the new project. Many were recruited via the VSO, enabling existing volunteers and those who had previously been volunteers to continue to be involved as active participants. Although some had already retired from volunteering and were uncertain whether they could contribute, the research project created an opportunity to resume their long-standing interest in, and commitment to, older peoples' well-being. As co-researchers they have been fully involved in developing the research design and in carrying out interviews and focus groups with participants. During the development of the research design we drew on the team member's own knowledge and understandings to explore notions of well-being. The discussions held over a series of training sessions led us to develop ideas about what contributes to older people's well-being so as to generate contextualised and holistic understanding. The team developed a topic guide which allows the style and content of the interview to develop according to how each participant engages with the interaction. In effect, this enables ethic of care principles, which we outline in detail below, to be woven into the fabric of the interviews.

Attentiveness

According to Tronto (1993), attentiveness to the needs of others is a prerequisite for care. This approach enables dialogue and recognises experiences from 'lay' and 'professional' positions. Attentiveness to differences within the team, in terms of their ages (60–87 years), the amount and type of support they might need and the level at which they wanted or felt able to be involved, led us to consider how to structure the project in such a way that different roles within the team could be developed. These include: conducting interviews and focus groups with participants, reviewing literature, coding interview data, advising and commenting on findings and analysis, transcribing data and administrative support, developing dissemination. We wanted to make involvement in the research a meaningful and rewarding experience for all and allow team members to use existing skills and develop new ones. In practice, we have found that attentiveness to the needs of the team requires attention to practical details such as timing and location of meetings (access to public transport) and producing accessible material (e.g. large-print format). It also requires flexibility to accommodate uninvited disruptions due to health issues which may come more frequently and be more difficult to deal with in later life. For some members, offering reassurance and support to carry out tasks and maintain active connections with the work has also been important. We have also needed to be aware that team members may be affected by the content of the interviews. Inviting other older people to talk about experiences that may detract from as well as contribute to well-being may prompt co-researchers' personal reflections that are difficult or troubling on aspects of their own lives.

Responsibility

Responsibility in this context means acting on the awareness gained from being attentive to the needs of the team members. Our responsibilities as the 'professionals' include the overall running and delivery of the project. Ultimately 'getting the job done' rests with us. This needs to be balanced with our responsibilities towards those we have 'invited' into the process to participate. We are committed to ensuring all team members can take part in ways they are comfortable with, but we also recognise that we do not start off with equal power in terms of shaping the conduct of the project. An ethic of care alerts us to what Kittay (1999) has called 'elusive equality' and to recognise the unhelpfulness of assuming equality when it does not exist. This approach helps us to identify the differences between us in relation to our roles and responsibilities and to reflect on how we handle this in practice. This has involved learning when we need to take the lead and provide the structure for the project to progress, at the same time allowing room for genuine input from team members. In this respect we are attempting to negotiate a 'shared responsibility' whereby team members take responsibility and have a commitment to the work and the team. Our responsibilities as researchers require us to take account of the potential impact of the research on participants and we also need to ensure that team members as co-researchers, as well as the participants, are treated with respect and not harmed in the research process. In practice this means a preparedness to take responsibility for what emerges from the research process, being attentive to any impact on team members as well as ensuring that we communicate clearly about the scope and expectations of the project.

Competence

Linked to both the above is the notion of competence. The inclusion of competence as one of the moral principles of care reminds us that good intentions are not enough: 'Intending to provide care, even accepting responsibility for it, but then failing to provide good care, means that in the end the need for care is not met' (Tronto 1993, p. 133). In the context of our research, setting up a participatory project with the aim of actively involving older people in a meaningful way requires the competent organisation of the process to meet that aim. This includes ensuring that the opportunities and roles we provide are appropriate and that the members of the team feel their contribution is recognised and valued. Ultimately participating in a project about well-being should certainly not detract from members' own well-being. It also means that we provide the training, support and back up for team members to carry out the tasks we ask of them and ensure they are not being disempowered, demoralised or disheartened by the role. These are ongoing processes that require constant review to assess whether we are all achieving what we hoped and anticipated. This also involves addressing constraints (financial and/or institutional) on our ability to be competent and to consider what responsibility we have to address or challenge these.

Responsiveness

'The fourth moral moment that arises out of caring is the responsiveness of the care-receiver to the care' (Tronto 1993, p. 134). Taking an open approach to our learning and building ongoing reflection as part of the research process creates ways of noticing how individual members of the team are responding to the work we are doing. So inviting feedback, hearing and listening to individual reactions is an important aspect of the project. We need to be aware that individual responses to taking part in the research will vary as people have different motivations and expectations of what taking part means in practice. Similarly, we need to be aware of the particular impact of being involved in the research, including the possibility of identifying with or being affected by the experiences of the participants. Issues and fears identified by the research participants resonate with some team members' own experiences and this requires sensitivity and care in thinking through appropriate ways to offer person-centred support. In practical terms this has led to a decision to work on data coding with a small sub-group to ensure we are aware of any personal impact this may have.

Trust

All of the other principles outlined above are predicated to a large extent on 'trust', without which the task of carrying out this kind of research would not be possible. The issue of trust increases in significance in relationships where power is unequal. Building trust between ourselves in developing our research partner-ship was crucial. Even though it was clear early on that there was much common ground between the VSO's value base and person-centred practice and the URC participatory approach, time was needed during the initial stages to establish our working relationships to take account of both the needs of the research and each organisation's working practices and to overcome any institutional barriers to working outside of 'usual' working arrangements. In relation to the team members, it has been equally important to build trust and create a safe environment for members to express their views, and to try out new experiences such as facilitating focus groups or conducting interviews.

Conclusion

As the project has progressed we can see that the way in which the research is being carried out is to some extent as important as the findings. A striking feature of our evolving relationship has been the harmony between the person-centred culture of practice of the VSO and the ethic of care framework that has informed the research approach. The principles outlined here offer context-specific ways of understanding and responding to both the ethical challenges of undertaking research and to the relational aspects of well-being identified by older people during the course of the work. This includes the significance of how we relate to others and the world around us for our sense of well-being. We argue that such an approach recognises the significance of care throughout our lives, and is relevant beyond contexts typically understood as examples of 'caring relationships'. It offers a principled framework within which to practise research as well as the potential for responsive policy making and offers practitioners ways of engaging with older people that include care as a key dimension of 'empowering' practice. Through our research partnership we see the potential for collaboration between academia, practice and intervention. By applying an ethic of care framework to research practice we can develop practice-based *and* academic knowledge, crossing the divide between theory and practice.

References

Barnes, M. (2006) *Caring and Social Justice*, Palgrave, Basingstoke.

Barnes, M. (2007) 'Participation, Citizenship and a Feminist Ethic of Care', in *Communities, Citizenship and Care: Research and Practice in a Changing Policy Context*, eds S. Balloch & M. Hill, Policy Press, Bristol, pp. 59–88.

Haylett, C. (2003) 'Remaking Labour Imaginaries: Social Reproduction and the Internationalising Project of Welfare Reform', *Political Geography*, Vol. 22, no. 7, pp. 765–88.

Kittay, E. F. (1999) *Love's Labor: Essays on Women, Equality and Dependency*, Routledge, New York and London.

McDowell, L. (2004) 'Work, Workfare, Work/Life Balance and an Ethic of Care', *Progress in Human Geography*, Vol. 28, no. 2, pp. 145–63.

Sevenhuijsen, S. (1998) *Citizenship and the Ethics of Care*, Routledge, London.

Sevenhuijsen, S. (2000) 'Caring in the Third Way: The Relation between Obligation, Responsibility and Care in Third Way Discourse', *Critical Social Policy*, Vol. 20, no. 1, pp. 5–37.

Sevenhuijsen, S. (2003) 'The Place of Care: The Relevance of the Feminist Ethic of Care for Social Policy', *Feminist Theory*, Vol. 4, no. 2, pp. 179–97.

Thorne, B. (1992) *Carl Rogers*, Sage, London.

Tronto, J. (1993) *Moral Boundaries: A Political Argument for an Ethic of Care*, Routledge, New York and London.

Ward, L., Barnes, M. & Gahagan, B. (2008) 'Cheers!? A Project about Older People and Alcohol', Health and Social Policy Research Centre, University of Brighton, UK, available at: <www.brighton.ac.uk/sass/research/publications> (accessed 22 December 2009).

Williams, F. (2001) 'In and beyond New Labour: Towards a New Political Ethics of Care', *Critical Social Policy*, Vol. 21, no. 4, pp. 467–93.

Williams, F. (2004) *Re-thinking Families*, Calouste Gulbenkian Foundation, London.

That Others Matter: The Moral Achievement—Care Ethics and Citizenship in Practice with People with Dementia

Tula Brannelly

There are opportunities in practice for practitioners to sustain the citizenship of the people with whom they work. These opportunities arise as a matter of everyday decision-making, in the ways that service users and their families are facilitated to participate in decisions affecting their lives. Citizenship also hinges on the organisation of services to meet the needs of service users and carers. In this article, a care situation which fails to meet the needs of one family is examined using an ethics of care. A social worker reflects on her role in the decision-making and the eventual lack of commitment from a wider team to provide good care. To answer yes to the question of whether others matter, we need to consider whether the moral acheivement has been accomplished; that is to show in practice, that others do matter.

Introduction

The ethics of care (Gilligan 1982; Tronto 1993; Sevenhuijsen 1998; Held 2006) is a political and philosophical theory which has 'radical political possibilities' (Sevenhuijsen 2003, p. 37). To explore one radical possibility this article focuses on the moral achievement in practice with people with dementia through discussion of the contributing factors and conflicts in good care (Tronto 1993).

One complicating factor in achieving care is when people are unable to determine care for themselves, as in the context of care for people with dementia who are vulnerable or marginalised because their voice may be lost in the practice of caring. The radical political possibility of the potential to support

Tula Brannelly has an interest in the effects of social policies on marginalised groups, particularly people who experience mental health problems. Research areas include practices and status associated with citizenship and the facilitation of citizenship through practice.

and sustain the citizenship of marginalised people can be achieved through relational caring: achieving care and social justice requires the application of care ethics (Barnes & Brannelly 2008).

This article draws on research with 50 people with dementia and their families, who were working with community psychiatric nurses and social workers, in a large UK city. The research used observation and interviews to examine the facilitation of participation and decisions regarding detention of older people with dementia, using an ethics of care analysis (Brannelly 2004, 2006).

Hearing the voice and preferences of people who are marginalised through disability can be problematic given both the experience of a disabling condition and the powerful relations within which care is embedded. This is further complicated by the potential for construction of carers as burdened and care receivers as burdensome (Barnes 2006). Also, the lack of professional guidance (Brannelly 2006) leads practitioners to risk aversion rather than meeting need. Potentially, care is not achieved as practitioners retreat to protectionist strategies which meet the needs of some but not all. Usually, this means that the needs that are met are those of practitioners and of carers, but not of people who need to be cared for. Therefore, the individualised practices through partnerships in care deny the participation of people most in need, and citizenship is compromised. An ethics of care offers answers to these issues.

Orme (2002) notes the lack of application of an ethics of care in practice, and this is particularly so in mental health practice. Of the 50 people with dementia in this research, 10 were placed in nursing homes and residential homes, either willingly or unwillingly. Overall, the individualised practice analysed with an ethic of care found that practitioners engaged with people with dementia and their carers in ways which demonstrated attentiveness, responsibility, competence and responsiveness. There were instances where this did not occur and these have been documented elsewhere (Brannelly 2006, 2007). This discussion examines where care for one woman with dementia resulted in oppressive practice, despite the practitioner involved demonstrating the values of an ethics of care.

Case Study

Parveen was a 38-year-old Pakistani woman who at the time of the research observation was hospitalised on a neurological ward. She had a diagnosis of dementia for the past four years, and a meeting was called to discuss discharge from hospital as she was terminally ill. Her immediate family, her husband and children, were present along with a number of professionals from the hospital, and community services. Parveen's mother was due to arrive from Pakistan to care for her daughter in her terminal illness. The community services outlined the reasons why it would be difficult for Parveen to return home but the social worker involved knew that it was unlikely that the family would agree that Parveen be admitted to a nursing home. Parveen had been cared for at home for the duration of her illness, and it was her and her family's preference that she returned home to die. The discussions eventuated in a plan which accommodated the community services' concerns and provided a set time period of days to arrange the necessary resources for Parveen to return home, which included the provision of equipment and regular nursing care 24 hours a day. In the intervening period, Parveen was to be admitted to a nursing home. Six weeks later, Parveen died in the nursing home.

On reflection, in the research interview the social worker commented on a number of aspects of the care that she found untenable. Having been attentive to Parveen and her family's needs, the social worker had fought hard to ensure that the place of death was of their choosing, in the acknowledgement of other family members' needs to provide care. Having had a long relationship with the family she accepted responsibility to provide good care; she had worked with the children to enable them to cope with their mother's long-term illness, especially her increasing disabilities which affected her communication with them. She had intimate knowledge of the relationships within the family, and the journey of illness that Parveen had experienced, having first been diagnosed with post-natal depression following the birth of her youngest child, later changed to a diagnosis of dementia and the implications of this for the family. She had been competent in ensuring the care received was good and that she responded to the changing needs of the family. That the wider care team did not share her commitment to good care was difficult, and the eventual outcomes were unsuitable. As the family were unable to provide care at the time of Parveen's death, this indicated a lack of meeting need, and a failure to care. The family were upset at the ongoing placement in the nursing home, particularly as the nursing home staff did not meet Parveen's cultural needs, not only for her daily requirements but most problematically at the time of her death.

An Ethic of Care

The theoretical perspective is informed by Tronto's (1993) and Sevenhuijsen's (1998, 2003) ethics of care, and in particular the 'integrity of care' (Tronto 1993, p. 136). Significantly, Tronto and Sevenhuijsen suggest that care is a disposition and a practice, and Tronto provides the following, broad definition:

> On the most general level we suggest that caring can be viewed as a species activity that includes everything we do to maintain, continue and repair our 'world' so that we can live in it as well as possible. That world includes our bodies, ourselves and our environment, all of which we seek to interweave in a complex, life-sustaining web. (Tronto 1993, p. 103)

Care as a practice takes into account the full context of caring, and the needs of all parties—considering the concerns of the care receiver as well as the skills of the care giver and the role of those taking care (Tronto 1993, p. 118). It is particularly important that the needs of *all* involved are identified. Often the needs of care givers and providers are not stated, or care is focused on one party rather than all. 'Caring about' is shaped culturally and individually, and so acknowledges the uniqueness and individuality of the care receiver rather than applying universalistic rules of care. 'Taking care of' recognises the strengths brought to the situation of all involved. Intimate knowledge is required so that complex of care giving is done well, and can only be recognised as having happened by the reaction of the care receiver.

Tronto (1993) identified four elements of the practice of care. *Attentiveness* requires that the practice of care is attentive to the needs of others, or those needs cannot be met. It is a difficult task and as such a moral achievement— 'That others matter is the most difficult moral quality to establish in practice' (Tronto 1993, p. 130). We might consider that professional agendas be put to one side so the needs of those requiring care are identified. An impact of inattentiveness is the unwillingness of one party to recognise the needs of others and thereby lack the opportunity to meet needs. For Parveen and her family, the wider professional consensus was that nursing home care would be adequate caring at her time of death. This resulted in a lack of urgency in arranging the necessary care at home. Weeks went by when there was the opportunity to remain attentive to the needs of the family, but the necessary arrangements were not made.

Where there may be conflict arising from the provision and receipt of care, or preferences may be for different outcomes, practitioners must discern each set of needs and take each into account to provide good care. Practitioners also need to state their responsibilities in such a situation, for example in a situation where a practitioner may be considering the use of mental health legislation if the person does not accept some form of help, and perhaps a carer feels that they are in crisis and cannot cope any longer. In terms of outcomes, whilst it may meet the immediate needs of the practitioner and the carer to detain a person to a place of safety, this is the least likely outcome preferred by the person needing care. Practitioners absorb detailed and intimate knowledge of families and the situated circumstances in which care is happening. This information is not passed on or written down but carried with the practitioner and the family. It is in the detail of this information where there is potential for opportunities to know what is an acceptable outcome for all involved. This requires creative use of power (Sevenhuijsen 2003b) as well as 'engagement in an ethical practice of complex moral judgements' (Tronto 1993, p. 157). It is in these circumstances that service users and families view care to be happening. In Parveen's situation, that the social worker persisted in facilitating arrangements for home care sustained and built trust in her care practice.

Responsibility is the second dimension of care, central to 'taking care of'. In most moral theory responsibility is aligned with obligation but Tronto argues that it is embedded in a set of implicit cultural practices, rather than a set of formal rules, and therefore responsibility arises out of the recognition of need because otherwise that need will not be met (Tronto 1993, p. 131). For Parveen, there was a difference in opinion regarding need—there was a need for Parveen to be cared for at the time of her death, but by whom was not of central importance to some of the agencies involved. Having the detailed knowledge from families, and arranging care which is acceptable and workable in that situated context, is likely to promote better care outcomes.

Competence: intending to provide care, even accepting responsibility for it, but then failing to provide good care means that in the end the need for care is not met (Tronto 1993, p. 133). So whilst Parveen's social worker had practised all the values of an ethic of care, the wider care team failed to provide good care. Caring work needs to be performed competently. From a perspective of care, we should not permit individuals to escape from responsibility for their incompetence by claiming to adhere to a code of professional conduct (Tronto 1993, p. 134). Where care is planned and interventions designed to promote care are implemented and effective, as well as acceptable, then competence is achieved. Competent care is reliant on resources to provide acceptable effective interventions and services, including skills and knowledge of practitioners.

Responsiveness recognises the experience of the care receiver as central to knowing that care has taken place. Within this are the concerns of vulnerability and inequality. Throughout our lives, all of us go through varying degrees of dependence and independence, of autonomy and vulnerability. Responsiveness requires that we remain alert to the potential for abuse that arises with vulnerability (Tronto 1993, p. 135), and the need to maintain a balance between care givers and care receivers. Therefore we only know that caring has been achieved when the care receiver is responsive to care. This is particularly important when people lacking voice makes it necessary to see the reaction to care, and therefore know whether care has been achieved. Parveen's family indicated the lack of care, not only in terms of not having the opportunity to care for her but also in the fact that the nursing home did not meet her cultural needs.

The integrity of care requires all elements to be present; Sevenhuijsen (1998) adds *trust* as the final element, in that caring relationships cannot exist without trust in order to use power creatively and positively in times of conflict. Care also requires that there is an intimate knowledge of the situation of caring, the complexities of providing care and the competencies of those providing care, as care is about making judgements about needs, conflicting needs, strategies for achieving ends and the responsiveness of care receivers (Tronto 1993, p. 137).

Challenging Social Practices with an Ethic of Care

Self-determination is an aspect of social inclusion (Barnes & Morris 2008), and participation in care promotes citizenship (Barnes 2006). Conflict or difficult decisions are likely to be encountered when people are not able to take responsibility for their own lives as a result of long-term cognitive difficulties or mental health problems. These include the use of medications, placement out of home such as in a residential home, or detention in mental health facilities

(Brannelly 2004). Caring is undertaken within families, by friends and within communities, but at times requires help from paid care givers, in the hope that as they are paid they can be trusted to respond in ways that are acceptable to those needing care. Care is complex when the preferences for care outcomes are different for each person involved, and where the practice of care is dependent on those actors.

With marginalised people, attentiveness to their voices and facilitation of participation through the integrity of care enables review to meet care needs. An ethics of care values interdependence rather than dependence and/or independence, thereby not positioning any person as burdensome and burdened, but recognising the reciprocity of giving and receiving care. Practice can be analysed using the values which provide the guidance required in situated and complex circumstances, and avoids meeting needs of one party at the expense of another. Rather than constructing care as the sharing of power, it has as a central tenet the rights and responsibilities involved in practice; foregrounding these in order to avoid oppression through practice.

Conclusion: That Others Matter—The Moral Achievement

The moral achievement occurs in practice when recognition of vulnerability and facilitation of participation become the starting point of care. Practitioners involved in relationships with people who require care must translate information gathered into clinical or social assessment and service planning in order to respond accordingly. This process helps to avoid oppression of practice. There are, therefore, many hurdles or potential conflicts and difficulties which may occur within the practice of care; or rather, there are many aspects and factors to consider and attend to for care to occur.

An ethics of care values the participation of all involved, including professional carers. This enables discussions of professional responsibility and potential outcomes, thereby centralising the experience of care rather than the needs of services. It also values the detailed and situated context of caring, which enables practitioners to better articulate why the outcomes that have been discussed and negotiated are required to happen. It accepts that care is part of families and communities (Barnes 2006), and that paid care givers contribute to enable care.

Experienced practitioners cite the perverse outcomes of care, such as those not intended by their involvement, as ethical dilemmas in practice. Based on the experiences of people with dementia and those involved in their care revealed in this research, my argument here is that an ethic of care strengthens the position for the negotiation of care between practitioners, service users and their families where there is intimate knowledge of the detailed care situation and what is required for the service user to experience care as good. The moral achievement is that others matter, and that the concerns of people who receive services are paramount in service provision. This serves to strengthen the voice of practitioners in the negotiations of care outcomes which are acceptable based on the detail and situated knowledge they have with service users and families. Care based on the ethics of care enables negotiations that are participative and therefore ensures that potentially marginalised voices are heard and responded to (Brannelly 2007, p. 100). Innes (2009) identifies citizenship and social inclusion as the way forward for the generation of theory, policy and practice related to people with dementia. Rather than considering rights and responsibilities to be a side issue, an ethics of care incorporates them in care provision. Citizenship is sustained when practice is based on the principles of an ethics of care which encompass the notions of humanness, autonomy, power and control, participation, equality and justice, and that others matter.

Acknowledgements

Thanks are due to Joan Orme and Annette Huntington who commented on earlier drafts of this article.

References

Barnes, M. (2006) *Caring and Social Justice*, Routledge, London.

Barnes, M. & Brannelly, T. (2008) 'Achieving Care and Social Justice for People with Dementia", *Nursing Ethics*, Vol. 15, no. 3, pp. 384–95.

Barnes, M. & Morris, K. (2008) 'Strategies for the Prevention of Social Exclusion: An Analysis of the Children's Fund', *Journal of Social Policy*, Vol. 37, no. 2, pp. 251–70.

Brannelly, T. (2004) 'Citizenship and Care for People with Dementia', unpublished PhD thesis, University of Birmingham.

Brannelly, T. (2006) 'Negotiating Ethics in Dementia Care: An Analysis of an Ethic of Care in Practice', *Dementia*, Vol. 5, no. 2, pp. 197–212.

Brannelly, T. (2007) 'Citizenship and Care for People with Dementia: Values and Approaches', in *Care, Community and Citizenship: Research and Practice in a Changing Policy Context*, eds S. Balloch & M. Hill, Policy Press, Bristol, pp. 89–101.

Gilligan, C. (1982) *In a Different Voice: Psychological Theory and Women's Development*, Harvard University Press, Boston.

Held, V. (2006) *The Ethics of Care: Personal, Political and Global*, Oxford University Press, New York.

Innes, A. (2009) *Dementia Studies*, Sage, London.

Orme, J. (2002) 'Social Work: Gender, Care and Justice', *British Journal of Social Work*, Vol. 32, no. 6, pp. 799–814.

Sevenhuijsen, S. (1998) *Citizenship and the Ethics of Care: Feminist Considerations on Justice, Morality and Politics*, Routledge, London.

Sevenhuijsen, S. (2003) 'The Place of Care: The Relevance of the Feminist Ethic of Care for Social Policy', in *Labyrinths of Care: The Relevance of the Ethics of Care Perspective for Social Policy* eds S. Sevenhuijsen & A. Švab, Peace Institute, Ljubljana, pp. 13–41.

Tronto, J. C. (1993) *Moral Boundaries: A Political Argument for an Ethic of Care*, Routledge, New York.

The Daily Grind of the Forgotten Heroines: Experiences of HIV/AIDS Informal Caregivers in Botswana

Odireleng Jankey and Tirelo Modie-Moroka

With the increasing number of people living with HIV/AIDS and the escalating costs of health care, there is an increasing demand for informal caregiving in the community. Currently, much emphasis is placed on individuals who are living with HIV/AIDS (in terms of the provision of social, psychological and economic support), but very little attention has been paid to the well-being and quality of life of informal caregivers. Lack of support and care for caregivers may have a negative impact on the quality of care and effective services for individuals living with HIV/AIDS. This paper is based on findings from a qualitative study that explored major sources of stress associated with caregiving among informal caregivers in a village in the southern part of Botswana. The paper suggests that informal caregivers are an integral part of the continuum of care. As a result, they need to be nurtured and supported for the betterment of those both infected and affected by HIV/AIDS. The paper concludes by discussing the implications for further research, policy and programme development.

Botswana and HIV and AIDS

Like many developing countries, Botswana has been hard hit by the HIV epidemic. Since the reporting of the first AIDS case in 1985, the spread of HIV/AIDS has continued to escalate (Government of Botswana 1997). At present, the spread of the HIV virus has reached epidemic proportions. Based on the Botswana HIV and AIDS Impact Survey II conducted in 2004, it was estimated that 17.1 per cent of

Dr Odireleng Jankey (PhD, MSW) is a lecturer in the Department of Social Work at the University of Botswana. She graduated from the University of Utah, USA with a PhD in Social Work in 2009. She has a Masters in Social Work with a research specialization. Dr Tirelo Modie-Moroka (PhD, MPH) is a Senior Lecturer at the University of Botswana, Department of Social Work and she graduated from the University of Pittsburgh, USA with a PhD in Social Work and a Masters in Public Health with a focus on Community and Behavioural Health Sciences in 2003.

the population was infected with HIV. In 2005, it was estimated that at least 270,000 people were living with HIV in Botswana. The Botswana AIDS Impact Survey III (BAIS III) recorded HIV prevalence rates of 17.6 per cent, with females having prevalence rates of 20.4 per cent compared to those of males at around 14.2 per cent.

Informal caregivers play a pivotal role in combating the spread of HIV and caring for those already affected. However, they experience physical (Ditirafalo *et al.* 2001), psychological (Bulmer 1987) and economic burdens (Dant & Gully 1994). At the first regional Southern Africa Development Community [SADC] Community-based Care conference (2001) it was recognized that HIV/AIDS 'creates a major additional burden on caregivers in the health care system and at home where women are the primary caregivers' (Van Praag 2001, p. 4). The conference concluded that caregivers would need 'concrete support systems to deal with the prevalent stresses' (2001, p. 4). Despite this recognition, the national strategic plan for HIV/AIDS (2003–09) in Botswana identified 'vulner-able' groups as youth and women, but did not mention 'caregivers' specifically as a distinct vulnerable group. Where mentioned, caregivers are ironically lumped together with people living with AIDS, which could mean that they do not receive targeted and specific interventions. This exclusion could indicate a lack of concern for them and their needs.

Theoretical Framework

The theoretical framework for this paper draws on both stress theory and self-in-relation theory. Stress theory may help to explain the process through which caregiving-related stress could result in the poor overall physical and psycholo-gical effects of those providing care. Cohen and Syme (1999) define stress as a situation in which environmental demands exceed the adaptive capacity of an organism, resulting in psychological and biological changes that may place people at risk of disease. In this paper, it is assumed that caregiving is stressful and therefore results in disequilibrium in the caregiver's life that can negatively impact the health of the caregivers.

This stress is further compounded by socialization into gender roles, which places women at the centre of unremunerated service. Self-in-relation theory suggests that, unlike men, women are socialized towards an ethic of care and responsibility (Miller 1987). Women are the primary caregivers in the home: for children, people with mental illness, the physically disabled, and the elderly. It is possible that women may conceptualize caring as a 'duty and obligation' in ways that men may not. Dant and Gully assert that 'women, faced with a perceived need to care ... feel that they have absolutely no choice whatsoever but to "carry on caring"' (1994, p. 6). Cohen and Syme also argue that 'women are given no choice but to be caregivers of society, without social support or reward, no matter what financial and personal sacrifices are involved' (1999, p. 33).

Jacques and Stegling contend that 'the sentimental cult of domestic virtues is the cheapest method at society's disposal of keeping women quiet without seriously considering their grievances or improving their position' (2002, p. 117).

While they may be motivated by a sense of empathy and compassion, the incongruence between the giving of care and the support they receive (while providing that care) creates a sense of misalliance and dissonance, which further deepens their physical, emotional and economic crises. In other words, their very ability to care and the quality of care that they are able to provide are shaped by factors such as gendered expectations and socio-economic conditions that result in stresses and burdens for these caregivers.

Method and Findings

This study was conducted among family and volunteer caregivers in Kopong, using a qualitative cross-sectional method of enquiry. Using qualitative methods, in-depth interviews were conducted to explore the experiences of caregivers providing care at home for people living with AIDS. The questions used to guide the interviews were a combination of open- and closed-ended probes.

Participants were recruited by word of mouth, advertisements via local media (local newspapers, television and radio interviews) and letters to local community-based organizations (churches, agencies and grassroots organizations). The recruitment period lasted from September to October 2008. The researchers explained the purpose of the study and obtained verbal consent from the caregivers. The interviews lasted an average of two hours.

Sample

Respondents were aged between 40 and 70 years old and provided 20 hours of care per week. Caregivers were more likely to be mothers, friends, aunts, non-relatives and volunteers from the community. Unemployed older women predominated as caregivers. Caregivers provided assistance with activities of daily living, informational and emotional support, childcare assistance and guardianship, transportation to medical appointments, discussions of health and social problems with healthcare providers, and organizing and/or administrating medications and treatments.

Caregiving responsibilities took an overwhelming toll on the physical and psycho-social well-being of caregivers. One respondent stated:

> We are mostly elderly women; we started with two men because men do not work for nothing. Youth also do not participate at all. Despite our old age, we work hard. Youth tell us that 'rona ga re na boithaopo jo bo senang sheleng [they don't volunteer where there is no money]'. We were 25 but now we are 21. It is women only.

Caregivers provide care in a context of poverty, fragmented government support, stigma and other challenges they face in old age.

In addition, urban dwellers and migrant labourers return to their villages of origin to be cared for by older relatives when they fall ill. The motivation to come home is to seek care, mostly from older relatives who are more self-sacrificing. Coming home is often accompanied by feelings of shame, blame and guilt, especially when the person has weak ties with the family and community. Society expects caregivers to provide care despite their disinclination to do so.

The Stress of Caregiving

Results suggest that though caregiving was a spiritually rewarding experience, often referring to it as a 'calling', oftentimes it was debilitating and emotionally exhausting. Caregivers were motivated by a spirit of servitude, though they had to contend with underlying feelings of anger, bitterness, disillusionment and unresolved fears. The study suggests that though caregiving is an act of servitude and volunteerism, the multiple roles that are added to women's work make it a daily grind, bringing ambivalence to the context of care. Despite this daily grind, the women who provide so much of the needed service remain forgotten in government programming for HIV/AIDS. As part of expectations of their gender roles in society women have obligations and responsibilities to provide care. As they take on the responsibilities of toiling through these multiple roles, society does not expect them to complain. That could be why in the event of death they are faced with an overwhelming sense of loss and guilt. They tend to blame themselves for not caring enough.

Caregivers stated that they were often beset by the fear of possible infection, but could not talk about that for fear that they would be labelled as stigmatizing patients. Moreover, caregivers felt stigmatized by the community as a result of their association with people living with AIDS. This stigmatization manifested itself by their being isolated by some community members and in a loss of friends. It was difficult for caregivers to reach for emotional support because of the stigma.

Some caregivers described themselves as possessing a sense of hardiness: 'ga ke pelo e lefafa ... ga ke tshosiwe ke balwetse [I am strong ... I am not scared of patients]'. This could be influenced by societal expectations that encourage women to be stoical and to 'hold the sharp end of a knife in the event of a crisis [mmangwana o tshwara thipa ka fa bogaleng]'. These expectations often fail to acknowledge that those who hold the sharp end of a knife will experience the deepest cut when the opposing force is greater. In this case, women caregivers put themselves in the firing line when they volunteer to provide care in the absence of a comprehensive, integrative and properly coordinated system of care.

They also put themselves in the firing line with respect to issues of privacy because the very care giving they provide violates basic principles and taboos in Botswana culture. In the study, women admitted that daily activities of bathing elderly sons or taking care of their fathers- or mothers-in-law were such cultural taboos that they would not speak about them with others—even those close to them.

Given the multiple roles that caregivers play in society, they often experience role conflict such as choosing between caregiving and livelihood activities in rural communities such as ploughing, weeding, bird scaring and harvesting. When the agricultural produce is lower than expected, some caregivers find themselves blaming people living with AIDS for their situation. Molelekwa (2000) found that there is an assumption that those members of the family who are not formally employed should automatically be caregivers to those in need of care. Their views about whether they are ready and willing to provide care are not sought. The assumption is that since they have 'nothing else to do' they could be caregivers, a role that is rarely, if at all, remunerated or appreciated. This lack of appreciation often creates tensions among caregivers, other family members and recipients of care, resulting in ambivalence and negative social support in caregiving.

Physical Effects of Caregiving

Caregiving is a physically demanding activity. Some caregivers reported health problems such as backache, headache and hypertension after assuming the caregiving role. Sims and Moss suggest that

> it is difficult for caretakers to achieve such a balance through employment or through socializing with friends and relatives because they have no time, there is no one else to take up the caregiving role, and friends and relatives often do not understand their problems and distance themselves from these women. (1991, p. 36)

Psycho-social Effects

It is evident that caregiving has negative psychological effects. The majority of caregivers worried about their patients and got frightened when they thought about caring for seriously ill patients under their care. This is consistent with Van Praag's findings (2001), who states that some HIV/AIDS care providers often describe feelings of having AIDS, while others have repeated worries about their next of kin's health. Caregiving also negatively affected some family relation-ships. Friction and conflicts result when family members compete for the attention of the caregiver or when they feel the caregiver is not doing enough for the patient (Schoen 1998).

Economic Stress

Caregiving leads to economic stress. Caregivers mentioned lack of financial support from the formal caregiving system; lack of food, clothing, and transportation; and diminished livelihood opportunities. Most of them could no longer work to provide for their families.

Caregivers receive a monthly allowance of P165.10 (US$23), no compensation from the state for a social service rendered and no recognition from society for their difficult labour. They are expected to provide care for the dependent person, meet the needs of the rest of the family and smooth over any hostility or resentment between the dependent relative and other family members. The wages of volunteer caregivers are too low to make any significant improvement in their lives. It is also difficult for caregivers to work, find employment or spend time on income-generating activities because they spend most of their time providing care. One of the respondents said that 'this ends up being our everyday job and yet we are not paid for it'.

Unresolved Historical Conflicts

The trend of family members abandoning AIDS patients could be an indication that all is not well in some families. There is evidence that some families may have unresolved familial conflicts and may seek to avenge or settle these historical scores when the other party is not well. When confronted with a sick family member, the crisis in the family seems to heighten, thereby placing the vulnerable patient at greater risk of negligence, anger and bitterness.

Caregivers may help in the alleviation of the patient's distress, but are not rightfully placed to resolve needling issues embedded in the family system. When patients are faced with a hostile family system and have to be taken care of by 'outsiders', it not only burdens the external caregivers but also deepens the stress the individual is experiencing. Caregivers also feel burdened by neglected patients and feel that while their role is restorative, they are unable to deal with the emotional pain of desertion that the patient is experiencing.

These sorts of burdens raise a range of moral questions about the nature of obligation, freedom, autonomy, beneficence, justice and responsibility. The ethic of botho/Botho Ethics is reflected in these findings: one is considered a person because of, with and through other people (Gaie 2007, p. 37). This means that caregiving is itself embedded in family principles of connectedness and togetherness. The women stated that this ethic that binds families together suggests or assumes that whether one has a poor relationship or has not spoken to a family member in years, one still has to be involved in the care of the person. Respondents are also aware of the reciprocal and often unconditional nature of caregiving. They know that they or other significant others may need care in the future. They understand and take seriously the mutuality and synchronicity among individuals and between individuals and society.

Positive Experiences of the Caregivers (Intervening Factors)

On the positive side, caregivers reported that the caregiving role had provided them with education and knowledge, which they were able to use and translate into benefits in their everyday lives. In addition, caregiving was regarded as a rewarding experience, especially if rendered to the neediest members of the community.

Conclusions

This study provides some useful insights into the experiences of caregivers. The most significant findings are that caregiving is provided mainly by elderly women who are predominantly peasant farmers; that caregiving in the context of material deprivation compounds the interpersonal experiences of the caregiving; and that older people experience serious physical, psychological and emotional stress. This study suggests a need to design interventions to support caregivers in their work. It suggests that changing the conditions under which care is given, whether through financial, social or psychological support systems, can work not only to relieve the stress and burden of caregivers but also to better the lives of those with HIV/AIDS who depend on them for care. This study also suggests that caregiving can be an ethically ambivalent practice in which cultural differences and factors such as gender, age, financial position, location and employment opportunities shape the possibilities for care being done well for those who need it. These and other factors can also determine the levels of physical, psychological, and economic stresses and burdens on those who provide care.

Further quantitative research is required to help clarify how social support could buffer the impact of caregiving stress on caregivers. One implication for research is that caregivers have developed coping mechanisms to deal with the stress of caregiving, but the potency of this mediation role remains untested. We need more empirical studies that would test the utility of coping theory for explaining the relationship between the stress of caregiving and the caregiver's well-being. Specifically, research is needed to ascertain the level of stress that caregiving has on caregivers, especially the elderly unpaid volunteers. Further enquiry is also needed to understand how cultural sensitivity, competence and knowledge about common practices are incorporated into their care plans and interactions with Batswana clients and their respective caregivers.

Armed with this knowledge, healthcare providers will be better prepared to anticipate difficulties faced by caregivers and thereby plan appropriate inter-ventions. There is, therefore, a need for management to design programmes that will reduce the stress levels of caregivers who provide care for HIV/AIDS patients not only in Botswana but in other places where similar factors impact on those who give and those who receive care. Innovative interventions should be designed to take into consideration the ethical dilemmas that are experienced by caregivers generally. Specifically, these interventions should give voice and legitimacy to the positive and negative experiences of caregiving.

References

Bulmer, P. (1987) *Psychological Perspective on AIDS Aetiology: Prevention and Treatment*, Lawrence Erlbaum Associates, London.

Cohen, S. & Syme, S. L. (1999) *Social Support and Health*, Harcourt Brace, New York.

Dant, H. & Gully, M. (1994) *Ideologies of Caring: Rethinking Community and Collectivism*, Macmillan, Basingstoke.

Ditirafalo, T., Mojapelo, D., Tau, M. & Doehlie, E. (2001) *Client Satisfaction and Provider's Perspective of Home-based Care in Kweneng District*, Gaborone, Botswana, unpublished.

Gaie, J. B. (2007) 'The Setswana Concept of Botho: Unpacking the Metaphysical and Moral Aspects', in *The Concept of Botho and HIV/AIDS in Botswana*, eds J. Gaie & S. K. Mmolai, Zapf Chancery, Eldoret, pp. 28–43.

Government of Botswana, Ministry of Health (1997) *HIV/AIDS, Medium Term Plan II 1997–2002*, Government Printer, Gaborone.

Jacques, G. & Stegling, C. (2001) 'AIDS and Home-based Care in Botswana: Panacea or Perfidy?', paper presented at the Third International Conference on Social Work in Health and Mental Health, Tampere, Finland.

Miller, J. B. (1987) *Towards a New Psychology of Women*, Beacon Press, Boston.

Molelekwa, T. (2000) 'An Assessment of Knowledge of Home-based Caregivers for AIDS Patients in the Context of Information Education and Communication (IEC)', unpublished thesis, Department of Social Work, University of Botswana.

Schoen, K. (1998) 'Caring for Ourselves: Understanding and Minimizing the Stress of HIV Caregiving', in *HIV & Social Work: A Practitioners Guide*, eds D. Aronstein & B. J. Thompson, pp. 527–36.

Sims, G. & Moss, T. (1991) *Long Term Care*, Brookings Institution, Washington, DC.

Van Praag, E. (2001) 'Lessons Learnt from Home-based Care Programme', paper presented at the First Southern Africa Regional Conference on Community Home-based for Persons Living with or Affected by HIV/AIDS, Gaborone, Botswana, 5–8 March, unpublished.

Index

Page numbers in **bold** refer to figures

INDEX

Noddings, Nel 52

northern and rural women caregivers 65–80; government policy 77–8; loss of primary industry 76; market forces 78; research 70–1; research results 71–2; research themes 72–4; threads across research themes 74–6

northern, rural and remote contexts 66–7; economic decline 67; research opportunity 69–70; service inadequacies 66

nursing 194–204; caring profession 194–5; females 196; foundations of ethic of care 195–7; future of care-based ethic 199–200; interpersonal caring 198–9; practice as ethic of care 197–8; socio-political forces, and 195

Nussbaum, Martha 40

obligation 44–9

parochialism 54

paternalism 54

paternalistic care 32

permanent visitors 98–9

personalisation 122–36; Austria 127–8; cash, and 134; choice, and 131–3; claims for 150; classification of schemes 133; comparative analysis 122–36; critical perspective 137–51; empowerment, and 131–3; equality, and 149; ethic of care, and 124–6; examples 126–9; France 128; governance, and 130–1; inflexible state services, and 132–3; Italy 127; meaning 138–9; Netherlands 126–7; normative cores 129; policy objectives, and 125–6; relegation of care, and 146; Sweden 128; undergovernance 131; United Kingdom 126; United States 129

personalisation agenda 109–21; age-related concerns 111; ageing population, and 113–16; being in control 114–16; disabled people 119; ethic of care perspective 111–13; independent living schemes 115; need for 110; older people, and 110–11, power dynamics 115; responsiveness, and 118; social care policy, and 110

personalisation schemes **134**

Peters, Heather 4

physical effects of caregiving 232

Physicians for Human Rights 47

Pithouse, Andrew 5

place, context of 65–80

planning and buying support 144–5

Pogge, Thomas 40

policy formulation 140

political ethic of care 158

Pratesi, Alessandro 4

privacy 189–91

productivity of care 94–108

professionalised care 169–70

psycho-social effects of caregiving 232

public policies 51

public services reform 138

punishment: children 13

Putting People First 141–4; care and protection 142; people addressed 141; values 143–4

Rank, Eva 160

Rees, Alyson 5

Reeves, Eric 46

recognition respect 86–7

relational autonomy 158

research practice 214–20; attentiveness 217; competence 218–19; developing relationship 215–16; older people's well-being 216–17; responsibility 218; responsiveness 219; trust 219

residential child care 165–79; central features 171–2; different voice 175–7; failure 167; government engagement 166; justice orientation 175; lifespace 171–2; love and right relationship 172–3; modernisation 167; professionalised care 169–70; rights 168–9; risks 168; shifting discourses of care 166–7

respect 85–6

responsibility 208, 218

responsiveness 209, 219

rights 168–9; importance of 33

risks 168

Robinson, Fiona 3

robocarers 88

Rummery, Kirstein 5, 90

SAPs 28

Sassen, Saskia 33

Schott, Robin May 17

second layer of research findings **72**

self-respect: gratitude, and 91

service cuts 67–8

Sevenhuijsen, Selma 137–8

Smith, Mark 5

social justice perspective 68–9

social politics: critical analyses 112

socio-economic inequalities 117–18

sociology of emotions 95

South Africa 18

Sprinzak, Ehud 18

Steckley, Laura 5

street-level bureaucracy 205–13; corrupted world of service, and 206–7; morality 210–11; policy making 210–11

stress of caregiving 231–2

Sweden; personalisation 128

symbols of care 95